Introduction to
Neurobiology

Introduction to Neurobiology

Heinrich Reichert, Ph. D.

Department of Zoology
University of Basel, Switzerland

Foreword by Corey S. Goodman

463 illustrations

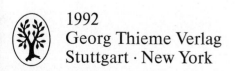

1992
Georg Thieme Verlag
Stuttgart · New York

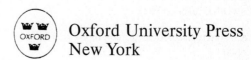

Oxford University Press
New York

Heinrich Reichert, Ph. D.
Department of Zoology
University of Basel
Rheinsprung 9
4051 Basel
Switzerland

Drawings by Brigitte Zwickel-Noelle

Translated by G. S. Boyan, Ph. D.
Department of Zoology
University of Basel
Rheinsprung 9
4051 Basel
Switzerland

This book is an authorized and updated translation of the German edition published and copyrighted 1990 by Georg Thieme Verlag, Stuttgart, Germany. Title of the German edition: Neurobiologie.

Library of Congress Cataloguing-in-Publication-Data
Reichert, Heinrich:
Introduction to Neurobiology / Heinrich Reichert. Foreword by Corey S. Goodman. [Drawings by Brigitte Zwickel-Noelle. Transl. by G. S. Boyan]. – Stuttgart ; New York : Thieme ; New York : Oxford Univ. Press, 1992
Dt. Ausg. u. d. T.: Reichert, Heinrich: Neurobiologie

© 1992 Georg Thieme Verlag, Rüdigerstrasse 14, 7000 Stuttgart 30, Germany

Typesetting by
Hofacker Digitale Druckvorbereitung,
7060 Schorndorf

Cover illustrations:
Photograph by Neher from „Wehner/Gehring, Zoologie"
Drawing by Gorman & Thomas, J. Physiol. 275 (1978) 357ff.

Printed in Germany by

ISBN 3-13-784701-X (GTV)
ISBN 0-19-521010-7 (OUP)

"Oxford" is a registered trademark of Oxford University Press.

Preface

This book is written for students who are interested in one of the most fascinating fields of modern science, namely the investigation of the nervous system and brain. This relatively new topic in the fundamental biological sciences is known as neurobiology. Modern neurobiology is an open science, with no restrictions placed on either methodological approaches or concepts, and one which is currently developing at an explosive pace.

It is not easy to do justice to these developments in an introductory textbook with its necessarily limited text, illustrations, and references. Nevertheless, I have attempted to present clearly and simply, based on appropriate examples, the principles of neurobiology that I consider to be most important. This could not be done without some generalizations with respect to content and some limit on the amount of detail presented. Some subjective selection of material from the many excellent pieces of neurobiological research was also necessary. Advanced neurobiolo-gists who require a more complete and detailed overview should consult the more extensive presentations available in the appropriate handbooks and specialized journals.

This book would have been unthinkable without the generous support of many local and international colleagues. Above all I wish to thank Rüdiger Wehner for many discussions, suggestions, and encouragement, and Wulf-Dieter Krenz for his critical review of the complete manuscript. Heartfelt thanks to Heinz Breer, José Campos-Ortega, Jean Jacques Dreifuss, Hans Hatt, Werner Rathmayer, and Herbert Zimmermann for their critical reading of individual chapters. I also wish to thank the excellent team at Thieme, particularly Brigitte Zwickel-Noelle for the outstanding illustrations, and Margrit Tischendorf for her personal involvement in the entire editorial process.

Basel, August 1992
Heinrich Reichert

Foreword

Neuroscience is the study of the brain; it is the study of the interactions, at the level of molecules as well as individual cells and vast arrays of cells, that control the ways in which we move, feel, think, and learn. Understanding how our mind works is one of the great frontiers of modern biology.

Neuroscience has undergone a revolution in the past 10 years which has transformed the ways in which we think about the brain—its development, its function, its plasticity, and its diseases and malfunctions. It is no longer a field based on descriptions and conjectures, but rather one based on discrete mechanisms, molecules, circuits, and models. Fueled by the advances in recombinant DNA and monoclonal antibody techniques, immortalized cell lines, and a variety of optical, staining, recording, imaging, and computer science technologies, the previously diverse disciplines of neuroscience—from the molecular and genetic to the integrative and cognitive—have become unified by common techniques and emergent principles. This revolutionary progress in neuroscience has created opportunities for discovery ranging from the basic understanding of how we think and perceive to how we learn, how disease can be prevented and how mental illness can be cured.

This remarkable influx of techniques and concepts from many different disciplines must be overwhelming for the beginning student. When today's senior neuroscientists took their first neurobiology course more than 20 years ago, life was much simpler; saltatory conduction, voltage clamp, and presynaptic inhibition were the most difficult concepts to grapple with in a largely physiological and anatomical field. They learned EPSP and IPSP without having to worry about c-DNA and NMDA. But today's students enter an exploding field with much greater breadth and depth, and for this they need the right introductory guide.

Some neurobiology books are perfect for medical students or graduate students, and others are ideal for the seasoned veteran, but what about the beginner? It takes a combination of concepts and principles sprinkled with just the right number of details and examples to match the needs of a student's first exposure to neuroscience. Heinrich Reichert has written just such a fresh treatment that seems as at ease with the molecular and cellular end of the field as it does with the integrative and cognitive. Given the recent impact of molecular advances emerging from genetic analysis in flies and worms and reverse genetics in frogs and mice, it is refreshing to see a textbook that presents the animal kingdom in its entirety, embracing evolution and diversity as the foundation for modern neuroscience. But in spite of the rush of excitement of the last decade that is amply captured in this book, today's student need not worry that this field has reached its twilight. There are still a few simple questions, like how do we think? how do we learn?, that await the next generation.

Corey S. Goodman
Professor, Department of Molecular
and Cell Biology
Howard Hughes Medical Institute
University of California
Berkeley, California, USA

Contents

3. Cellular Neurobiology: Synaptic Transmission 51

6. Systems Integration 148

7. Development 176

8. Maintenance and Repair 211

9. Processes Dependent on Experience 225

1. Nervous Systems: Introduction and Comparative Overview

Nervous Systems are Neuron Systems

Around 1890 the Spanish neuroanatomist Ramón y Cajal made a series of significant discoveries using a histological staining technique developed earlier by the Italian physician Golgi. These discoveries were based on his ability to demonstrate the extensive, and oddly branched, individual elements of all nervous systems. These basic elements are the individual nerve cells, the neurons.

Cajal's discoveries led to the establishment of the "neuron doctrine," which states that the nervous system, like all other organs, is composed of individual cells, in this case, of neurons. These neurons process and exchange signals with one another at specific points of contact which the English neurophysiologist Sherrington called synapses. The concept of a "reticular" organization, in which the cells of the nervous system were supposedly fused into a multicellular, syncytium-like continuum, therefore had to make way for the extension of cell theory to the nervous system. This discovery that nervous systems are really systems of neurons provided the spark for an explosive development in the scientific investigation of nervous systems, and signalled the birth of modern neurobiology.

What has become more and more obvious during the last hundred years is just how significant this discovery was. During this time neurobiology has become established as a multidisciplinary science, founded on the conviction that an understanding of the nervous system requires experimental studies at all levels of biological organization. Thus, studies on biochemical and biophysical aspects of brain function are just as much part of the repertoire of neurobiological research as are studies on neuronal circuitry and the behavior of whole animals. However, despite the diversity of research methods and conceptual approaches, modern neurobiology is based on one unifying principle: a complete understanding of the subcellular molecular level as well as the supra-cellular integrative level of organization starts and ends at the cellular, neuronal level. At the heart of neurobiological research is the neuron. Neurons are the fundamental components of structure and function in all nervous systems. Their performance potential is breathtaking. While in the primitive nerve net of coelenterates they can control only the simplest reactions, in the form of the complexly organized human brain they represent the greatest problems *and* the greatest hopes of our world.

Invertebrate Nervous Systems

The origin of the first neurons

When did the first neuron arise during evolution? This question is particularly difficult to answer, mainly because in many respects nearly all cell types display neuron-like properties. Cells produce electrical potentials across their cell membranes. Intense physical stimuli can produce changes in these potentials. Evoked potential changes are conducted spatially. Indeed, communication between single cells is a prerequisite for metazoic organization. The distinctive feature of a neuron, however, is that it is specialized to apply all these cellular properties toward information processing.

Although even prokaryotic cells display properties like excitability, receptor function, effector control and coordination, one can not, by definition, regard single cells as specialized nerve cells. This applies equally to the groups of cells one finds at the organizational level of Porifera, where neither specialized nerve cells nor a specialized nervous system are found. Real nerve cells and a real nervous system are, however, unequivocally present in the coelenterates. How this came about in evolution must remain open, or as Nauta put it "nerve cells seem to have sneaked into phylogeny."

Coelenterates: a nerve net

With the coelenterates we reach the organizational level of specialized tissue. These animals consist of an epithelial-like ectoderm, in which specialized sensory and muscle cells occur, and a similarly epithelial-like endoderm, which contains nutritive cells and muscle cells, as well as secretory cells. In addition, specialized nerve cells of ectodermal origin occur. These are mostly arranged in a diffusely distributed, two-dimensional *nerve net* (Fig. 1.**1**). In the more highly evolved coelenterates, the nerve cells can be grouped into special anatomical aggregates which may constitute a nerve ring or ganglia.

The sensory inputs to the nerve net of a coelenterate can come from various types of sensory cells. Chemoreceptors, photoreceptors, tactile receptors, and the specialized receptors of the statocysts are all present. Coordinated motor behavior, as evidenced by the elegant, oriented swimming behavior of jelly-fish, is produced by motoneurons which innervate muscle fibers. Sensory information can be transmitted in reflex-like manner directly from sensory cells to motoneurons. It can also be processed by interneurons—these are neurons which function like neither a sensory cell nor a motoneuron. In addition, neuronal activity can also be spontaneously generated and then processed further. Remember, though, that all this occurs on the basis of a diffusely distributed nerve net; a real central nervous system (CNS) has not formed in these animals. Nevertheless, the development here of inter-neuronal networks marks the beginnings of a significant development which progresses throughout all higher animal groups.

Platyhelminths and nemathelminths: the beginnings of a bilaterally symmetrical central nervous system

The flatworms are the simplest creatures to develop organs, and the first to possess a real CNS. These simply organized Bilateria have a distinct longitudinal body axis, and possess a more or less specialized head region. Sensory cells are found all over the body surface, but are especially prevalent in the head region, where some are aggregated in specialized structures, for example, simple "eyes" which consist of cupshaped agglomerations of photoreceptor cells. In more highly developed, free-living species, we find collections of nerve cells in the head region which give the appearance of a head ganglion or brain (Fig. 1.**2a**). Bilaterally symmetrical *nerve cords* exit this ganglion and innervate the entire body. In keeping with the heterogeneity of the Platyhelminth group, a variety of different types of nerve cords are produced. These nerve cords can assume a segment-like structure as a result of the more or less regular array of cross-connections.

A low level of cephalization is also found in the roundworms. In these animals the anterior end of the nervous system is generally an esophageal ring from which two main nerve cords, one dorsal and the other ventral, project posteriorly (Fig. 1.**2b**). Interestingly, muscle processes project into these nerve cords and so obtain their motor innervation in an unconventional way. The motor repertoire of free-living platyhelminths and nemathelminths is restricted to simple movements like crawling, swimming, and simply oriented reflex behavior.

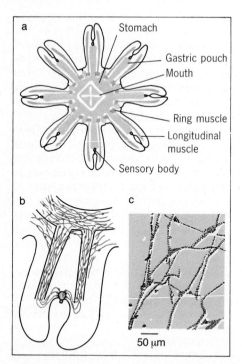

Fig. 1.**1**   The nervous system of coelenterates. **a** Ephyra of *Aurelia,* general view. **b** Ephyra of *Aurelia,* partial view of the nerve net, the musculature and a sensory structure. **c** Partial view of the nerve net of *Cyanea* following removal of the epithelial cells (after Claus and Friedemann, Horridge and Mackie)

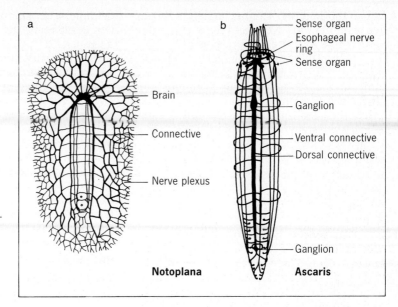

Fig. 1.2 The nervous system of platyhelminths and nemathelminths. **a** Brain and ventral plexus of *Notoplana*. **b** Esophageal ring, nerve cord and sensory organs of *Ascaris*. (after Hadenfeldt, and Goldschmidt and Voltenlogel)

Annelids: segmentation and cephalization advance

The organization of the CNS of annelids reflects the segmented body plan of these animals. The nervous system consists of a metamerically organized, ladder-like chain of ganglia at whose anterior end there is a distinct *brain* (Fig. 1.3). The process of increasing cephalization usually involves the fusion of several anteriorly situated segmental ganglia. The dorsally situated brain is connected to the ventral chain of segmental ganglia via circumesoph-

ageal connectives. Each segmental ganglion, which typically consists of about 1000 neurons, is organized in a bilaterally symmetrical way. Both ganglionic halves are linked to one another by commissures and to neighboring ganglia by connectives. Peripheral nerves—typically three pairs—project from each ganglion and innervate the segmental body wall. All ganglia have a structure which is characteristic for higher invertebrates; the neuronal cell bodies lie in a peripheral layer, the neuronal processes (dendrites and axons) lie in a neuropil in the

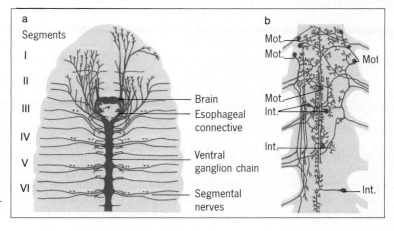

Fig. 1.3 The nervous system of annelids. **a** Brain, ganglion chain and nerve bundles in the anterior end of *Lumbricus*. **b** Motoneurons (Mot.) and interneurons (Int.) in the ventral ganglion chain of *Lumbricus* (after Hess, Zawarzin and Retzius)

core of the ganglion. In some annelids, distinctive giant neurons occur, and these play an important role in fast escape responses.

A multitude of chemoreceptors, photoreceptors and mechanoreceptors are found, some in the individual body segments, and others in differentiated sensory organs, particularly at the head end. There is a primitive somatosensory system, and in some species there are also well-defined eyes. In the more highly evolved polychaetes structured optic ganglia are formed. Along with the formation of sensory organs there is an increase in the specialization of different brain regions. In some species the brain can reach a degree of complexity approaching that found in simple arthropods and molluscs. In some brains there are specializations for neurosecretion. The first indications of a stomatogastric system occur in the wall of the anterior gut.

The motor behavior of annelids consists of, among other things, a range of coordinated movements in which crawling, swimming, digging, and locomotion via parapodia, all depend on the utilization of large regions of body wall musculature. The central nervous control of these behaviors is based on phenomena such as neuronal oscillators, local reflexes, central and peripheral inhibition, and reciprocal excitation and inhibition, all of which are also employed by higher animal species.

Arthropods: complex brains and specialized segmental ganglia

The representatives of the largest invertebrate group have a CNS with the same basic organization as in the annelids:

— a ventral nerve cord comprising bilaterally symmetrical segmental ganglia which innervate the periphery via nerves, and are linked to one another via paired connectives;
— an anterior, dorsally situated brain which is connected to the ventral nerve cord via neck connectives;
— a stomatogastric system which innervates the anterior gut.

The most important differences between the nervous systems of the arthropods and annelids involve specializations in the body organization of arthropods—the articulated appendages and the fusion of originally unitary,

metameric segments into the functional entities comprising the head, thorax, and abdomen.

The tendency of the head region to increase in size and importance leads to the formation of a complex brain consisting of extensively fused cerebral ganglia (Fig. 1.4). In higher arthropods well-defined brain regions can be identified, and these are often associated with the processing of information from specialized sensory organs. In insects, for example, we find a *protocerebrum* which receives visual sensory input from both compound eyes and from the simple ocelli, a *deutocerebrum* which receives sensory input from the antennae, and a *tritocerebrum* which receives input from the head surface. These brain structures together contain about 90% of the neurons in the central nervous system, which in the larger Crustacea amounts to about one million nerve cells. The fine structure of the brain represents a high order of organizational complexity consisting of cell body regions, fiber bundle regions, multiple neuropil centers, and aggregates of neurosecretory cells. The development of efficient compound eyes is associated with the formation of complexly organized optic lobes. In the higher arthropods there are brain regions which consist of associative neuropil, such as the corpora pedunculata of insects.

The requirement for accurate motor control of the articulated body appendages, especially the thoracic legs, has led to an increasing specialization of the ventral segmental ganglia. The thoracic ganglia typically contain more interneurons, more efferently projecting motoneurons, and larger numbers of afferent sensory fibers, than do the abdominal ganglia. This can also apply to the terminal ganglion, as this ganglion is often associated with specialized structures on the posterior end of the animal. In addition there is a tendency toward fusion of the segmental ganglia into fewer (in some cases single) ganglia. One such ganglion, the subesophageal, which is itself formed from several ganglia and controls the mouthparts, is generally found enclosed in the head capsule. The control of neuromuscular activity is surprisingly fine-tuned. Excitatory as well as inhibitory neurones are involved, and complex, multineuronal, innervation patterns of muscle fibers occur. The differential control of the segmental appendages is made possible by a variety of segmental sensory structures. These in-

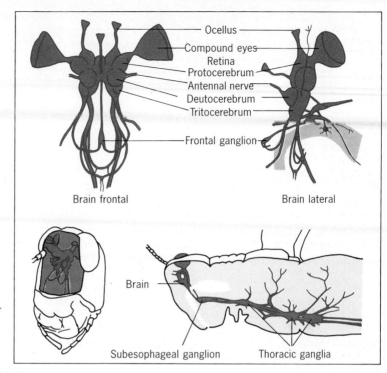

Brain frontal   Brain lateral

Fig. 1.**4**   The nervous system of insects: CNS of *Locusta*. Frontal and side views of the various brain regions (top). Brain and ventral ganglia in relation to the head and body (bottom) (after Albrecht, Williams and Wilson)

clude strand receptors, muscle receptor organs, chordotonal organs, and campaniform sensilla. On the body surface, an exoskeleton, various mechanoreceptors, and olfactory sensilla are found. The segmental specializations of the arthropod nervous system allow complex motor activity to be generated. This includes flying, running, jumping, manipulation, and sound production.

Molluscs: a diversity of organizational types

The gastropods, bivalves, and cephalopods exhibit a huge diversity of neural systems. In the simplest representatives the nervous systems are not much more complex than in some flatworms, while others, like the squid, have brains which rank as the most highly developed among all invertebrates. The basic organization of the CNS comprises about five pairs of ganglia which are arranged around the gut, generally near the head, and are linked to one another by connectives and commissures. It is usually possible to distinguish cerebral, buccal, pleural, pedal, and abdominal ganglia. In addition there are smaller peripherally situated ganglia, and often a peripheral nerve net as well. This basic organizational plan can vary considerably among individual molluscan species, to the extent that the various ganglia can change their position and even fuse with one another (Fig. 1.**5**).

There are various levels of organization among the sensory receptor structures, from simple isolated sense cells up to complex sense organs. Some species have a specialized osphradial organ in the mantle cavity which monitors the osmolarity of sea water. The behavioral repertoire of the various molluscs is as diverse as is the structure of their nervous systems. Locomotory activity ranges from literally a snail's pace, up to the extraordinarily fast jet-propelled escape response of cephalopods, which is controlled by a giant fiber system. The cephalopods, which are among the fastest animals in the ocean, have a particularly efficient visual sytem. They possess a complex CNS consisting of approximately 10^8 neurons, which, with its association areas, has advanced integrative capabilities, and in particular an amazing learning capacity. Seen from a neurobiological perspective, they are indeed comparable to the lower vertebrates.

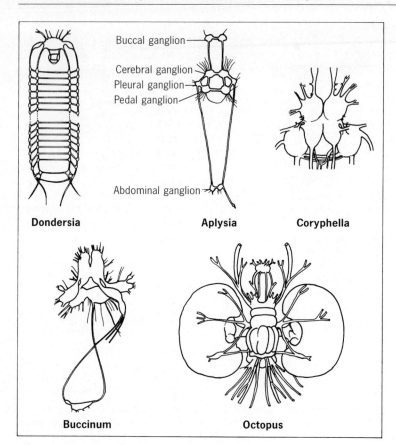

Buccal ganglion

Cerebral ganglion
Pleural ganglion
Pedal ganglion

Abdominal ganglion

Dondersia   **Aplysia**   **Coryphella**

Buccinum   **Octopus**

Fig. 1.**5** The nervous system of molluscs. Schematic representation of the central nervous systems of *Dondersia, Aplysia, Coryphella, Buccinum,* and *Octopus* (after Bullock and Horridge)

Vertebrate Nervous Systems

Evolution

The nervous systems of the most primitive vertebrates have about the same complexity and performance as the nervous systems of the most highly evolved invertebrates. It is safe to assume that the predecessors of the vertebrates had even simpler neural structures. In some larval Tunicata (Urochordata) for example, a dorsal tubular nervous system consisting of only a few hundred neurons has developed. Acranians (Cephalochordata) have a dorsal neural tube, but virtually no differentiated brain. By contrast, among the most highly evolved vertebrates there is a fantastic increase in complexity. In the simplest terms, this becomes apparent as an enormous increase in the number of neurons which make up the nervous system. One estimate is that the human ner-

vous system has 10^{12} neurons. The majority of these neurons occur in the brain, where the trend toward cephalization, which began with the platyhelminths, culminates. More than 99.999% of these neurons are interneurons. Thus, the intermediate nerve net which began at the level of the coelenterates has attained its phylogenetic summit.

Basic organizational plan: a dorsal nerve cord with cerebral ganglia

Despite the diversity of organizational plans found among vertebrate nervous systems, it is possible to recognize certain common characteristics. The nervous system has central and peripheral components. The central nervous system (CNS) consists of a dorsally situated, tube-shaped nerve cord, which arises via invagination from a single layer of ectodermal epithelium. At the anterior end this tube is transformed into a group of enlarged and thickened vesicles. These anterior, vesicle-like extensions, produce the *cerebral ganglia,* which represent the actual brain, and are enclosed in the skull. The posterior tube-shaped section becomes the *spinal cord,* which is surrounded by the bones of the vertebral column.

The organization of the spinal cord can be considered primitive in many respects (Fig. 1.**6a**). The neuronal cell bodies, which derive from the inner layer of the neural tube, remain within the central part of the spinal cord. From there they send their axonal processes, which serve to conduct signals over long distances, into peripheral tracts. Simplifying, one can consider that the neurons in the dorsal half of the neural tube process sensory information,

and the neurons in the ventral half process motor information. This is reflected in the organization of the serially repeating nerve pairs which run out from the spinal cord. These divide near the spinal cord into a dorsally situated sensory root which receives afferent axons from sensory neurons, and a ventrally situated motor root which contains the efferent axons of motoneurons. In most vertebrates both roots rejoin after a short distance to form a single spinal nerve which then divides again into various branches. The cell bodies of the sensory neurons do not lie in the spinal cord like those of the motoneurons, but rather in special spinal ganglia which are part of the sensory nerve roots (dorsal root ganglia).

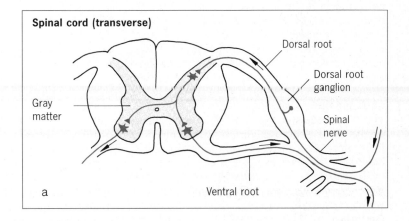

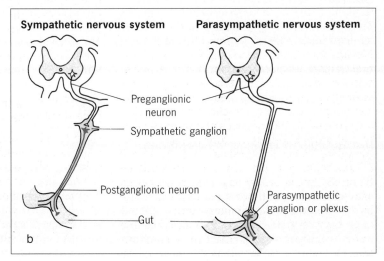

Fig. 1.**6** Organization of the spinal cord of vertebrates, schematic. **a** Cross-section of the spinal cord, dorsal root ganglion and spinal nerves. **b** Spinal cord with preganglionic and postganglionic neurons of the autonomic nervous system

The visceral motoneurons which innervate the intestines and internal organs also occur together in ganglia (Fig. 1.6b). These ganglia of the *autonomic nervous system,* together with all peripherally located nerve fibers, form the peripheral components of the nervous system. A typical function of the autonomic nervous system involves relaying signals from the spinal cord to the visceral motoneurons in the peripheral ganglia. In primitive vertebrates the ganglia of the autonomic nervous system are located near the innervated target organs. In more highly evolved vertebrates this is the case only for the parasympathetic part of the autonomic nervous system. The ganglia of the sympathetic part of the autonomic nervous system are, by contrast, arranged in a ladder-like manner along the vertebral column.

In the course of evolution the spinal cord and peripheral nervous system have, in many respects, developed from being independent segmental reflex centers into structures which are subservient to higher cerebral centers. However, this evolutionary conversion is modest compared with the dramatic changes which the cerebral ganglia themselves undergo during phylogenesis. This development has as its starting point structures which, in the most primitive vertebrates, consist of little more than three morphologically distinguishable swellings of the neural tube: the rostrally situated *prosencephalon,* the adjacent *mesencephalon,* and the *rhombencephalon* which carries over into the spinal cord. During the course of phylogenesis all three structures (and particularly the prosencephalon in the most highly developed vertebrates) undergo an extremely prolific further differentiation. Moreover, it is the dorsal regions of the cerebral ganglia, those connected with particular sense organs, that continue to develop most strongly.

Organization of an idealized vertebrate brain

It is clear that a division of the brain into gross anatomical components must be somewhat arbitrary. In fact neural structures run seamlessly into one another, neural connections and tracts form a continuum both from an anatomical viewpoint and in terms of information processing. Nevertheless, subdivision of the brain is still useful (Fig. 1.7).

The rhombencephalon resembles the spinal cord in its basic features and arises from it without a precise borderline. The organization of this most caudal brain region remains remarkably constant among vertebrates. The posterior half of the rhombencephalon is termed the *myelencephalon* or medulla oblongata. The anterior half is called the *metencephalon.* The metencephalon can be further subdivided into a ventrally situated pons and a pronounced dorsal structure, the *cerebellum.* The cerebellum consists of two hemispheres and its size varies considerably among different species. Some fish have an extremely enlarged cerebellum (up to 90% of the brain mass), while in most amphibians it is very small. The cerebellum is assumed to have originally processed sensorimotor vestibular information. In higher vertebrates further sensory modalities are also served, so that the cerebellum forms a sensorimotor integration center which processes information from practically all sense organs in order to control complex motor acts.

Anterior to the rhombencephalon lies the *mesencephalon.* This is the most rostral part of the neural tube that is still segmentally organized, and it has segmental nerves projecting from it. Its dorsal region, the tectum, processes visual information in lower vertebrates. In mammals the tectum is differentiated into two paired structures, the superior and inferior colliculi. While the superior colliculi continue to be part of the visual system, the inferior colliculi participate in the processing of auditory information. In the ventral part of the mesencephalon lie important motor centers which are formed from larger aggregations of neuronal cell bodies, and so are anatomically described as bodies or nuclei.

Anterior to the mesencephalon lies the *diencephalon,* which is the unpaired part of the prosencephalon. In simplified form, two main functions are ascribed to this brain region:

— the processing of mainly sensory information arising from the rest of the nervous system, and the transmission of this information to the telencephalon;

— the overall control of the pituitary, and with it the endocrine system and many visceral functions.

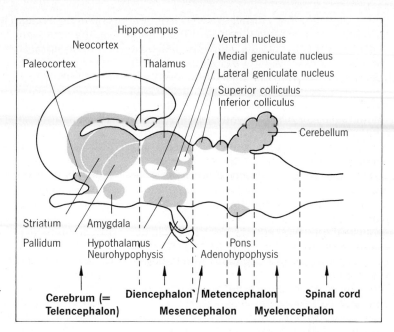

Fig. 1.**7**   Simplified schematic representation of the various regions of the vertebrate brain (after Nauta and Feirtag)

The latter function is carried out by the ventral part of the diencephalon, the *hypothalamus.* The hypothalamus initiates and monitors the release of hormones from the pituitary, a ventral appendage consisting of a posterior neurohypophysis (a part of the brain) and an anterior adenohypophysis (an endocrine gland of epithelial origin). The various nuclei of the hypothalamus play important roles in functions such as nutrient uptake, drinking, temperature regulation, sexual drive, and different emotional states.

The former function is performed by the dorsal part of the diencephalon, the *thalamus.* The structural basis for the processing and transmission of sensory information is found in the many thalamic nuclei. In mammals, the ventral nucleus processes somatosensory input, the medial geniculate nucleus, auditory input, and the lateral geniculate nucleus, visual information. Little is known about the function of the other "association nuclei" of the thalamus. In mammals in particular, the thalamus is in close contact with novel and spatially dominant structures in the telencephalon. These are the neocortex and the newer parts of the striatum.

Brain size and complexity culminate in the mammalian telencephalon

The anterior part of the prosencephalon is known as the *telencephalon,* cerebrum, or cerebral hemispheres. Originally the telencephalon was simply an olfactory processing center. During evolution the telencephalon has progressed from being a thin-walled rostral bulge of the neural tube to a structure which dominates the rest of the brain (Fig. 1.**8**). In mammals, the cerebrum makes up by far the largest part of the brain. Its outer rind, the stratified *cerebral cortex,* may be extensively wrinkled and convoluted, leading to an enormous enlargement of the cortical fields.

The cerebral cortex can be divided into various regions. Let us begin with the most rostral structure of the telencephalon. This region is a terminal swelling called the bulbus olfactorius and processes olfactory information. The olfactory tract runs caudally from the bulbus olfactorius to the olfactory cortex. Histologically, these three structures have a relatively primitive organization, and never consist of more than three layers. The olfactory cortex is present in all vertebrates and is therefore sometimes termed the *paleocortex*. In fish, the olfactory cortex makes up most of the cortex. Further cortical areas join onto the paleocortex, and these extend out in a dorsocaudal direction due to a massive cortical expansion. In mammals the most complex and largest region of the brain, the *neocortex,* is found here. In evolutionary terms this is the newest part of the brain. The neocortex consists of six layers. Five layers contain neuronal cell bodies, and one, the most peripheral, comprises nerve fibers. (Regions of the brain which consist largely of cell bodies are termed "gray matter"; those comprising mainly nerve fibers are termed "white matter"). In mammals a special structure known as the *hippocampus* originates medially on the edge of the cortex where it rolls inward and folds on itself. This region of the cortex only has one cell body layer. The hippocampus is, among other things, important for learning processes.

Further important neuron aggregations are located deep in the cerebral hemispheres. The largest such complex is the *corpus striatum,* sometimes also called the *basal ganglia.* This structure consists of the histologically distinct striatum and globus pallidus regions. The striatum can be further subdivided into the nucleus caudatus and the putamen. The corpus striatum has important functions in the control of movement. Below the olfactory cortex lies the amygdala, which consists of a collection of several brain nuclei. The amygdala and the hippocampus comprise the major components of the limbic system. They embody the close relationship between the telencephalon and the hypothalamus.

Cerebral function and regional specialization

The cerebral cortex has a microarchitecture which is remarkably uniform across wide regions. It is composed of repeated column- or band-shaped groups of neurons which are arranged orthogonally to the cortical layers. These aggregations are assumed to represent the elementary subunits of cortical function. Despite this homogeneous organization based on similar subunits, certain areas of the cortex become specialized to process different types of information. A morphologically distinct part of the cortex which is specialized in this way is termed a *cortical field.* The sensory and motor cortical fields are those which have been most extensively studied.

A given sensory field often contains a topographic representation of the particular sensory information which it is specialized to process. Somatosensory cortical fields can form a topographic representation of the body surface (Fig. 1.**9**). Visual cortical fields can topographically represent the retina and thereby the visual surroundings. Auditory receptive fields

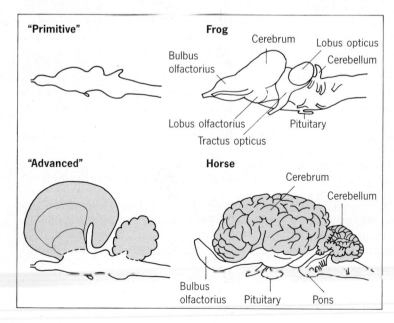

Fig. 1.**8** Evolutionary development of the telencephalon, greatly simplified (left). Comparison of the brain of frog and horse shows the increase in the cerebrum (right) (after Romer)

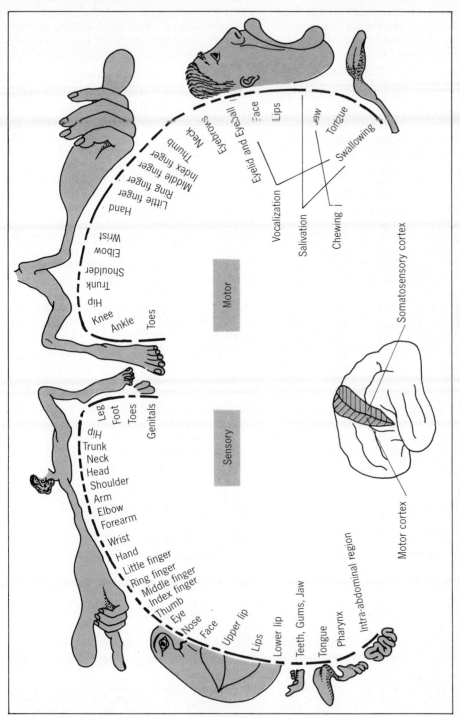

Fig. 1.9   Topographic representation of the somatosensory and motor fields on the cortical surface of the human brain (after Penfield and Rasmussen)

represent different sound characteristics in a spatially organized way. In a similar way there are motor fields on the cortical surface which relate to the topography of the body musculature. Within these motor fields there are giant pyramidal cells which project as far as the spinal cord, and can directly influence motoneurons there.

Two organizational principles which apply to the sensory and motor cortical fields are worth mentioning:

— There are multiple cortical representations for each major sensory modality and for the somatic motor system. These fields are often spatially adjoined to one another and are arranged so that they partially overlap. Each one of these multiple fields is concerned with different aspects of sensory information or motor control. Both parallel and serial (hierarchical) integrative processes are involved.
— The topographic images are not 1:1 representations but are instead "distorted" by a weighting process. The size of the cortical area which is allocated to a given peripheral body structure translates into the "importance" of this structure (more accurately, to the number of nerve fibers which connect

this structure with the brain). The cortical areas which are concerned with the snout in the pig, with the ear in the bat, or with the hand in the human, are overproportionately large.

In primitive mammals a large part of the cortex consists of sensory and motor fields. By contrast, in higher mammals and particularly primates, large parts of the cortex cannot be unambiguously attributed to either sensory or motor functions. These cortical areas are sometimes referred to as *association fields* and most probably serve higher cognitive processes as well as learning and memory functions. In humans there are in addition, distinctive, species-specific, regional specializations. These include, for example, those cortical regions which participate in the generation of language.

The description of a brain in terms of anatomically distinct subunits should not give the impression that we are dealing with a multicomponent system like, say, a stereo system. The subunits of the brain are in reality collections of neurons and nerve fibers whose job it is to process information. The brain is an enormous, cellularly organized, multiply crosslinked information-processing system.

References

General reviews

Alexander, R. M. 1979. The invertebrates. Cambridge University Press, London.

Angevine, J. B., Cotman, C. W. 1981. Principles of neuroanatomy. Oxford University Press. London.

Barrington, E. J. W. 1979. Invertebrate structure and function. Wiley, New York.

Bullock, T. H., Horridge, A. 1965. The structure and function of the nervous system in invertebrates. Freeman, San Francisco.

Bullock, T. H., Orkand, R. O., Grinnell, A. 1977. Introduction to nervous systems. Freeman, San Francisco.

Cajal, S. Ramón y. 1911. Histologie du système nerveux de l'homme et des vertèbres. Maloine, Paris.

Carpenter, M. B., Sutin, J. 1983. Human neuroanatomy, 8th ed. Williams & Wilkins, Baltimore.

De Armond, S. J. 1989. Structure of the human brain: a photographic atlas, 3rd ed. Oxford University Press, London.

Gupta, A. P. 1987. Arthropod brain: its evolution, development, structure, and functions. Wiley, New York.

Hydén, H. 1976. The neuron. Elsevier, Amsterdam.

Lentz, T. 1968. Primitive nervous systems. Yale University Press, New Haven.

Nauta, W. J. H., Feirtag, M. 1986. Fundamental neuroanatomy. Freeman, New York.

Northcutt, R. G. 1981. Evolution of the telencephalon in non-mammals. Ann. Rev. Neurosci. 4: 301–350.

Popper, K. R., Eccles, J. C. 1977. The self and its brain. Springer, Berlin.

Romer, A. S., Parsons, T. S. 1977. The vertebrate body. Saunders, Philadelphia.

Sarnat, H. B., Netsky, M. G. 1981. Evolution of the nervous system. Oxford University Press, London.

Sherrington, C. 1906. The integrative action of the nervous system. Yale University Press, New Haven.

Udin, S. B., Fawcett, J. W. 1988. Formation of topographic maps. Ann. Rev. Neurosci. 11: 289–328.

Williams, P. L., Warwick, R. 1975. Functional neuroanatomy of man. Saunders, Philadelphia.

2. Cellular Neurobiology: Signal Generation

The Neuron: a Cell Like Any Other?

Neuronal specialization

Just like other cells, neurons must fulfill metabolic functions, participate in the exchange of substances, and possess mechanical stability. They have the same genes, the same biochemical mechanisms, and the same organelles, as do other cells. However, neurons differ from other cells in one important respect. They process information. To this end they have developed various specializations which support their function as information-processing units. These specializations include a cellular structure with highly branched processes, a cell membrane which can generate and conduct electrical signals, and points of synaptic contact where information can be passed on from one cell to another.

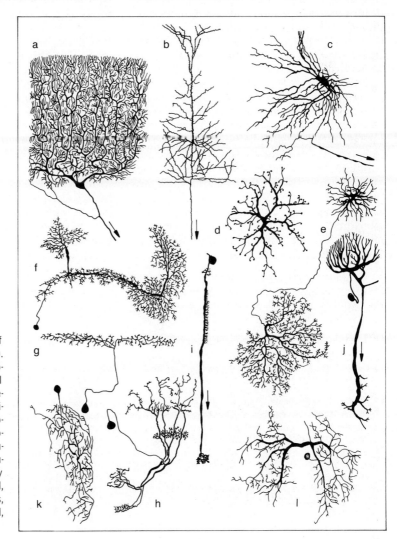

Fig. 2.1 Anatomical diversity of neurons. **a** Purkinje cell (human). **b** Pyramidal cell (rabbit). **c** Motoneuron (cat). **d** Horizontal cell (cat). **e** Horizontal cell (cat). **f** Premotor interneuron (locust). **g** Visual amacrine cell (fly). **h** Multipolar neuron (fly). **i** Visual monopolar neuron (fly). **j** Visual interneuron (locust). **k** Premotor interneuron (crayfish). **l** Mechanosensory interneuron (crayfish) (after Cajal, Fisher and Boycott, Burrows, Strausfeld, O'Shea and Rowell, and Reichert)

The extensive and branched structure of a neuron serves intercellular communication

The functioning of the nervous system depends on information flow in complex circuits which are made up of numerous neurons. Each single neuron contributes to information processing in several ways. As a receiver unit, it takes up signals from other neurons and converts these signals into propagated electrical activity. As a sender unit, it conducts this electrical activity to other locations and then transfers the electrically encoded information to receiving neurons. The processes of signal conversion and conduction are based on cell structures whose anatomical diversity is amazing (Fig. 2.1). There are neurons which consist of little more than a spherical cell. Others have thin cellular processes which can be 10 000 times longer than the diameter of the cell soma. Others again have forms which resemble a fireworks display or the branches of a tree. Some researchers assume that of the 10^{12} neurons in the human brain no two have exactly the same form. Indeed, in many cases neurons can be individually identified on the basis of their structure alone. The diversity of neuronal forms mirrors the many possibilities of interneuronal communication. This is because the structure of a neuron embodies the path of signal transfer in neuronal networks.

Despite this anatomical diversity there are some structural properties which most neurons have in common (Fig. 2.2). All neurons have a *cell body* which contains the nucleus and important organelles such as the Golgi apparatus, endoplasmic reticulum, polysomes, mitochondria and fibrillar elements. Various neuronal processes project out from this cell body, or from a single branch which connects the cell body with the region of arborization. Many neurons have a particularly long process which often projects to distant regions of the nervous system. This process is termed the *axon*. The other, shorter, processes of a neuron are called *dendrites*. Many neurons do not have axons. In these anaxonal or amacrine neurons all the nerve processes are dendrites. Since there is an exception to every rule, neurons with very short axons are also found. To deal with this situation, the term *neurite* is often used to describe any neuronal process.

A few decades ago the difference between dendrites and axons appeared to be very important. This is because one assumed, based on Cajal's "doctrine of dynamic polarization," that the dendrites and cell body were the input regions of a neuron, and the axon and axon terminals were the output regions. We now know that this is not always true. Signals can be transferred from axons to dendrites, from axons to axons, from axons to cell bodies, from dendrites to dendrites, from dendrites to axons, from dendrites to cell bodies, and from cell bodies to cell bodies. In addition, points of contact between different axonal and dendritic regions can be arranged in a reciprocal or a serial manner.

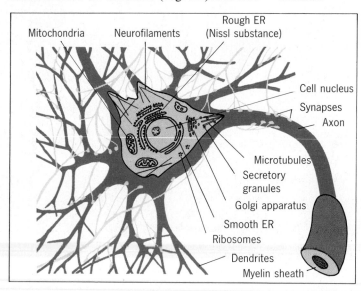

Mitochondria   Neurofilaments   Rough ER (Nissl substance)

Cell nucleus
Synapses
Axon

Microtubules
Secretory granules
Golgi apparatus
Smooth ER
Ribosomes
Dendrites
Myelin sheath

Fig. 2.**2**   Structural organization of a neuron, schematic (after Stevens)

Signal transfer between neurons occurs at synapses

Synapses are specialized points of contact between neurons where signal transfer takes place (Fig. 2.3). A typical neuron makes between 100 and 10 000 synapses. The term "synapse" goes back to Sherrington who postulated, based on functional considerations, that the transfer of signals between neurons must be different from the conduction of signals along neuronal processes. At all synapses there is a synaptic cleft between the presynaptic and the postsynaptic cell.

At electrical synapses, electrical signals are transmitted across the synaptic cleft via special molecular contact points. In this way, signals are transmitted directly, though generally in attenuated form, from one cell to the next. At chemical synapses a change in electrical potential in the presynaptic cell causes the release of a chemical neurotransmitter. This diffuses through the synaptic cleft, binds to receptors in the membrane of the postsynaptic cell, and then causes changes in this cell. Neurotransmitter is stored in membrane-bound vesicles in the presynaptic terminal. It is released as a result of the fusion of these synaptic vesicles with the presynaptic membrane.

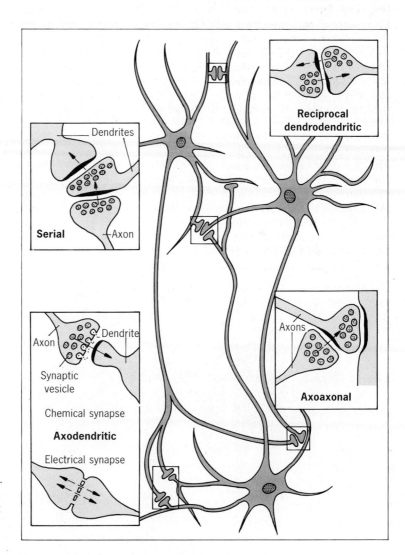

Fig. 2.**3** Sites of synaptic contact between neurons, schematic. Insets show the different types of synaptic contact sites (after Snyder)

The consequence of synaptic transmission is often a potential change in the postsynaptic cell. This potential change can influence the activity of the postsynaptic cell in either an excitatory or an inhibitory way. Since a given neuron generally receives synaptic input from many other neurons, its overall electrical response is determined by the integration of all excitatory and inhibitory postsynaptic potentials (PSPs).

The neuronal soma is important in cell maintenance

In addition to the usual metabolic chores which the soma of every cell has to carry out, the neuronal cell body must also perform several important specialized functions. Neurons carry out a particularly intensive synthesis of macromolecules. Large quantities of special membrane proteins, membrane lipids, and supporting cytoskeletal elements are required to construct and stabilize the membranous regions of the cell's extensive neurites. All these molecules have to be synthesized by a cell body, which typically makes up only about one-tenth of the total neuronal volume. In many neurons, neuropeptides, which are often utilized as transmitter substances, must also be synthesized in the cell body. Because of the increased rate of protein synthesis, a concentration of rough endoplasmic reticulum known as

the Nissl substance is often found near the cell body.

Since the biosynthesis of protein takes place almost exclusively in the cell body, special intracellular transport systems have been developed in order to bring synthesized molecules to distant dendritic and axonal regions. Conversely, degradation products from the dendrites and axons are transported back to the lysosomal system of the cell body for molecular reprocessing.

The high rate of biosynthetic activity in neuronal cell bodies is not just directed toward the specialized mass production of a few types of macromolecules. The diversity in the structure and function of neurones is also based on a molecular diversity. More genetic information is used in the nervous system than in any other organ of the body. About 200 000 different mRNA sequences are expressed in the human brain.

The cell membrane is electrically excitable

The ability of nerve cells to process information would be unthinkable without the special properties of the neuronal cell membrane. Electrical signals in a neuron spread along the cell membrane. The properties of the presynaptic and postsynaptic membrane enable and influence the transmission of information from one cell to another. Synaptic integration is based on the electrical properties of the

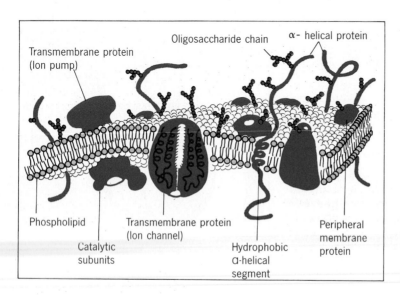

Transmembrane protein (Ion pump)

Oligosaccharide chain   α- helical protein

Phospholipid

Catalytic subunits

Transmembrane protein (Ion channel)

Hydrophobic α-helical segment

Peripheral membrane protein

Fig. 2.**4**   Schematic organization of the neuronal cell membrane which consists of a lipid bilayer and membrane proteins (after Bretscher)

neuronal membrane. Additionally, the cell membrane plays important roles in growth and in target recognition during embryonic development.

Like other cell membranes, the neuronal cell membrane is made up of a lipid bilayer into which various membrane proteins are incorporated (Fig. 2.4). Intrinsic proteins are those embedded in the membrane. Some of these membrane proteins extend completely through the membrane. Peripheral membrane proteins are attached to the membrane surface. Many of these proteins are glycoproteins whose oligosaccharide chains project out into the extracellular space and form an extracellular matrix there.

For simplicity, one can classify the membrane proteins either as structural proteins, receptors, enzymes, pumps, or channels, although these different classes are not mutually exclusive. Structural proteins contribute to the maintenance of the cellular structure and the formation of connections among neurons. Receptors allow the recognition of specific signal-transmitting molecules. Enzymes facilitate chemical reactions in or near the membrane. Receptors and enzymes, for example, control the production of a postsynaptic signal during transmission at chemical synapses. Pumps, by using metabolic energy, can establish ionic gradients or gradients of other molecules across the membrane. Channels allow charged ions and molecules passage through the hydrophobic lipid bilayer of the membrane. The electrical activity in nerve cells results from the interaction between ion pumps and ion channels. Ion pumps and ion channels, working together, generate electrical phenomena such as resting potentials, action potentials and synaptic potentials.

Potential Difference across the Cell Membrane

Measurement and significance of the resting potential

Neurons, like all other living cells, have an electrical potential difference between the two sides of the plasma membrane. This potential difference can be measured by inserting a fine microelectrode into a nerve cell and then comparing the intracellular potential with the potential of a reference electrode in the extra-

cellular fluid (Fig. 2.5). For "resting" neurons, that is for neurons which are not generating or transmitting signals, one measures a constant negative potential difference; the inside of the cell is negative compared with the cell's external environment whose potential is set at 0. This potential difference, termed the *resting potential,* generally lies between –50 and –80 mV. The resting potential forms the basis for the generation, processing, and conduction of electrical signals in the nerve cell. In order to understand how the resting potential is produced, one has to understand two interrelated phenomena:

– the inequality of ion concentrations on the two sides of the membrane,
– the selective permeability of the cell membrane for different types of ions.

Both are the result of the diverse molecular properties of transmembrane proteins.

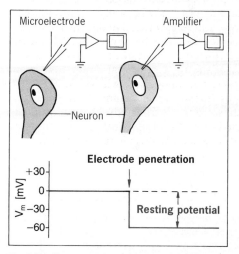

Fig. 2.**5**   Measurement of the potential difference across a cell membrane. A microelectrode connected to an electronic amplifier is inserted through the membrane into the cell. The measured constant negative potential difference is the resting potential. V_m = membrane potential

Ion pumps establish concentration gradients

The ionic composition of the intracellular and extracellular fluids is complex and can also vary considerably among species. For neurons, the most important inorganic ions are Na^+, K^+, Ca^{2+}, Mg^{2+}, Cl^-, and HCO_3^-. Numerous organic anions such as negatively charged amino acids and polypeptides are also found, but only intracellularly. For simplification these are collectively referred to as A^-. If the ionic composition of the intracellular milieu of a neuron is compared to that of the extracellular milieu (Table 2.1), it becomes obvious that the concentrations of all the important ions on both sides of the membrane are unequal. Indeed, there are considerable *concentration gradients* across the cell membrane for these ions. For K^+ ions the intracellular concentration is considerably higher than the extracellular. By contrast, for Na^+ and Cl^- ions the intracellular concentration is considerably lower than the extracellular. How are these different ionic distributions generated? The answer lies in the amazing capacity of a group of membrane-bound transport proteins to selectively pump ions from one side of the membrane to the other. With the help of metabolic energy, these *ion pumps* can selectively transport ions across the cell-membrane, from a region of lower concentra-

Tab. **2.1**   An example of the composition of intracellular and extracellular fluids

	Intracellular concentration (mmol)	Extracellular concentration (mmol)
K^+	124	2
Na^+	10	145
Ca^{2+}	5	2
	($< 10^{-7}$ unbound)	
Mg^{2+}	14	1
Cl^-	2	77
HCO_3^-	12	27
A^-	74	13
other	(84)	(36)

tion, to one of higher concentration. The energy for this transport of ions against a concentration gradient is in most cases obtained by hydrolysis of ATP.

The most important and best characterized of these ion pumps is a Na^+–K^+-exchange pump, called the Na^+–K^+-ATPase. This ion pump has the particularly important function of establishing opposing concentration gradients for K^+ ions and Na^+ ions across the cell membrane. How important this task is can be seen from the fact that up to 70% of the energy consumed by an active nerve cell is used for

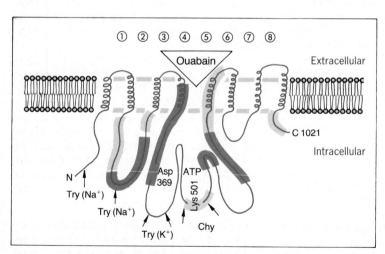

Fig. 2.**6**   Molecular organization of a Na^+–K^+–ATPase. A model for the catalytic subunit of the ion pump. Hydrophobic regions of the molecule which extend through the membrane are labeled with the numbers 1–8. Molecular regions are shown where trypsin (Try) and chymotrypsin (Chy) act when Na^+ or K^+ are bound to the molecule. Aspartate at position 369, and lysine at position 501 are probably involved in the binding and hydrolysis of ATP. The glycoside ouabain inhibits the ion pump (after Cantley)

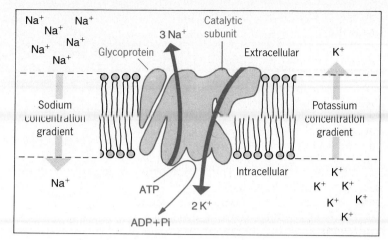

Fig. 2.**7**   Schematic representation of ion transport via the Na⁺–K⁺·ATPase. As a result of ATP-dependent ion transport, oppositely directed concentration gradients for Na⁺ and K⁺ are built up across the cell membrane. P_i = inorganic phosphate

driving the Na⁺–K⁺-exchange pumps. The Na⁺-K⁺-ATPase consists of a catalytic subunit, which extends through the cell membrane, and of an associated glycoprotein (Fig. 2.**6**). The ion pump selectively binds Na⁺ ions and ATP on the cytoplasmic side, and K⁺ ions on the extracellular side of the membrane. Hydrolysis of an ATP molecule produces a conformational change in the pump which is not yet fully understood, but results in three Na⁺ ions being transported into the cell, and two K⁺ ions being transported out of the cell (Fig. 2.**7**). A different membrane-bound ion pump is able to transport Ca^{2+} ions from the inside to the outside of the cell, again by hydrolysis of ATP. Other ion pumps are responsible for the transport of Cl^- and HCO_3^- ions across the cell membrane.

The concentration gradients established by the ATP-dependent ion pumps can serve as sources of energy for other, ATP-independent, transport processes. For example, some ion pumps do not use ATP directly as an energy source, but rather the Na⁺ ion concentration gradient established by the Na⁺–K⁺ ion pump. Since the concentration of Na⁺ ions is considerably higher outside the cell, the influx of Na⁺ ions is energetically favorable and can be coupled to a simultaneous cotransport of other ions against their concentration gradient.

The concentration gradients of various ions across the cell membrane provide a source of readily available energy. This energy source can be used to generate a potential difference between the two sides of the membrane.

Ion channels are responsible for selective permeability

A lipid bilayer has a negligible permeability to ions. In artificial membranes made up of lipid bilayers, measured permeabilities to ions are 10^{-9} times smaller than to water molecules. This is because the electrically charged and hydrated ions diffuse through the hydrophobic lipid bilayer with difficulty. In biological membranes, an increased permeability to ions is achieved due to numerous *ion channels* that are incorporated into the lipid bilayer. Most ion channels consist of barrel-shaped assemblies of polypeptide subunits which extend through the membrane, and thus form a lipid-free hydrated *pore* (Fig. 2.**8**). The ionic permeability of a membrane possessing such ion channels can be 10^4–10^5 times higher than one consisting only of lipid molecules.

There are many different types of ion channels. They all facilitate the diffusion of ions through the cell membrane. But not all ions can pass through a given ion channel with the same ease. Most ion channels have a *selective permeability* to different types of ions. There are two main reasons for this:

— The diameter of a channel pore can be quite small. At its narrowest point, such a pore may be only a few ångstroms wide. Larger ions or molecules are sterically hindered in their diffusion through such a channel. In this way the ion channel functions like a molecular sieve.

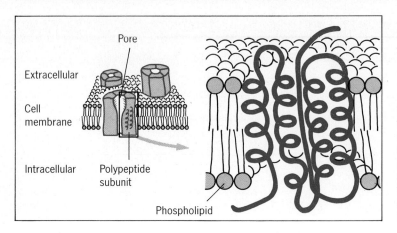

Fig. 2.**8** Schematic representation of the ion channels in the lipid bilayer of the cell membrane. The ion channels are generally composed of barrel-shaped assemblies of polypeptide subunits which form a hydrophilic pore in the membrane (after Unwin and Bretscher)

— The polypeptide chains which line the pore often have electrically charged regions. These can function like electrostatic barriers. Depending on the sign of the charge and the spatial distribution of these charged regions, either positive or negative ions can preferentially pass through the pore.

Although no ion channel is totally selective, it is often possible to achieve a considerable degree of ionic selectivity. Thus certain potassium channels have a 100-fold higher permeability for potassium ions than for sodium ions. Likewise there are channels which have a high specific permeability for Na^+, Cl^-, or Ca^{2+} ions. These are called sodium, chloride or calcium channels. There are even various subclasses of ion channels which all selectively allow the passage of the same ion species, but differ in other molecular properties. All these ion channels have one thing in common: they make a high flow rate of specific ions through the otherwise impermeable cell membrane possible. Flow rates of more than 10^6 ions per second through a single channel can be reached. Since every neuron possesses many channels, it is clear that a considerable flux of ions through the membrane can be achieved.

Electrochemical gradients and the Nernst equation

In the presence of open, selectively permeable ion channels in the cell membrane, a concentration gradient for ion species X across the cell membrane will produce a flow of ions from one side of the membrane to the other. This flux, J_x, for the ion species X through the membrane is given by

$$J_x = P_x \, ([X]_1 - [X]_2)$$

where P_x is the total permeability of the cell membrane for this ion species, and can be considered as the sum of the unitary permeabilities of all the ion channels for ion X. $[X]_1$ and $[X]_2$ are the concentrations of ion X on each side of the membrane. $([X]_1-[X]_2)$ is, therefore, the concentration gradient for this ion.

A flux of ions through the membrane transports electrical charge from one side of the membrane to the other. This ionic current can lead to a separation of electrical charge on both sides of the membrane, and this in turn produces an electrical potential across the cell membrane. In order to understand how this comes about, consider the hypothetical cell shown in Figure 2.**9**. In this cell there are opposing concentration gradients across the membrane for K^+ and A^- ions on the one hand, and for Na^+ and Cl^- ions on the other. Despite these concentration gradients, both sides of the membrane are initially electrically (and osmotically) neutral.

Assume that ion channels which are selectively permeable only to K^+ ions are now incorporated into the membrane. These channels are impermeable to all other ions. As a result, there is a flux of K^+ ions across the cell membrane from inside to outside (Fig. 2.10). Initially this flux is driven exclusively by the concentration gradient for K^+ ions according to the equation above. However, with every K^+ ion that flows down its concentration gradient from inside to outside, a surplus positive charge accumulates on the cell's exterior side. This additional positive charge cannot be neutralized because the negatively charged Cl^- and A^- ions cannot pass through the K^+-selective ion channels. The cell's exterior therefore becomes positively charged compared with the cell's interior.

The accumulation of surplus positive charge on the outside of the membrane results in the formation of an electrical *potential difference across the cell membrane* which opposes any further diffusion-driven outward flow of positively charged K^+ ions. This is because the electrical potential difference produces an electrical gradient which opposes the concentration gradient, and via electrostatic interactions, drives K^+ ions from the outside to the inside. This potential difference increases until an *equilibrium* is reached at which the concentration gradient for K^+ ions is just balanced by an opposing electrical gradient for K^+ ions (Fig. 2.11). At equilibrium, the concentration gradient drives the same number of K^+ ions outward per unit time as flow inward driven by the potential difference. In the terminology of thermodynamics, the electrochemical potential for K^+ ions is the same on both sides of the membrane. The resulting electrical potential difference across the membrane is termed the *equilibrium potential* or E_K for K^+ ions. (The equilibrium potential is actually a potential difference; according to convention the electrical potential inside the cell V_i is measured relative to the electrical potential outside V_o).

The equilibrium potential for a single diffusible ion species can be described by the Nernst equation. This equation was derived by Nernst from the laws of thermodynamics. It states that the equilibrium potential for an ion X depends on the absolute temperature, the

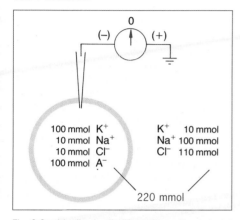

Fig. 2.**9**   Idealized cell with a cell membrane impermeable to ions. There is no potential difference across the membrane. The cell is in osmotic equilibrium. A^- = large organic anions

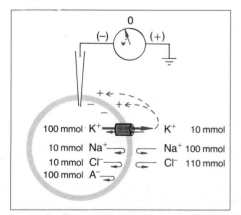

Fig. 2.**10**   The same idealized cell as in Figure 2.**9** immediately after the hypothetical implantation of ion channels which are selectively permeable to K^+ ions. A potential difference across the membrane results from the diffusion-dependent flow of K^+ ions from inside to outside

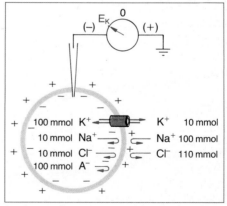

Fig. 2.**11**   The same idealized cell seen in Figure 2.**10**, now having reached an equilibrium state. The outward directed concentration gradient for K^+ ions is balanced by an oppositely directed electrical gradient. The potential difference across the membrane is equal to the equilibrium potential for K^+ ions (E_K)

valency of the diffusing ion, and the concentrations of the ion on both sides of the membrane:

$$E_X = V_i - V_o = \frac{RT}{zF} \times \ln \frac{[X]_o}{[X]_i}$$

R is the gas constant, T the absolute temperature (in degrees Kelvin), F the Faraday constant (96 500 coulomb/g equivalent charge) and z is the valency of ion X. $[X]_o$ and $[X]_i$ are the concentrations of ion X on the outside and inside of the membrane respectively. (For precise measurements, the concentration terms in the equation must be replaced by activity terms). For most neurobiological applications this equation can be simplified by expressing T as 293 °K (20 °C), RT/F as a constant in millivolt units, and by converting ln to log. For a univalent positive ion X:

$$E_x = 58\,mV \times \log \frac{[X]_o}{[X]_i}$$

Thus, if the initial concentration of K^+ ions inside the cell is 0.1 Mol, and the concentration of K^+ ions outside is 0.01 Mol, then

$$E_K = 58\,mV \times \log \frac{[K^+]_o}{[K^+]_i}$$

$$E_K = 58\,mV \times \log \frac{0,01}{0,1}$$

$$E_K = -58\,mV$$

$$E_K = 58\,mV \times (-1)$$

Given a concentration gradient for K^+ ions of 10:1, cell inside against cell outside, a potential difference of –58 mV (inside negative) is formed across the cell membrane, provided that the membrane possesses ion channels which are exclusively permeable to K^+ ions. Interestingly, compared with the total number of K^+ ions inside the cell, only very few have to diffuse through the cell membrane from inside to outside to create this potential. To understand this in a quantitative way, the capacity of the cell membrane to separate electrical charges must be taken into consideration.

The cell membrane has an electrical capacitance

The lipid bilayer that makes up the cell membrane does more than just seal off the cell and anchor transmembrane proteins. Because the membrane forms a very thin, electrically isolating layer which separates two conducting fluids, it invariably also functions as an electrical capacitor. Just like any other capacitor the cell membrane is able to separate charges and thereby create an electrical potential. Quantitatively this property is described by the capacitance C of the cell membrane, which is the amount of electrical charge Q necessary to produce an electrical potential V according to the equation

$$C = Q/V$$

For most cell membranes the capacitance per square centimeter is about 1 μF (microfarad).

This relatively high capacitance of the cell membrane is crucial for the generation of the membrane potential. Under physiological conditions the ionic composition of the extracellular and intracellular compartments always remains electrically neutral (principle of electrical neutrality). There is no excess of dissolved positive or negative charges in either of the two compartments. By contrast, the lipid bilayer of the cell membrane, which has a diameter of only a few nanometers, can accumulate ions of different sign on both its sides. The cell membrane can be considered roughly equivalent to a two-plate capacitor whose capacitance is inversely proportional to the distance between the plates. The entire electrical potential difference between the inside and outside of the cell is determined by the separated ionic charges which accumulate at the cell membrane and so charge up the cellular capacitor (Fig. 2.12).

How much charge has to be separated on the two sides of the cell membrane to produce a potential of –58 mV? From Q = CV and a capacitance of C = 1 μF/cm² one can calculate that per cm²

$$Q = 5.8 \times 10^{-8}\ coulomb$$

must accumulate on the membrane surface. Since one Coulomb comprises 6.25×10^{18} elementary charges, this corresponds to

$$Q = 3.6 \times 10^{11}\ elementary\ charges.$$

A cell body of 50 μ diameter has a membrane surface area of $A = 7.85 \times 10^{-5}$ cm². Thus,

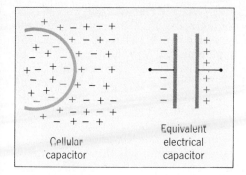

Fig. 2.**12**   The cell membrane as the cellular equivalent of a two-plate capacitor. A potential difference between the inside and the outside of the cell occurs when the cellular capacitor is charged

there must be a charge separation on this membrane surface of

$$Q \times A = 3.6 \times 7.85 \times 10^6 = 27.5 \times 10^6$$

elementary charges.

About 30 million K^+ ions have to leave the inside of the cell and accumulate on the outside of the membrane in order to generate a membrane potential of -58 mV. For a 0.1 molar concentration of K^+ ions inside the cell, this corresponds to *less than 10^{-5}* of the approximately 40×10^{11} K^+ ions present in the cell. Thus, the equilibrium potential for K^+ ions can be established without creating any significant change in the intracellular ion concentration.

If a change in membrane potential occurs, the thermodynamically stable equilibrium potential E_K readjusts itself via ion flux in the appropriate direction. This is because every deviation of the actual membrane potential V_m from the equilibrium potential E_K evokes an electromotive force

$$EMF = V_m - E_K$$

which opposes the deviation and produces an ionic current through the membrane until the equilibrium potential is reestablished. The changes in intracellular ion concentrations necessary for this type of readjustment are again minimal. To compensate for even a 100 mV deviation of the membrane potential from the equilibrium potential in our hypothetical cell, only

$$27.5 \times 10^6 \text{ ions} \times \frac{100 \text{ mV}}{58 \text{ mV}} = 47 \times 10^6 \text{ ions}$$

have to flow from one side of the membrane to the other. This ion flux is so small that the cell could "readjust" to thousands of perturbations of this type without creating major changes in its internal K^+ concentration. We shall see that such perturbations occur often, and are even employed to transmit signals over long distances.

The resting potential is not a simple thermodynamic equilibrium potential

The Nernst equation accurately describes the membrane potential of a cell that is exclusively permeable to K^+ ions. The membrane potential of nonneuronal glia cells, which have a high intracellular concentration of K^+ and are readily permeable only to K^+ ions, can indeed be largely described by the Nernst equation. The membrane potential of a real neuron, however, can only be *approximated* by the equilibrium potential for K^+ ions as described by the Nernst equation (Fig. 2.**13**). This is because the cell membrane of a real nerve cell is not only permeable to K^+, but also to other small inorganic ions. There are two reasons for this.

— Real K^+ channels, in real nerve cells, are partially permeable to other ionic species, particularly to other cations.
— Real neurons have other ion-selective channels in their cell membrane apart from K^+ channels, and these are selective for Na^+, Ca^{2+}, or Cl^- ions.

For both of these reasons a neuron has permeabilities to all these ions which are not insignificant, even when the cell is at rest. Real neurons are really only impermeable to the larger organic anions like amino acids and proteins.

The fact that a neuron is also permeable to ions other than K^+ ions has important consequences for the generation of the membrane potential. The membrane potential V_m is based on a *steady-state equilibrium,* rather than a simple thermodynamic equilibrium. Several different ionic species contribute to this steady state, and unlike a stable thermodynamic equilibrium state, it needs metabolic energy to be maintained.

This becomes obvious if we consider the changes in membrane potential which result when a few Na^+-selective ion channels are incorporated into the cell membrane of our hypothetical neuron (Fig. 2.**14**). Na^+ ions can now flow into the cell. This flux is, on the one hand, driven by the concentration gradient for Na^+,

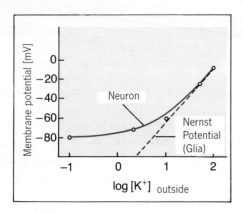

Fig. 2.**13**   The membrane potential of a nerve cell is only approximated by the Nernst potential (equilibrium potential) for K^+ ions. The dependence of the membrane potential on the external K^+ concentration is shown for a typical neuron. The membrane potential for glia cells generally corresponds to the Nernst potential for K^+ ions

since the concentration of Na^+ ions is higher in the extracellular medium than it is in the intracellular. But the ion flux is also driven by an electrical gradient. Given a concentration difference of 10:1 between the outside and inside of the cell, the equilibrium potential for Na^+ is

$$E_{Na} = +58\,mV \times log \frac{[Na^+]_o}{[Na^+]_i}$$

$$E_{Na} = +58\,mV \times log\,10$$

Thus for a membrane potential of $Vm = -58\,mV$, which corresponds to the equilibrium potential for K^+, there is an electromotive force of

$$EMF = V_m - E_{Na} = -58\,mV - (+58\,mV) = -116\,mV$$

(directed inward) acting on the Na^+ ions. An influx of Na^+ ions depolarizes the cell by driving the membrane potential toward the equilibrium potential for Na^+. However, as the membrane potential V_m begins to deviate from the equilibrium potential for K^+, it causes an electromotive force

$$EMF = V_m - E_K$$

for K^+ ions, which opposes the depolarization. The resulting flux of K^+ ions out of the cell drives the membrane potential toward the equilibrium potential for K^+, and tends to repolarize the cell. A steady-state equilibrium is rapidly established where a depolarizing flux

of positively charged Na^+ ions into the cell is exactly counteracted by a hyperpolarizing outward flux of positively charged K^+ ions. The membrane potential V_m that is established by these ionic fluxes differs from an equilibrium potential in that it depends not only on the relative concentrations of these ions, but also on the individual permeabilities of these ions.

Assuming steady-state equilibrium conditions, the *Goldman equation* provides a quantitative description of the way the membrane potential depends on the different permeabilities of the various ions. In its general form, the equation is given as

$$V_m = \frac{RT}{F} \times ln\,\frac{\Sigma_{k=1,n}\,z_k P_k [X_k]_o + \Sigma_{l=1,m} z_l P_l [Y_l]_i}{\Sigma_{k=1,n}\,z_k P_k [X_k]_i + \Sigma_{l=1,m} z_l P_l [Y_l]_o}$$

for n different positively charged ionic species X, and m different negatively charged ionic species Y, with their respective valencies z and total permeabilities P, (o = outside, i = inside). The Goldman equation can be derived from the principles of thermodynamics and electrochemistry given the simplifying assumptions that: (a) the passage of an ionic species through the membrane occurs by simple diffusion as the result of a potential gradient; and (b) the different ionic fluxes through the membrane are independent of one another.

In most cases, the membrane potential of a nerve cell can be described adequately if K^+, Na^+, and Cl^- ions are considered in the Goldman equation. Under steady-state equilibrium conditions the magnitude of the membrane potential of a cell is then given by

$$V_m = 58\,log\,\frac{P_K [K^+]_o + P_{Na}[Na^+]_o + P_{Cl}[Cl^-]_i}{P_K [K^+]_i + P_{Na}[Na^+]_i + P_{Cl}[Cl^-]_o}$$

We can see from this equation that the greater the permeability of the membrane for a particular ionic species, the more the equilibrium potential of that ionic species determines the membrane potential V_m. If we take the (hypothetical) extreme case of $P_{Na} = P_{Cl} = 0$, then the equation above reduces to

$$V_m = 58\,log\,\frac{[K^+]_o}{[K^+]_i} = E_K$$

In reality P_{Na} and P_{Cl} are never equal to 0. Typical measurements for the various ionic permeabilities in a resting neuron (squid giant fiber) are $P_K : P_{Na} : P_{Cl} = 1 : 0.04 : 0.45$.

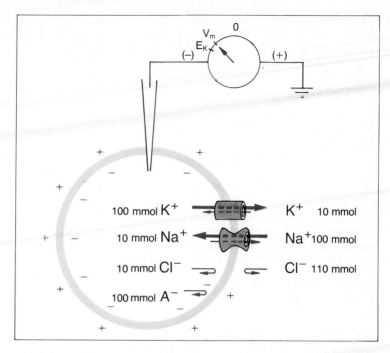

Fig. 2.14   The membrane potential is determined by a steady-state equilibrium. The same idealized cell as in Figure 2.**11** following addition of Na^+-selective ion channels. A steady-state equilibrium becomes established in which the inflow of Na^+ ions is balanced by an outflow of K^+ ions. The resulting stable membrane potential V_m is determined by the concentration gradients and the permeabilities of both ionic species

Thus, even though the resulting *resting potential* of a neuron generally lies near the K^+ equilibrium potential, it is not a thermodynamic equilibrium potential. Ionic fluxes must always occur across the cell membrane if the resting potential is to be maintained. These ionic fluxes would lead to a gradual decline in the ionic concentration gradients, particularly for Na^+ and K^+ ions, if metabolic energy were not continually invested to drive the compensatory Na^+–K^+ ion pumps. Thus, the Na^+–K^+ ion pumps play an important indirect role in the maintenance of the resting potential. But this is still not the whole story. Since every cycle of the Na^+–K^+ ion pump transports three Na^+ ions out of the cell for every 2 K^+ ions it transports into the cell, this results in one net positive charge being moved outward with each cycle. In this way the active Na^+–K^+ ion pumps also contribute directly to the membrane potential. They are *electrogenic*. One can show that the electrogenic contribution of the Na^+–K^+ ion pumps to the resting potential is proportional to P_{Na}/P_K under steady-state equi-

librium conditions. In neurons with a relatively high Na^+ permeability this can account for up to 20% of the total value of the resting potential.

The electrical properties of the cell membrane can be represented by equivalent circuits

In its resting potential the neuron has at its disposal a cellular source of energy which can be used to generate electrical signals. In order to describe the processes of signal generation at the cell membrane quantitatively, an electrical analog *equivalent circuit* which reproduces the electrical behavior of the cell membrane is useful. Such an equivalent circuit could be very simple if the membrane potential were only dependent on the diffusion of a single ionic species like K^+ (Fig. 2.**15**). The diffusion-dependent ion flux responsible for the potential across the cell membrane can be viewed simply as an electrical current carried by K^+ ions. This current flows through ion-selective membrane channels each of which has a unitary conductance g_K for K^+ ions. These membrane channels can be represented as approximating an ohmic resistor R_K with a total summed conductance $G_K = \Sigma g_K = 1/R_K$. The driving force for the ionic current can be represented as a battery in series with this conductance, with a voltage corresponding to the equilibrium potential E_K for K^+ ions. Finally, the characteristics of the lipid bilayer which allow the membrane to separate charges can be represented by a capacitor with a capacitance of C_m connected in parallel.

Since, however, the resting potential is determined by a steady-state equilibrium of independent K^+, Na^+, and Cl^- ion currents, the equivalent circuit for the membrane potential must in fact contain three different summed conductances G_K, G_{Na}, and G_{Cl}, and three different batteries with voltages E_K, E_{Na}, and E_{Cl}. These batteries must also have the correct polarities. In addition, in a steady-state equilibrium the K^+ and Na^+ currents produced by active Na^+–K^+ pumps also have to be considered along with the diffusion-dependent ionic currents I_K, I_{Na}, and I_{Cl} flowing through ion-selective channels (Fig. 2.16).

Describing the membrane potential with the aid of such electrical analog circuits is particularly useful for analyzing changes in current and voltage in a nerve cell. This is important because the propagation of neuronal signals depends on such changes in current and voltage, as well as on their spatial and temporal manifestations.

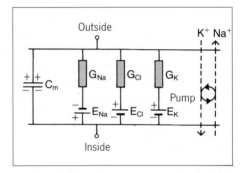

Fig. 2.**15**   Equivalent circuit for the electrical behavior of a hypothetical cell membrane permeable only to K^+ ions. The circuit consists of a resistor, a battery and a capacitor. G_K represents the total conductance of the membrane for K^+ and corresponds to the conductance of all K^+-selective ion channels. C_m represents the capacitance of the membrane. E_K is a voltage source whose potential represents the equilibrium potential for K^+ (after Hille)

Fig. 2.**16**   Equivalent circuit for a neuronal cell membrane which is selectively permeable to Na^+, K^+, and Cl^-. The total conductance and the electromotive driving force for each ionic species are represented by a resistor and a battery. C_m is the capacitance of the membrane and is represented by a capacitor. A Na^+–K^+ ion pump maintains the concentration gradients across the membrane

Neurons Generate and Conduct Electrical Signals

Origin and significance of neuronal signals

Neurons use electrical signals to process and transmit information. These signals are temporal changes in the potential across the cell membrane. Such signals, which are "disturbances" of the resting potential, arise as a result of ionic currents flowing into or out of the cell. These ionic currents are evoked either at the synapses of a nerve cell by the activity of other presynaptic neurons, or, in specialized receptor cells, by specific sensory stimuli. *Excitatory postsynaptic potentials* (EPSPs) and *inhibitory postsynaptic potentials* (IPSPs) can be evoked at a synapse as a result of ionic currents through the membrane of the postsynaptic cell. The potential changes resulting in the specialized sensory cells are called *receptor potentials*.

Postsynaptic potentials and receptor potentials are graded in amplitude and time course, and spread passively along the cell membrane without signal amplification. These *electrotonic* potentials can conduct information, in analog form, about the amplitude and time course of a given input, be it a synaptic input or the input from sensory cells. This capacity for analog information coding and conduction is limited by the fact that the conversion of the transmembrane current into an electrotonic voltage signal is not distortion-free. The temporal properties of an electrotonic potential will be slowed and its amplitude attenuated due to the electrical resistance and capacitance properties of the cell membrane.

Membrane resistance and membrane capacitance determine the time course of an electrotonic signal

Signal conduction in the processes of a nerve cell and in a cable consisting of a metallic conducting core are basically similar, but they differ quantitatively in two important ways.

- The conductance of a typical nerve cell is about 10^7 times less than that of a metallic cable. All the currents in nerve cells are carried by ions, whereas those in metallic conductors are carried by free electrons. Ions have a smaller mobility, and occur in lower concentration in the nerve cell, than do electrons in a metal wire.
- Current flow decreases much more in a nerve cell than in a cable. The membrane of a nerve cell is a comparatively poor insulator. The cell membrane is leaky to ions mainly because of the ion channels it has incorporated in it. Thin nerve processes also have a relatively high internal resistance to ionic currents, and so a certain proportion of the ionic current in a nerve fiber will not spread

longitudinally but instead "leak" out through the membrane. These factors result in a relatively large attenuation of the voltage signal as it passes along the nerve fiber. Added to this is the fact that the cell membrane has a relatively high capacitance. As ionic current propagates along a nerve cell longitudinally, capacitive currents are diverted to recharge the membrane capacitance. As a result, fast signals in particular become slowed and attenuated as they propagate.

In order to understand these two processes, it is helpful to construct an electrical equivalent circuit for a patch of cell membrane and then apply the laws of electrodynamics to the analysis of neuronal signal generation. What effect does an ionic current which flows across the cell membrane have on the membrane potential? If the cell membrane were composed only of resistive elements, then it could be represented by a simple resistor in an equivalent circuit (Fig. 2.**17**). A current pulse which flows across the membrane is represented by the resistive current I_R flowing across the resistor after the current source is turned on. According to Ohm's law, the membrane potential V_m then has exactly the same time course as the current pulse

$$V_m = RI_R$$

If the cell membrane were composed only of capacitive elements, then it could be represented by a single capacitor in an equivalent circuit (Fig. 2.**18**). Switching on a current source causes a capacitive current I_C to flow across the capacitor, and since $V = Q/C$, this

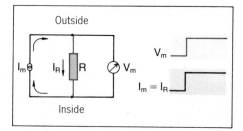

Fig. 2.**17**   Current–voltage relationship for a hypothetical membrane consisting only of resistive elements. Switching on a current source causes the total membrane current I_m to flow as a resistive current I_R across the resistor R. This produces a membrane potential V_m which has the same time course as I_m

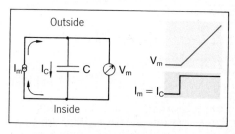

Fig. 2.**18**   Current–voltage relationship for a hypothetical membrane consisting only of capacitive elements. Switching on a current source causes the total membrane current I_m to flow as a capacitive current I_C and charges the capacitor C. This produces a membrane potential V_m which increases at a constant rate

leads to a change in membrane potential according to

$$\frac{dV_m}{dt} = \frac{1}{C}\frac{dQ}{dt} = \frac{I_C}{C}$$

A constant current pulse would produce a constantly changing membrane potential, and the time courses of current and voltage would therefore differ very strongly.

A real cell membrane, as described above, has both resistive and capacitative elements which run in *parallel* in an electrically equivalent circuit (Fig. 2.**19**). This has the important consequence that the voltage changes generated by the capacitative and resistive elements of membrane must always be the same. How would the membrane potential change on application of a constant rectangular current pulse? Since in the very first instant a voltage has yet to develop across the membrane, no current can flow across the resistor. The total current, in the form of the capacitative current I_C, is therefore available to charge up the capacitor. So initially, the voltage will increase like that in a purely capacitative equivalent circuit.

However, as soon as the capacitor begins to charge and a voltage difference occurs, a partial resistive current I_R driven by this voltage difference flows across the resistor. This, in turn, means that less capacitative current is available to charge the capacitor ($I_R + I_C = I_m =$ const.). The rate at which the capacitor charges will decrease. As the voltage at the capacitor continues to increase, more and more resistive

current flows across the resistor, until finally a voltage is reached which will cause the total current, now following Ohm's law as $I_m = I_R = V_m/R$, to flow across the resistor. The capacitor does not charge further. A new constant membrane potential has established itself. The established voltage is now that of a purely resistive equivalent circuit.

The time course for the voltage that develops across the membrane in response to a constant rectangular current pulse is exponential. It can be described as

$$\Delta V_m(t) = I_m R(1-e^{-t/\tau})$$

The parameter τ is called the time constant of the membrane and is defined in terms of the membrane resistance and membrane capacitance as

$$\tau = RC$$

The time constant is equivalent to the time following application of a rectangular current pulse at which the membrane potential reaches 63% of its final value (because $1 - (1/e) \approx 63/100$). For most neurons τ lies between 1 and 20 ms. The longer the time constant, the longer a change in membrane potential requires to reach its new plateau value, and the greater will be the distortion during the generation of an electrotonic signal.

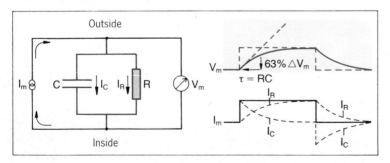

Fig. 2.**19**   Current–voltage relationship for a cell membrane consisting of resistive as well as capacitative elements. Switching on a current source causes the total membrane current I_m to flow initially as a capacitative current I_C across the capacitor C. The capacitative current I_C then decreases continually while the resistive current I_R increases, until the total current flows as a resistive current across the resistor R. This produces a membrane potential V_m which approaches the maximum value $I_m R$ exponentially with a time constant $\tau = RC$. After switching off the current source, the capacitor C discharges across the resistor R, with I_C and I_R having opposite signs

Electrotonic potentials decrease during spatial conduction

During the conduction of an electrotonic signal along the processes of a neuron, we encounter the problem of signal decrement. This is due to the fact that during the longitudinal spread of an ionic current along the processes of a neuron, a portion of this current is lost.

A quantitative analysis of these events is possible by using an equivalent circuit which takes into account the membrane resistance as well as the internal resistance for each unit of length of a neuronal process (Fig. 2.20). The external resistance of the extracellular fluid is neglected. The cell membrane has a certain, albeit small, permeability to ions for every unit of length. Thus, during the spread of an ionic current along a neuronal process, a portion of the total current will always flow across the membrane resistance to the outside and therefore be lost for further signal propagation. An equiv-

alent resistive current loss is repeated for each unit of length. Therefore, with increasing distance an exponential decline in ionic current, and in the potential change produced by the current occurs. The decrement of the membrane potential with distance x from the point of origin is given by

$$V_m(x) = V_o e^{-x/\lambda}$$

V_o is the potential change at the point of origin and λ is the *length constant* of the nerve process. The length constant corresponds to the distance over which a potential decreases to 37% of its original value (because $1/e \approx 37/100$). λ depends on the relationship between the membrane resistance r_m and the internal length resistance of the nerve process r_i according to

$$\lambda = \sqrt{(r_m/r_i)}$$

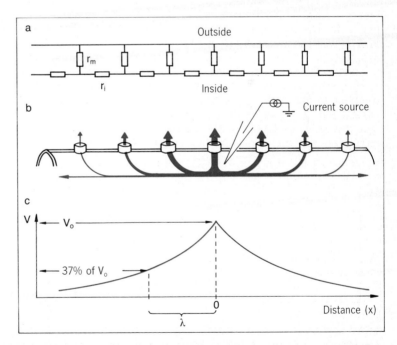

Fig. 2.**20**   Attenuation of an electrotonic signal during propagation. **a** Equivalent circuit of a hypothetical nerve fiber consisting of membrane resistances r_m and internal resistances r_i. **b** Current loss as a result of membrane conductance. During the spread of an ionic current, a certain percentage of the current flows across the membrane per length unit. **c** Exponential decrease of the potential change with distance from the source. V_o is the potential change at the source. λ is the length constant and gives the distance over which the potential change has declined to about 37% of its original value

The more ion channels there are per unit of length in the membrane, the smaller r_m will be. The smaller the diameter of a nerve process, the larger r_i will be. For most neurons λ is 0.1 – 1.0 mm. Since the length constant determines how far potentials can be electrotonically conducted, it is clear that for most neurons passive, electrotonic, signal transmission is only possible over short distances.

Apart from the resistive current loss mentioned above there is also a capacitative current loss during signal propagation. This is because for every unit of length, a portion of the ionic current must be used to recharge the membrane capacitance during the spread of a potential change. Membrane capacitance therefore must be considered in any realistic representation of the equivalent circuit of a nerve process. The transmission properties of such a *cable model* are complex and cannot be explained using just simple exponential laws (Fig. 2.21). Quantitatively, these events, which are similar to those involved in signal transmission in an undersea cable, can be described by solving the "cable equation"

$$V(x, t) = \lambda^2 \frac{\delta^2 V}{\delta x^2} - \tau \frac{\delta V}{\delta t}$$

(Jack et al., 1983). Qualitatively, both signal decrement and signal distortion increase with distance from the point of origin of a potential change, and both processes affect fast signals more strongly than slow ones.

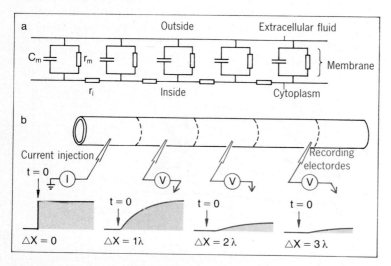

Fig. 2.**21a,b**   Cable model for signal propagation in a neuron. **a** Equivalent circuit of a nerve fiber whose membrane is represented by resistive elements r_m and capacitative elements C_m connected in parallel, and whose cytoplasm is represented by internal resistances r_i. **b** Spread of potential change along a nerve fiber. Potential changes caused by current application at one site are attenuated and temporally distorted with increasing distance from the source

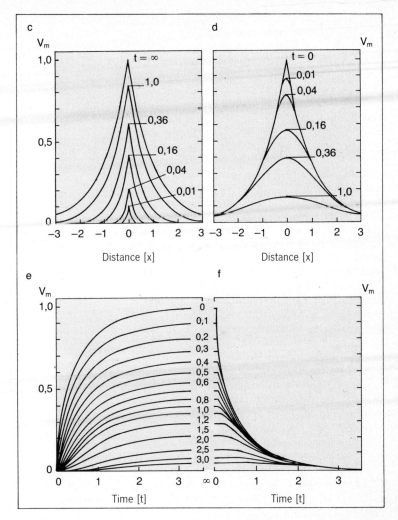

Fig. 2.**21c – f**   Theoretical distribution of the changes in electrotonic potential in a nerve fiber following the beginning (**c,e**) and end (**d,f**) of a constant current pulse applied at site $x = 0$. The spread of the potential changes at various times is shown in **c** and **d**. The time course of the potential changes at various sites along the nerve fiber is shown in **e** and **f**. The time (t) is given in units of the time constant τ, and the distance (x) in units of the length constant λ. Potential changes are normalized with respect to the maximum potential change (after Hodgkin and Rushton)

Neuronal integration is based on passive electrotonic potentials

The passive electrical properties of neurones, represented by τ and λ, are important for the cellular integration of synaptic inputs. They determine the time course of synaptic potentials, and how efficiently these potentials are conducted from their point of origin to their spatially distant sites of action. In this way the resistive and capacitive properties of a neuron

contribute to *neuronal integration*. They influence the processes by which a neuron converts all incoming signals into a response.

The time constant is important because most synaptic potentials are evoked by relatively short-duration synaptic currents. The longer the time constant of the synaptic membrane, the longer the duration of the synaptic potentials elicited by such currents. If their duration is sufficiently long, then several syn-

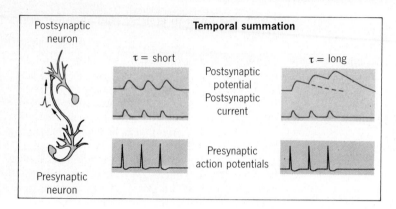

Fig. 2.**22**   Synaptic integration via temporal summation. The potential changes which are evoked in a postsynaptic cell by repetitive activity in a presynaptic neuron can temporally overlap and their amplitudes summate. However, this happens only when the time constant of the postsynaptic membrane is sufficiently long

aptic potentials that are elicited within a short space of time by the same presynaptic neuron can temporally overlap. A *temporal summation* results (Fig. 2.**22**). This can, for example, cause the amplitudes of successive EPSPs to summate such that the threshold of the neuron for the release of synaptic transmitter, or for the generation of an action potential, is reached. Temporal summation can also play a role in receptor cells.

   The length constant of a neuron is important because it influences the spread of signals and thus the development of *spatial summation* (Fig. 2.**23**). In spatial summation, synaptic potentials which are evoked at spatially different locations in a neuron can summate. If the length constant of a neuron is very short, then synaptic potentials evoked in dendritic branches distant from one another decrease to such an extent during propagation that a summating interaction is barely possible. To all intents and purposes the two synaptic potentials then act in isolation from one another.

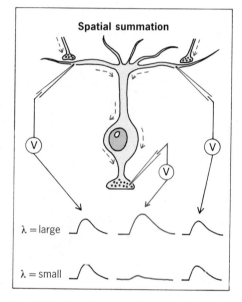

Fig. 2.**23**   Synaptic integration via spatial summation. Synaptic potentials evoked at different sites in a neuron can summate at a distant site. The chances for summation become weaker the smaller the length constant λ of the neuron

There are limits to electrotonic signal conduction

As long as a neuron is small in relation to its length constant (and as long as the signals transmitted by this neuron are slow compared with the time constant), then electrotonic signal conduction will be sufficient for cellular information processing. This is the case for many neurons in the brain. These neurons carry out all their signal conduction on the basis of electrotonically transmitted synaptic potentials. Examples of such neurons are the horizontal cells, the bipolar cells, and many of the amacrine cells in the retina of vertebrates, as well as the "nonspiking" premotor interneurons of arthropods (Fig. 2.24). Like most neurons in more complex nervous systems, these neurons are small and have only a short axon, or even no axon at all.

Not all neurons, however, can rely on electrotonic potentials. Many animals are much larger than the length constants of their neurons! They must, therefore, possess neurons which can transmit signals over relatively long distances. Since electrotonic potentials are not appropriate for this, a second mechanism is used to conduct signals in neurons with a longer axon. This mechanism is based on the transformation of passively spreading electrotonic potentials into actively evoked, all-or-nothing pulsed potentials called *action potentials*. Action potentials can be conducted quickly, without temporal distortion or decrement, and over long distances.

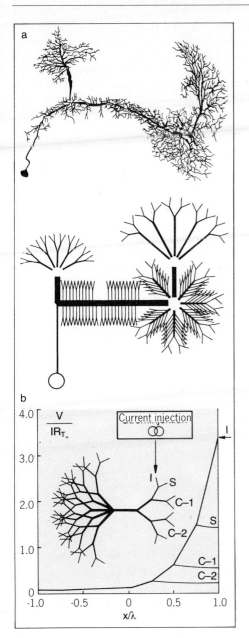

Fig. 2.**24**   Electrotonic signal propagation. **a** A premotor interneuron of the locust which produces exclusively passively transmitted potentials. The electrotonic behavior of the interneuron (above) can be described quantitatively in terms of the equivalent cylinder model (below). **b** Equivalent cylinder model and calculated distribution of potential changes in different regions of the model as a result of constant current injection at the site l. x = distance, λ = length constant, S = first-order branches, C-1 = second-order branches, C-2 = third-order branches (after Siegler and Burrows, and Rall)

Action Potentials Allow a Rapid and Reliable Transfer of Signals over Larger Distances

Principle and significance

Many neurons, in particular those that must transmit signals over relatively large distances, are equipped with special excitatory mechanisms. These mechanisms allow the neuron to carry out a rapid and regenerative depolarization and repolarization of the membrane in response to a suprathreshold depolarization of the membrane potential. The form of this explosion-like wave of depolarization and repolarization, termed the action potential, is stereotyped. Starting from the negative resting potential, positive potential levels can be reached in less than a millisecond. Afterward the membrane potential can return to values near those of the resting potential, again within milliseconds (Fig. 2.25). Action potentials propagate in a regenerative manner along a neural process, without attenuation or distortion. They are therefore ideally suited to signal conduction over longer distances.

What are these properties of the action potential based on? The answer takes us once again into molecular dimensions. This is because the "macroscopic" properties of the action potential are determined by the "microscopic" properties of a special class of transmembrane proteins.

Some ion channels open and shut in a voltage-dependent manner

There are ion channels which have either an open or a shut configuration depending on the membrane potential. Such *voltage-dependent or voltage-gated ion channels* generally belong to a class of transmembrane proteins which can have different quasi-stable configurations. Each configuration is stable in the face of small thermal molecular motion. Transitions from one configuration to another are facilitated by various *gating mechanisms*. Such gating mechanisms can be activated by extracellular ligand binding, by changes in intracellular ion concentrations, by intracellular messenger substances, or by potential changes across the membrane. More than one of these factors can influence the gating mechanism of an ion channel. A voltage-dependent ion channel, for example, can also be influenced by the intracellular Ca^{2+} concentration.

The transition of a voltage-dependent ion channel from a quasi-stable closed form to a quasi-stable open form can only be described statistically. This is because the actual conformational change involves energetically unfavorable transition forms and requires stochastically occurring suprathreshold thermal

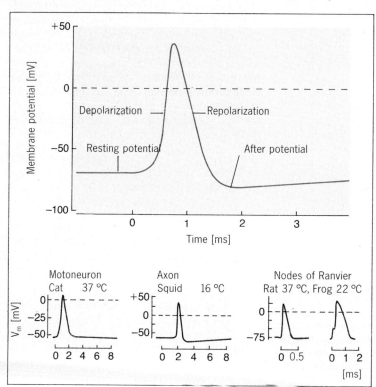

Fig. 2.**25**   The action potential. A general scheme for the course of an action potential (above). Real action potentials recorded in different neurons (below) (after Hille)

movements in the channel region. A *relaxation time,* similar to the half-life of a radioisotope, is used to describe the transition rate from one configuration to another. The configuration that has the lowest total energy at any given membrane potential is statistically the most probable form (Fig. 2.26). This stochastic nature of the conformational change applies generally to structural transitions in gated ion channels.

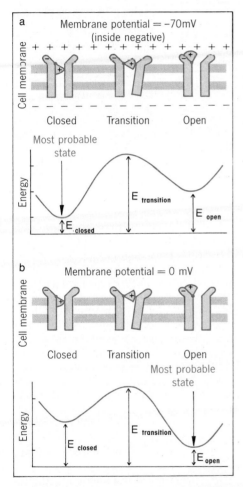

Fig. 2.**26**   Schematic representation of the gating behavior of a hypothetical voltage-dependent ion channel which can assume several conformations. **a** At the resting potential the closed conformation of the ion channel has the lowest energy and is therefore the most probable state. **b** During a strong depolarization the open conformation has the lowest energy and is thereby the most probable state (after Alberts et al.)

The properties of individual gated ion channels in neuronal membranes can be determined with a high resolution current measurement technique called the *patch clamp* method (Fig. 2.27). This involves placing a microelectrode on the surface of the neuron and, by using simple suction, achieving a tight seal (with a resistance in the gigaohm range) between the microelectrode tip and the membrane region under the microelectrode. The result is that all the current flowing through that small patch of membrane reaches the microelectrode, and from there a sensitive current-measuring device. The potential of the isolated patch of membrane can be set and held at a defined value via a feedback circuit. Further, a few simple mechanical manipulations permit the microscopically small membrane patch to be freed from the nerve cell and oriented so that either the former cell exterior or the former cytoplasmic side now faces outward. This allows current measurements to be made from isolated membrane fragments under conditions where the ionic surround can be changed and precisely controlled. Developed by Sakmann and Neher, this potentiostatic measurement on small membrane patches makes it possible to measure the *elementary currents* through single ion channels, and therefore the voltage-dependent kinetic properties of single molecules.

There are many different types of voltage-gated ion channels, all of which have different molecular properties. In order to understand the fundamentals of action potential generation, we need only to consider two of these channel types: these are the *voltage-gated Na+ channel* and the *voltage-gated K+ channel.*

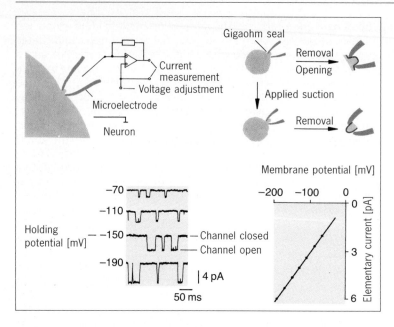

Fig. 2.**27**   Potentiostatic measurement of the elementary currents which flow through single ion channels. The patch clamp technique. Schematic representation of the recording technique (above). Voltage dependence of the elementary current through open ion channels (below)(after Neher and Sakmann)

Conformational changes in a voltage-gated Na⁺ channel constitute the molecular basis of the action potential

The major component of the voltage-gated Na^+ channel consists of a glycoprotein with a molecular weight of about 260 kDa. The primary structure of the protein segment of this molecule has been determined using recombinant DNA techniques. The protein is a single polypeptide chain consisting of four internally homologous transmembrane domains which are interconnected by smaller nonhomologous sequences. Each one of these four domains consists of six helical subregions which probably span the cell membrane (Fig. 2.**28**). Other voltage-gated ion channels appear to have a related structure given the high degree of homology in their primary amino acid sequences. Further small glycoprotein subunits can be added to the large protein unit in different neurones. The major protein alone can generate a functional Na^+ channel. Following injection of the mRNA for the major protein into a nonneural cell (an oocyte), this cell can translate the mRNA into protein, and then incorporate this functional-channel protein into its own membrane.

The four transmembrane domains of the major protein are thought to be arranged around a central pore region in the membrane, and to change their configuration in a voltage-dependent manner, leading to opening or closing of the channel. The molecular basis of the ion selectivity of the Na^+ channel is still not clear. The amino acid sequence of the major protein unit is surprisingly similar in all animal species studied to date. Nevertheless, there are subtle differences in the structural, physiological, and pharmacological properties of the voltage-dependent Na^+ channels in different animal species, as well as in different neurons of the same species. The following description of the properties of the voltage-dependent Na^+ channel must therefore be viewed as a simplification.

The different quasi-stable configurations in which voltage-gated Na^+ channels occur can be summarized as *closed, open,* and *inactivated.* At the resting potential, the channel mainly occurs in its closed form. This is because at the resting potential the closed form is energetically the most stable. As the membrane potential becomes less negative, that is, as the neuron is depolarized, the open form then becomes energetically more favorable.

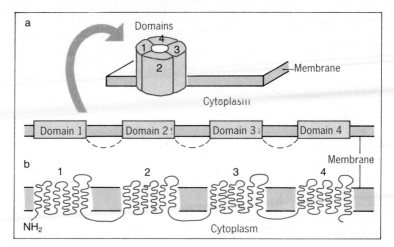

Fig. 2.**28** Molecular organization of the voltage-dependent Na⁺ channel. **a** The major protein consists of four linked domains which are arranged around a central pore in the membrane. **b** Each domain (1–4) contains six helical motifs which presumably extend through the membrane (after Noda et al.)

Thus, when the neuron is depolarized the channel switches from the closed to the open configuration (Fig. 2.**29**). In the open configuration the channel selectively allows Na⁺ ions to diffuse according to their electrochemical gradient.

The changes in the total energy of the two conformational states are induced by the large changes in the electrical field across the membrane which arise from a depolarization. For example, when a membrane with a diameter of about 10 nm is depolarized from –70 mV to –20 mV, this corresponds to a change in the electrical field across the membrane of 50 000 V/cm! Such intense electrical fields can exert quite large forces on the protein region of the Na⁺ channel. These forces can affect the polarizable chemical bonds and the charged amino acid residues in such a way that a conformational change from closed to open is energetically favored. The Na⁺ channel therefore possesses a type of potential sensor that reacts to changes in the electrical field, and then evokes conformational changes in the ion channel. The shift in membrane charge during such conformational changes is small, but can be measured as a capacitative *gating* current.

A short time after transition from the closed to the open configuration, the Na⁺ channel switches spontaneously to a third, inactivated configuration, despite the continued depolarization. Once the channel is in its inactivated configuration it is impermeable to Na⁺ ions, and thus is functionally closed. However, this inactivated configuration differs from the initial closed form, in that the channel cannot immediately switch to an open form again. Put another way: even on strong depolarization, the inactivated form has only a small probability of switching to the open configuration. In order to open again, the channel must first be brought into its closed, but not inactivated, form. This happens when the membrane potential is repolarized to values near the resting potential. A subsequent depolarization can then once again lead to a rapid opening of the ion channel.

A transient inward Na⁺ current depolarizes the neuron

The membrane regions of a neuron capable of generating action potentials possess many Na⁺ channels. In nonmyelinated axons, values of between 35 and 500 Na⁺ channels per square micrometer are found. In response to a sufficiently large depolarization of the membrane, some of these channels will switch to their open configuration. Driven by their concentration and electrical gradients, Na⁺ ions will then flow into the neuron through the open channels. A Na⁺ current, in the picoampere range, will flow through each open channel before the channel switches to its inactivated config-

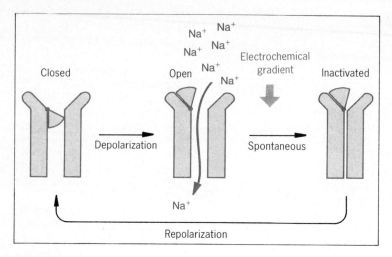

Fig. 2.**29** Schematic representation of the gating behavior of the voltage-dependent Na^+ channel. The channel goes from a closed to an open conformation when the neuron is depolarized. Subsequently the channel inactivates spontaneously

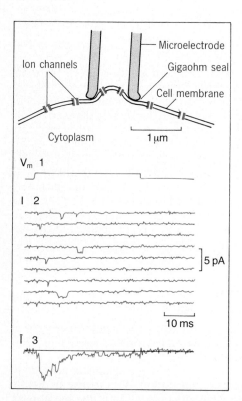

Fig. 2.**30** Characterization of the voltage-dependent Na^+ channel with the patch clamp technique. Single ion channels open and close in a stochastic manner in response to repeated depolarizing voltage steps (1), resulting in a corresponding fluctuation in the elementary currents flowing through the open channels (2). The total current flowing through many such statistically fluctuating channels has a continuous course (3) (after Sigworth and Neher)

uration. Thus, every single channel allows a Na^+ current to pass in an all-or-nothing manner. However, the total inward Na^+ current flowing through many Na^+ channels, all of which open in a statistically fluctuating manner, has a more continuous time course, and reaches much higher values (Fig. 2.**30**). This total inward Na^+ current causes a further depolarization of the membrane. As a result, other Na^+ channels which were previously closed switch to an open configuration. This results once more in an increased Na^+ inward current, which causes a further depolarization, and so on (Fig. 2.**31**).

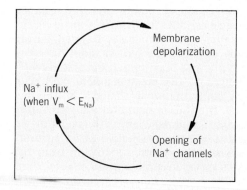

Fig. 2.**31** Self-amplifying cycle which leads to the rapid opening of many voltage-dependent Na^+ channels on initiation of an action potential

Through this regenerative *self-amplifying process,* most of the Na⁺ channels can switch to their open state in less than 1 ms. The permeability of the membrane to Na⁺ ions becomes much higher than to K⁺ ions, and the peak value of the Na⁺ inward current reaches 1 mA per square centimeter of membrane surface. The inward flowing Na⁺ ions drive the membrane potential toward the equilibrium potential for sodium, E_{Na}, which lies near +50 mV, inside positive with respect to outside. Thus the membrane potential can change from –70mV to almost +50 mV in less than 1 ms (Fig. 2.32).

However, the membrane potential does not generally reach +50 mV. This is because very soon after they have opened, the Na⁺ channels switch spontaneously to their inactivated, functionally closed, state. As a result, the Na⁺ permeability, having reached its maximum value, falls back to its small initial value, so that the membrane potential is repolarized once more to the value of the resting potential.

Not every depolarization produces an action potential. There is a *threshold level* of depolarization which must be exceeded for the regenerative opening of the Na⁺ channels to occur. If the depolarization remains below this threshold level then no action potential is generated. This is because small depolarizations result in only a few Na⁺ channels switching to an open configuration. Accordingly, the Na⁺ influx is also initially small leading to only a small additional depolarization. However, since the membrane possesses a certain resting conductance for K⁺ ions, every depolarization away from the resting potential evokes a repolarizing outward K⁺ current. This leads to competition between inflowing Na⁺ and outflowing K⁺ ions. If the outward K⁺ current dominates, the resulting membrane potential moves back again to the resting potential, and the evoked depolarization remains subthreshold. If the inward Na⁺ current dominates, that is if sufficient Na⁺ channels are opened by the evoked depolarization, then the self-amplifying, autocatalytic cycle that leads to further Na⁺ channels opening is initiated. Once the depolarization exceeds this threshold level, then a stereotyped action potential is generated, which no longer depends on the amplitude of the suprathreshold depolarization. The action potential is an all-or-nothing response.

The above described depolarization of the membrane potential from –70mV to positive values, and its repolarization back to –70mV, all within a few milliseconds, result in an action potential of the type seen in the myelinated axons of vertebrates. The properties of this type of action potential are largely determined by the characteristics of the voltage-dependent Na⁺ channels. In many neurons

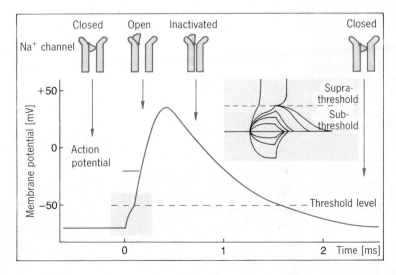

Fig. 2.**32**   Time course of an action potential. The opening of a few Na⁺ channels leads to an initial depolarization. If this depolarization exceeds a threshold value then a rapid regenerative opening of many other Na⁺ channels follows, resulting in the depolarizing phase of an action potential. Since the Na⁺ channels spontaneously inactivate, the repolarization of the membrane occurs automatically

that produce action potentials, an even shorter duration action potential can be achieved due to the additional influence of a voltage-gated K+ channel.

An outward K+ current increases the repolarization rate of the action potential

At the resting potential, the voltage-gated K+ channel is mostly in its closed configuration. Depolarization of the membrane results in a transition to the open configuration. In these respects the channel resembles the voltage-gated Na+ channel. However, the voltage-dependent K+ channel differs from the voltage-gated Na+ channel in three ways.

– The transition of the K+ channel from the closed to the open configuration is slower than for the Na+ channel.
– The K+ channel does not switch spontaneously from an open configuration to an inactivated and functionally closed form.
– The open K+ channel can only be changed to a functionally closed form when the membrane potential is repolarized to values near that of the resting potential.

Given these properties, the following will occur during a depolarization when voltage-gated Na+ channels as well as voltage-depen-

dent K+ channels are present in the membrane (Fig. 2.33). Initially, Na+ channels will open as a result of suprathreshold depolarization, Na+ influx occurs, and this will further depolarize the membrane, as a result of which more Na+ channels will open, and so on. On its own this autocatalytic sequence would depolarize the membrane up to positive values. However, even before the maximum depolarization is reached, Na+ channels begin to inactivate. This would normally lead to a slow repolarization of the membrane, except that the initial depolarization also causes an opening of K+ channels, albeit with slower kinetics. The K+ conductance increases considerably, and following its electrochemical gradient, there is a large K+ efflux out of the cell. This leads to a rapid repolarization of the neuron toward the equilibrium potential for K+ ions, E_K. As a consequence of the transient large increase in the K+ conductance, the repolarization can even lead to an afterpotential that is more negative than the resting potential. The repolarization of the membrane potential results in the voltage-dependent K+ channels moving from an open to a closed configuration. The initial conditions are thereby reestablished, and the membrane potential is once again at the resting potential. The end result of this interaction of Na+ and K+ channels is a rapid action potential of about 1 ms duration.

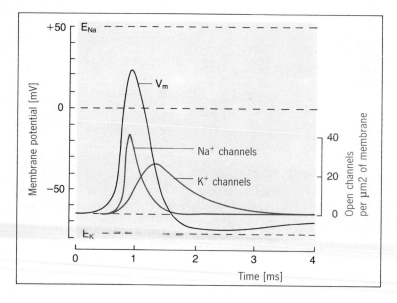

Fig. 2.**33**   Form of an action potential generated by voltage-dependent Na+ and K+ channels. The variation of the membrane potential with time, as well as the number of open channels per µm² of membrane surface are shown for a given axon region (after Hodgkin and Huxley, and Hille)

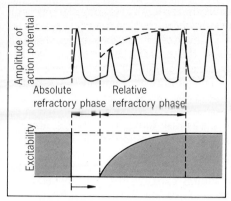

Fig. 2.**34** Refractory phases following an action potential (after Eckert)

Although such an action potential is very short, a second action potential cannot occur immediately after the first. The membrane remains in a *refractory state* for some milliseconds following the generation of an action potential because many Na⁺ channels are still in their inactivated form, and Na⁺ channels cannot be reopened from their inactivated state. This means that another action potential can only be evoked after the membrane is repolarized, and the Na⁺ channels switch, according to their own kinetics, from an inactivated to a closed configuration. Once in the closed configuration they can then be activated again. The refractory state can be divided into an *absolute refractory period,* during which no action potential can be evoked, and a subsequent *relative refractory period,* during which the amplitude of the action potential generated does not yet reach its maximum value (Fig. 2.**34**).

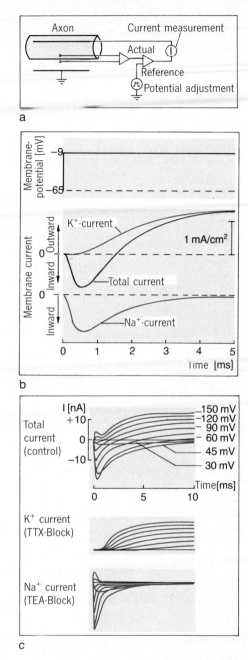

Fig. 2.**35** Measurement of "macroscopic" ionic currents using the voltage clamp technique. **a** Simplified representation of the apparatus required to control membrane potential, and measure the transmembrane currents flowing at a given potential value. **b** Response of an axon membrane to a depolarizing voltage step under voltage clamp conditions. The total current is the ionic current that is measured under normal conditions. K⁺ current is the ionic current that is measured when the extracellular Na⁺ is replaced by choline. The Na⁺ current is the calculated difference between the total current and the K⁺ current. **c** Pharmacological separation of the component ion currents of an axon membrane under voltage clamp conditions. A series of different voltages are applied under control conditions, during TTX block of Na⁺ channels, and during TEA block of K⁺ channels (after Hodgkin and Huxley, and Hille)

Classic voltage clamp experiments provide a phenomenological description of ionic currents during the action potential

Measurements on single ion channels allow the current and voltage relationships that occur in a neuron during the generation of an action potential to be predicted. These predictions can be tested if the time- and voltage-dependence of the ionic current across the whole cell membrane is measured. On a historical note, it is interesting that Hodgkin and Huxley had already carried out a phenomenological "verification" of the ion channel concept in the 1950s, at a time when there was still no method available for studying the molecular behavior of ion channels. In their pioneering experiments, Hodgkin and Huxley employed the *voltage clamp* technique on a particularly fortuitous preparation, the squid giant axon. Voltage clamp consists of a feedback amplifier which measures the actual value of the membrane potential via a first intracellular electrode, and then compares this with a predetermined reference value (Fig. 2.**35a**). Whenever the actual value deviates from the reference value, then the necessary current required to reestablish the reference value is injected into the cell via a second intracellular electrode. In this way the membrane potential can be controlled at all times, and the transmembrane currents flowing at a given potential value can be measured.

The currents measured under voltage clamp include ionic and capacitative currents. We will only consider the ionic currents here since the capacitative currents generally only last a few microseconds. Figure 2.**35b** shows that with a voltage jump from the resting potential to a holding potential near 0 mV (in this case –9 mV), there is an initial inward-directed ionic current, which changes over after a few milliseconds to an outward-directed ionic current. This total current can be experimentally subdivided into its individual current components. Replacement of the Na^+ ions in the extracellular solution results in only a delayed outward current component being measured. Subtraction of this K^+ current from the total current reveals an early inward-directed current component. The same result can be obtained using pharmacological agents (Fig. 2.**35c**). When the Na^+ channel is selectively blocked by tetrodotoxin (TTX) for example, the remain-

ing current is carried by K^+ ions. This K^+ current has slower activation kinetics, reaches a maximum only after a few milliseconds, and remains at this maximum for as long as the holding voltage is applied. The converse result is achieved by pharmacologically blocking the K^+ channels with tetraethylammonium (TEA). The resulting current component is carried by Na^+ ions, has fast activation kinetics, and decays to zero of its own accord after a few milliseconds.

The Na^+ and K^+ currents measured in the voltage clamp experiments have exactly the "macroscopic" properties expected given the "microscopic" properties of the individual voltage-dependent Na^+ and K^+ channels. Nevertheless, it must be emphasized that the time course of the total ionic current for Na^+ or K^+ ions does not correspond to the time course of the ionic current through a single ion channel. The current through an ion channel proceeds in an all-or-nothing manner. The course of the total current, by contrast, depends on the number of ion channels open at any time, and is therefore determined by the *probability* that an individual ion channel is open.

A variety of different ion channels participate in the generation of action potentials

The generation of action potentials in many axons is based on the properties of the voltage-gated Na^+ and K^+ channels described above. In most neurons, however, other types of ion channel with voltage-dependent gating behavior can also occur. These are found mainly (but not exclusively) in the dendrites or the cell body. The generation of the depolarizing phase of the action potential can involve, for example, Ca^{2+} ion channels. In some neurons the Ca^{2+} component of the action potential even predominates. The inflow of Ca^{2+} ions during the action potential can itself exert an influence on other types of ion channels, in particular on different types of K^+ channels. A summary of the properties of some of the many different ion channels with voltage-dependent gating behavior is shown in Table 2.**2**.

It seems that neurons possess a whole spectrum of different ion channels in their cell membranes, all of which are capable of influencing the production of regenerative signals. In addition, different types of ion chan-

Table 2.**2**   **Properties of voltage-gated ion channels**

Channel type	Current	Function	Blocked by
Sodium channel	I_{Na}	Fast depolarization during action potential	Tetrodotoxin (TTX) Saxitoxin (STX)
Potassium channel	I_K	Repolarization during action potential regulation of high-frequency firing rate	Tetraethylammonium (TEA) 4-aminopyridine
Calcium channel	I_{Ca}	Medium-fast depolarization; long duration action potentials	Co^{2+}, Ni^{2+}
Sodium, calcium channel, "bursting"	I_B	Burst generating; slow depolarization, depolarizing afterpotential	–
Calcium-dependent potassium channel	$I_{K(Ca)}$	Role in intracellular Ca^{2+} signalling; controls low frequency firing of action potentials	Ba^{2+}, TEA
Early, transient potassium channel	I_A	Regulates low frequency firing of action potentials, maintains relationship between depolarization and firing rate	4-Aminopyridine TEA
Inward rectifying potassium channel	I_{IR}	Important in the generation of plateau potentials	Rb^+, Cs^+

nels can be incorporated into spatially discrete regions of a neuronal cell membrane. This makes it possible for dendrites, cell body, and various axon regions to have completely different excitable properties. In the extreme case, different regions of one and the same neuron can even be electrically isolated from one another, resulting in several separate functional compartments within the one cell.

Signal propagation in millisecond pulses

Despite the many types of ion channels, the amplitude and time course of the action potential generated by a given neural process are largely stereotyped. Generally, only the interval between successive action potentials varies. The *frequency of the action potentials* is therefore used for *information coding* (a pulse-coded analog system). The great advantage in using action potentials for signal conduction is that an action potential propagates as a wave of excitation across large distances, without attenuation. Local currents spread out electrotonically along the membrane from each active region and depolarize neighboring membrane regions. As a result of these local depolarizations the Na$^+$ channels which are still closed immediately adjacent to the propagating action potential, switch to the open configuration. This leads to a powerful and rapid depolarization of this membrane region, which itself then depolarizes neighboring membrane regions, and so on (Fig. 2.**36**). The action potential spreads regeneratively along a neural process, without

loss of amplitude, rather like a flame along a burning fuse. Since the amplitude of an action potential exceeds the threshold for the regenerative opening of Na$^+$ channels many times (4–5 times), this type of transmission possesses a considerable *safety factor*.

The fact that action potentials have refractory periods has two important consequences for propagation.

– Although depolarizing currents spread out in both directions along the cell membrane from the site of the largest Na$^+$ ion conductance, the action potential cannot "run backward." This is because the membrane region that has just generated an action potential cannot produce another during the absolute refractory period.

– The maximum frequency of action potentials in a neuron is limited. A fast action potential lasts about 1 ms. Because of the refractory period, a further action potential can normally only be elicited after another millisecond. This limits the maximum frequency of action potentials to about 500 Hz (in exceptional cases 1000 Hz for specialized neurons).

During the spread of an action potential, each membrane region becomes a signal amplifier that converts a suprathreshold depolarization into a signal of approximately 100 mV lasting 1 ms. However, the *velocity of spread* of an action potential is determined by the passive electrotonic properties of the neurite, rather than by

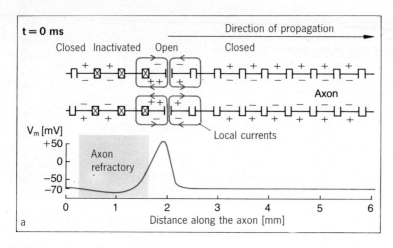

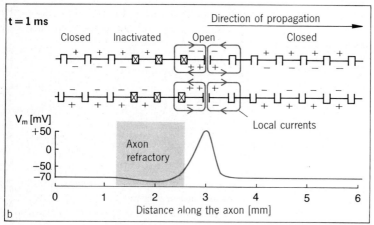

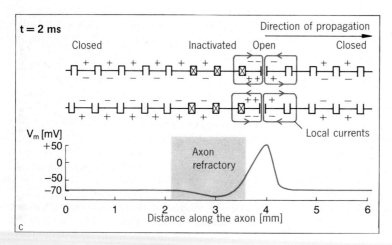

Fig. 2.**36** Propagation of an action potential along an axon. Conformational changes in the Na$^+$ channels, local ionic currents, and spatial extent of the action potential, are shown at three consecutive intervals in **a,** **b,** and **c.** The axon is refractory immediately after the action potential. The propagation of the regenerative action potential occurs without decrease in amplitude (after Alberts et al.)

the active amplification mechanism. This is because the conduction velocity is determined by the rate at which local currents depolarize the membrane in front of an active region to threshold. A quantitative description of conduction velocity has to take into account the cable properties of the neurite, which depend on λ and τ. As a simplification, the larger the length constant, the more local currents can spread along the membrane, and the quicker the depolarization of a membrane region to threshold will be (Fig. 2.37). Since the length constant $\lambda = \sqrt{r_m/r_i}$, then either an increase in the membrane resistance r_m, or a decrease in the internal longitudinal resistance r_i, will produce a faster propagation of the action potential. Larger axons generally conduct action potentials more quickly than small ones because r_i decreases with increasing axon radius (r_i is inversely proportional to the axon radius squared). Some invertebrates have therefore developed giant fibers in order to achieve a high conduction velocity. In the squid the diameter of such a giant axon can be as large as 1 mm, which results in conduction velocities near 20 m/s. An alternative strategy for attaining a high conduction velocity is to increase r_m. This strategy has been perfected by the vertebrates.

The conduction velocity can be increased by myelination and localized concentrations of ion channels

Many axons in the vertebrate nervous system are wrapped in a myelin sheath. Myelin is produced by specialized glia cells, the oligodendrocytes, in the CNS, and by glia-like cells, the Schwann cells, in the peripheral nervous system. Glia cells use their own plasma membrane for the spiral-like wrapping around axons (Fig. 2.38a,b). Every myelinated axon is enveloped by several glia cells, with each glia cell wrapping an axon region about 1 mm in length. Myelin-free areas, the nodes of Ranvier, are found at regular intervals between those axon segments that are enveloped by glia cell membrane.

Myelin consists of up to 70% of phospholipids, glycolipids, and cholesterol. Since ion channels are almost completely absent in the membrane of the myelin sheath, it is a very good electrical insulator. This increases the membrane resistance of the axons, and lowers the membrane capacitance in the internodal regions. The cable properties of the myelinated axonal regions are thereby improved, and a significant increase in length constant is attained. Transmembrane currents can virtually only occur at the naked nodes of Ranvier in myelinated axons. In addition, almost all the Na^+ channels that occur in the axon are concentrated at these nodes (more than 1000 channels/μm^2). Thus, when an action potential is evoked at a node of Ranvier, local currents flow quickly, largely unattenuated, to the next node and evoke a new action potential there. Action potential production jumps via this *saltatory propagation* mode from one node to the next (Fig. 2.38c). Since the length constant of a neuron is increased by myelination, this type of signal propagation is significantly faster than in unmyelinated axons (Fig. 2.38d). Conduction velocities of up to 100 m/s are reached in myelinated axons having an axon diameter of maximally 10–20 μm. An unmyelinated axon would have to have a diameter of several millimeters to be able to conduct this fast. If the human spi-

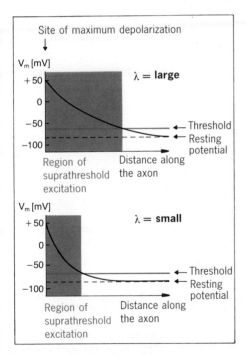

Fig. 2.**37** Electrotonic properties of the axon determine the conduction velocity of the action potential. Local currents spread out from the site of the action potential (the site of maximum depolarization). The longer the length constant of the axon, the greater is the area of the nerve fiber these local currents depolarize above threshold

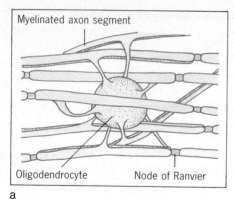

Myelinated axon segment

Oligodendrocyte   Node of Ranvier

a

nal cord contained only unmyelinated neurons, then it would have to be several meters in diameter in order to provide the same conduction velocities for the same number of axons. Myelination saves space without sacrificing performance. This type of excitatory conduction also saves metabolic energy, since ion fluxes only occur in the small membrane regions at the nodes. Since myelination significantly accelerates action potential propagation, it is not

Myelin

Axon

Cell nucleus   Extracellular space
Schwann cell

N

N
+ + +
N
C   C
+ + +   N + + + C   C
N
Po   PLP   MBP   MAG

b   Proteins of the myelin sheath

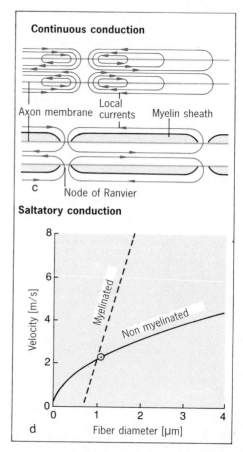

Continuous conduction

Axon membrane   Local currents   Myelin sheath

c   Node of Ranvier

Saltatory conduction

Velocity [m/s]

Myelinated

Non myelinated

d   Fiber diameter [µm]

Fig. 2.**38 a,b** Myelination and saltatory conduction. **a** An oligodendrocyte contributes to the myelination of several axons. **b** Cross-section through a Schwann cell and through an axon enveloped with myelin from that cell. The myelin sheath is shown at increasing magnifications to demonstrate the layer-like organization of the myelin, and to illustrate the location and configuration of important myelin proteins. P_0 = protein zero, PLP = proteolipid protein, MBP = myelin basic protein, MAG = myelin-associated glycoprotein, N = N-terminal group, C = C-terminal group

Fig. 2.**38c** During continuous conduction the entire region of the axon is depolarized by local currents and induced to generate an action potential. During saltatory conduction, local transmembrane currents flow mainly through the nonmyelinated membrane regions at the nodes of Ranvier. In addition, almost all the Na^+ channels of the axon are concentrated at the nodes. The initiation of the action potential therefore jumps from one node to another.

Fig. 2.**38d** Theoretical relationship between fiber diameter and conduction velocity for myelinated and nonmyelinated fibers (after Lembke, Morell and Norton, and Rushton)

surprising that the loss of the myelin sheath leads to serious impairment of neuronal function. This becomes dramatically obvious in multiple sclerosis, a disease which involves demyelination of whole areas (plaques) of the human CNS.

It is interesting to consider the spatial dimensions of an action potential in neurons with a high conduction velocity. A typical action potential 1 ms long and propagating at 100 m/s, extends along 10 cm of axonal membrane, and involves approximately 100 nodes at once. Temporally action potentials are very short events, but spatially they can be quite large.

References

General Reviews

Barchi, R. I. 1988. Probing the molecular structure of the voltage-dependent sodium channel. Annu. Rev. Neurosci. 11: 455-496

Betz, H. 1990. Ligand-gated ion channels in the brain: The amino acid receptor superfamily. Neuron 5:383-392

Catteral, W. A. 1988. Structure and function of voltage-sensitive ion channels. Science 242: 50-61

Cooke, I. and Lipkin, M. (eds.) 1972. Cellular Neurophysiology: A Source Book. Holt, Rinehart, Winston

Glover, C. M. and Hames, B. D. (eds.) 1989. Frontiers in Molecular Biology: Molecular Neurobiology. IRL Press, Oxford

Hammond, C. and Tritsch, E. 1990. Neurobiologie Cellulaire. Doin Editeurs, Paris.

Hille, B. 1992. Ionic Channels of Excitable Membranes. 2nd edition, Sinauer, Sunderland.

Jack, J. J. B., Noble, D., and Tsien, R. W. 1983. Electric Current Flow in Excitable Cells. Oxford University Press, New York

Jan, L. Y. and Jan, Y. N. 1989. Voltage-sensitive ion channels. Cell. 56: 13-25

Junge, D. 1981. Nerve and Muscle Excitation, 2nd edition, Sinauer, Sunderland

Kandel, E. R. (ed.) 1977. Handbook of Physiology, Sec. 1: The Nervous System, Vol. 1: Cellular Biology of Neurons. American Physiological Society, Bethesda

Katz, B. 1966. Nerve, Muscle and Synapse. McGraw-Hill, New York

Keynes, R. D. and Aidley, D. J. 1981. Nerves and Muscles. Cambridge University Press, Cambridge

Koester, J. and Byrne J. H. (eds.) 1980. Molluscan Nerve Cells. Cold Spring Harbor, New York

Kupferman, I. 1980. Role of cyclic nucleotides in excitable cells. Annu. Rev. Physiol. 42:629-641

Matthews, G. G. 1986. Cellular Physiology of Nerve and Muscle. Blackwell, Palo Alto

Morell, P. and Norton, W. T. 1980. Myelin. Sci. Am. 242: 88-118.

Morell, P. (ed.) 1984. Myelin, 2nd edition. Plenum, New York

Nicholls, J. G., Martin, A. R. and Wallace, B. 1992. From Neuron to Brain, 3rd edition, Sinauer, Sunderland

Ottoson, D. 1983. Physiology of the Nervous System. Macmillan, London

Roberts, A. and Bush, B. M. H. (eds.) 1981. Neurones without Impulses. Cambridge University Press, Cambridge

Sakmann, B. and Neher E. (eds.) 1983. Single-Channel Recording. Plenum, New York

Shepherd, G. M. 1988. Neurobiology, 2nd edition, Oxford University Press, New York

Strichartz, G., Rando, T. and Wang, G. K. 1987. An integrated view of the molecular toxicology of sodium channel gating in excitable cells. Annu. Rev. Neurosci. 10: 237-268

Tsien, R. W. 1983. Calcium channel in excitable cells. Annu. Rev. Physiol. 45: 341-358

Unwin, N. 1989. The structure of ion channels in membranes of excitable cells. Neuron 3: 665-676.

Original Publications

Agnew, W. S., Levinson, S. R., Brabson, J. S. and Raftery, M. A. 1978. Purification of the tetrodotoxin binding component associated with the voltagesensitive sodium channel of Electrophorus electricus electroplax membrane. Proc. Natl. Acad. Sci. USA 75: 2606-2610.

Almers, W. and Levinson, S. R. 1975. Tetrodotoxin binding to normal and depolarized frog muscle and the conductance of a single sodium channel. J. Physiol. 247: 483-509.

Almers, W., Stanfield, P. and Stuhmer, W. 1983. Lateral distribution of sodium and potassium channels in frog skeletal muscle: Measurements with a patchclamp technique. J. Physiol. 336: 261-284.

Arbuthnott, E. R., Boyd, I. A. and Kalu, K. U. 1980. Ultrastructural dimensions of myelinated peripheral nerve fibres in the cat and their relation to conduction velocity. J. Physiol. 308: 125-127.

Armstrong, C. M., Bezanilla, R. and Rojas, E. 1973. Destruction of sodium conductance inactivation in squid axons perfused with pronase. J. Gen. Physiol. 62: 375-391.

Armstrong, C. M. and Bezanilla, F. 1974. Charge movement associated with the opening, and closing of the activation gates of Na channels. J. Gen. Physiol. 63: 533-552.

Armstrong, C. M. and Hille, B. 1972. The inner quaternary ammonium ion receptor in potassium channels of the node of Ranvier. J. Gen. Physiol. 59: 388-400.

Baker, P. F., Blaustein, M. P., Hodgkin, A. L. and Steinhardt, R. A. 1969. The influence of calcium on sodium efflux in squid axons. J. Physiol. 200: 431-458.

Baker, P. F., Blaustein, M. P., Keynes, R. D., Manil, J., Shaw, T. I. and Steinhardt, R. A. 1969. The ouabainsensitive fluxes of sodium and potassium in squid giant axons. J. Physiol. 200: 459-496.

Baker, P. F., Foster, R. F., Gilbert, D. S. and Shaw, T. I. 1971. Sodium transport by perfused giant axons of Loligo. J. Physiol. 219: 487-506.

Baker, P. F., Hodgkin, A. L. and Ridgway, E. B. 1971. Depolarization and calcium entry in squid giant axons. J. Physiol. 218: 709-755.

Baker, P. F., Hodgkin, A. L. and Shaw, T. I. 1962. Replacement of the axoplasm of giant nerve fibres with artificial solutions. J. Physiol. 164: 330-354.

Baker, P. F., Hodgkin, A. L. and Shaw, T. I. 1962. The effects of changes in internal ionic concentrations on the electrical properties of perfused giant axons. J. Physiol. 164: 355-374.

Bostock, H. and Sears, T. A. 1978. The internodal axon membrane: Electrical excitability and continuous conduction in segmental demyelination. J. Physiol. 280: 273-301.

Bostock, H., Sears, T. A. and Sherratt, R. M. 1981. The effects of 4-amino-pyridine and tetraethylammonium ions on normal and demyelinated mammalian nerve fibres. J. Physiol. 313: 301-315.

Brinley, F. J. 1980. Regulation of intracellular calcium in squid axons. Fed. Proc. 39: 2778-2782.

Bunge, M. B., Bunge, R. P. and Ris, H. 1961. Ultrastructural study of remyelination in an experimental lesion in adult cat spinal cord. J. Biophys. Biochem. Cytol. 10: 67-94.

Caldwell, P. C., Hodgkin, A. L., Keynes, R. D. and Shaw, T. I. 1960. The effects of injecting "energy rich" phosphate compounds on the active transport of ions in the giant axons of Loligo. J. Physiol. 152: 561-590.

Chiu, S. Y., Ritchie, J. M., Rogart, R. B. and Stagg, D. A. 1979. A quantitative description of membrane currents in rabbit myelinated nerve. J. Physiol. 292: 149-166.

Chiu, S. Y. and Ritchie, J. M. 1981. Evidence for the presence of potassium channels in the paranodal region of acutely demyelinated mammalian nerve fibres. J. Physiol. 313: 415-437.

Cole, K. S. and Curtis, H. J. 1939. Electric impedance of the squid giant axon during activity. J. Gen. Physiol. 22: 649-670.

Conner, J. A. and Stevens, C. F. 1971. Voltage clamp studies of a transient outward membrane current in gastropod neural somata. J. Physiol. 213: 21-30.

Conti, F., De Felice, L. J. and Wanke, E. 1975. Potassium and sodium ion current noise in the membrane of the squid giant axon. J. Physiol. 248: 45-82.

Conti, F., Hille, B., Neumcke, B., Nonner, W. and Stämpfli, R. 1976. Measurement of the conductance of the sodium channel from current fluctua-

tions at the node of Ranvier (frog). J. Physiol. 262: 729-742.

Conti, F. and Neher, E. 1980. Single channel recordings of K^+ currents in squid axons. Nature 285: 140-143.

Curtis, H. J. and Cole, K. S. 1940. Membrane action potentials from the squid giant axon. J. Cell. Comp. Physiol. 15: 147-157.

Dahlström, A. 1971. Axoplasmic transport (with particular respect to adrenergic neurones). Phil. Trans. R. Soc. Lond. B 261: 325-358.

Dipolo, R., Requena, J., Brinley, F. J., Mullins, L. J., Scarpa, A. and Tiffert, T. 1976. Ionized calcium concentrations in squid axons. J. Gen. Physiol. 67: 433-467.

Eckert, R. and Lux, H. D. A voltage-sensitive persistent calcium conductance in neuronal somata of Helix. J. Physiol. 137: 218-244.

Ellisman, M. H., Agnew, W. S., Miller, J. A. and Levinson, S. R. 1982. Electron microscope visualization of the tetrodotoxin binding protein from Electrophorus electricus. Proc. Natl. Acad. Sci. USA 79: 4461-4465.

Fenwick, E. M., Marty, A. and Neher, E. 1982. Sodium and calcium channels in bovine chromaffin cells. J. Physiol. 331: 599-635.

Frankenhaeuser, B. and Hodgkin, A. L. 1956. The after-effects of impulses in the giant nerve fibres of Loligo. J. Physiol. 131: 341-376.

Frankenhaeuser, B. and Hodgkin, A. L. 1957. The action of calcium on the electrical properties of squid axons. J. Physiol. 137: 218-244.

Garrahan, P. J. and Glynn, I. M. 1967. The incorporation of inorganic phosphate into adenosine triphosphate by reversal of the sodium pump. J. Physiol. 192: 237-256.

Goldman, D. E. 1943. Potential, impedance and rectification in membranes. J. Gen. Physiol. 27: 37-60.

Gorman, A. L. F. and Thomas, M. V. 1977. Changes in intracellular concentration of free calcium ions in a pacemaker neurone, measured with metallochromic indicator dye arsenazo III. J. Physiol. 275: 357-376.

Grossman, Y., Parnas, I. and Spira, M. E. 1979. Differential conduction block in branches of a bifurcating axon. J. Physiol. 295: 283-305.

Grossman, Y., Parnas, I. and Spira, M. E. 1979. Ionic mechanisms involved in differential conduction of action potentials at high frequency in a branching axon. J. Physiol. 295: 307-322.

Hagiwara, S. and Harunon, H. 1983. Studies of single calcium channel currents in rat clonal pituitary cells. J. Physiol. 336: 649-661.

Hagiwara, S. and Tasaki, I. 1958. A study on the mechanism of impulse transmission across the giant synapse of the squid. J. Physiol. 143: 114-137.

Hamill, O. P., Marty, A., Neher, E., Sakmann, B. and Sigworth, F. J. 1981. Improved patch-clamp techniques for high-resolution current recording from cells and cell-free membrane patches. Pflügers Arch. 391: 85-100.

Hille, B. 1971. The permeability of the sodium channel to organic cations in myelinated nerve. J. Gen. Physiol. 58: 599-619.

Hodgkin, A. L. 1937. Evidence for electrical transmission in nerve. I, II. J. Physiol. 90: 183-210, 211-232.

Hodgkin, A. L. 1939. The relation between conduction velocity and the electrical resistance outside a nerve fibre. J. Physiol. 94: 560-570.

Hodgkin, A. L. 1954. A note on conduction velocity. J. Physiol. 725: 221-224.

Hodgkin, A. L. and Horowicz, P. 1959. The influence of potassium and chloride ions on the membrane potential of single muscle fibres. J. Physiol. 148: 127-160.

Hodgkin, A. L. and Huxley, A. F. 1939. Action potentials recorded from inside a nerve fibre. Nature 144: 710-711.

Hodgkin, A. L. and Huxley, A. F. 1952. Currents carried by sodium and potassium ions through the membrane of the giant axon of Loligo. J. Physiol. 116: 449-472.

Hodgkin, A. L. and Huxley, A. F. 1952. The components of the membrane conductance in the giant axon of Loligo. J. Physiol. 116: 473-496.

Hodgkin, A. L. and Huxley, A. F. 1952. The dual effect of membrane potential on sodium conductance in the giant axon of Loligo. J. Physiol. 116: 497-506.

Hodgkin, A. L. and Huxley A. F. 1952. A quantitative description of membrane current and its application to conduction and excitation in nerve. J. Physiol. 117: 500-544.

Hodgkin, A. L., Huxley, A. F. and Katz, B. 1952. Measurement of current-voltage relations in the membrane of the giant axon of Loligo. J. Physiol. 116: 424-448.

Hodgkin, A. L. and Katz, B, 1949. The effect of sodium ions on the electrical activity of the giant axon of the squid. J. Physiol. 108: 37-77.

Hodgkin, A. L. and Keynes, R. D. 1955. Active transport of cations in giant axons from Sepia and Loligo. J. Physiol. 128: 28-60.

Hodgkin, A. L. and Keynes, R. D. 1956. Experiments on the injection of substances into squid giant axons by means of a microsyringe. J. Physiol. 137: 592-617.

Hodgkin, A. L. and Rushton, W. A. H. 1946. The electrical constants of a crustacean nerve fibre. Proc. R. Soc. Lond. B 133: 444-479.

Huxley, A. F. and Stämpfli, R. 1949. Evidence for saltatory conduction in peripheral myelinated nerve fibres. J. Physiol. 108: 315-339.

Kamb. A., Tseng-Crank, J. and Tanouye, M. A. 1988. Multiple products of the Drosophila Shaker gene may contribute to potassium channel diversity. Neuron 1: 421-430.

Landowne, D. and Ritchie, J. M. 1970. The binding of tritiated ouabain to mammalian non-myelinated nerve fibres. J. Physiol. 207: 529-537.

Latorre, R. and Miller, C. 1983. Conduction and selectivity in potassium channels. J. Memb. Biol. 71: 11-30

Levinson, S. R. and Meves, H. 1975. The binding of tritiated tetrodotoxin to squid giant axon. Phil. Trans. R. Soc. Lond. B 270: 349-352.

Ling, G. and Gerard, R. W. 1949. The normal membrane potential of frog sartorius fibers. J. Cell. Comp. Physiol. 34: 383-396.

Llinás, R. and Nicholson, C. 1975. Calcium role in depolarization–secretion coupling: an Aequorin study in squid giant synapse. Proc. Natl. Acad. Sci. 72: 187-190.

Lux, H. D. and Nagy, K. 1981. Single channel Ca^{2+} currents in Helix pomatia neurons. Pflügers Arch. 291: 252-254.

Marmont, G. 1949. Studies on the axon membrane. J. Cell. Comp. Physiol. 34: 351-382.

Meech, R. W. 1974. The sensitivity of Helix aspersa neurones to injected calcium ions. J. Physiol. 237: 259-277.

Miller, C. 1989. Genetic manipulation of ion channels: A new approach to structure and mechanism. Neuron 2: 1195-1205

Moody, W. J. 1981. The ionic mechanism of intracellular pH regulation in crayfish neurones. J. Physiol. 316: 293-308.

Moore, J. W., Blaustein, M. P., Anderson, N. C. and Narahashi, T. 1967. Basis of tetrodotoxin's selectivity in blockage of squid axons. J. Gen. Physiol. 50: 1401-1411.

Mullins, L. J. and Brinley, F. J. 1967. Some factors influencing sodium extrusion by internally dialyzed squid axons. J. Gen. Physiol. 50: 2333-2355.

Mullins, L. J. and Noda, K. 1963. The influence of sodium-free solutions on the membrane potential of frog muscle fibers. J. Gen. Physiol. 47: 117-132.

Nakajima, S. and Takahashi, K. 1966. Post-tetanic hyperpolarization and electrogenic Na pump in stretch receptor neurone of crayfish. J. Physiol. 187: 105-127.

Nishsi, S. and Koketsu, K. 1960. Electrical properties and activities of single sympathetic neurons in frogs. J. Cell Comp. Physiol. 55: 15-30.

Nishi, S. and Koketsu, K. 1968. Early and late afterdischarges of amphibian sympathetic ganglion cells. J. Neurophysiol. 31: 109-118.

Noda, M., Shimizu, S., Tanabe, T., Takai, T., Kayano, T., Ikeda, T. Takahashi, H. Nakayama, H., Kanaoka, Y., Minamino, N., Kangawa, K., Matsuo, H., Raferty, M. A., Hirose, T., Inayama, S., Hayashida, H., Miyata, T. and Numa, S. 1984. Primary structure of Electrophorus electricus sodium channel deduced from cDNA sequence. Nature 312: 121-127.

Obaid, A. L., Socolar, S. J. and Rose, B. 1983. Cell-to-cell channels with two independently regulated gates in series: Analysis of junctional conductance modulation by membrane potential, calcium and pH. J. Memb. Biol. 73: 68-89.

Overton, E. 1902. Beiträge zur allgemeinen Muskel- und Nervenphysiologie. II. Über die Unentbehrlichkeit von Natrium- (oder Lithium-) Ionen für den Kontraktionsakt des Muskels. Pflügers Arch. 92: 346-386.

Papazian, D. M., Schwarz, T. L., Tempel, B. L., Jan, Y. N. and Jan, L. Y. 1987. Cloning of genomic and complementary DNA from Shaker, a putative potassium channel gene from Drosophila. Science 237: 749-753.

Quick, D. C., Kennedy, W. R. and Donaldson, L. 1979. Dimensions of myelinated nerve fibers near the motor and sensory terminals in cat tenuissimus muscles. Neuroscience 4: 1089-1096.

Rasminsky, M. and Sears, T. A. 1972. Internodal conduction in undissected demyelinated nerve fibres. J. Physiol. 227: 323-350.

Ritchie, J. M. 1982. On the relation between fibre diameter and conduction velocity in myelinated nerve fibres. Proc. R. Soc. Lond. B 217: 29-35.

Reichert, H., Plummer, M. and Wine, J. J. 1983. Identified nonspiking local interneurons mediate nonrecurrent lateral inhibition of crayfish mechanosensory interneurons. J. Comp. Physiol. 151: 261-276.

Rushton, W. A. H. 1951. A theory of the effects of fibre size in medullated nerve. J. Physiol. 115: 101-122.

Russell, J. M. 1983. Cation-coupled chloride influx in squid axon. Role of potassium and stoichiometry of the transport process. J. Gen. Physiol. 81: 909-925.

Schachner, M. 1982. Cell type-specific antigens in the mammalian nervous system. J. Neurochem. 39: 1-8.

Siegler, M. V. S and Burrows, M. 1979. The morphology of local nonspiking interneurons in the metathoracic ganglia of the locust. J. Comp. Neurol 183: 121-148.

Sigworth, F. J. and Neher, E. 1980. Single Na^+ channel currents observed in cultured rat muscle cells. Nature 287: 447-449.

Skou, J. C. 1964. Enzymatic aspects of active linked transport of Na^+ and K^+ through the cell membrane. Prog. Biophys. Mol. Biol. 14: 133-166.

Sokoloff, L. 1977. Relation between physiological function and energy metabolism in the central nervous system. J. Neurochem. 29: 13-26.

Sokolove, P. G. and Cooke, I. M. 1971. Inhibition of impulse activity in a sensory neuron by an electrogenic pump. J. Gen. Physiol. 57: 125-163.

Takeshima, H., Nishimura, S., Matsumoto, T., Ishida, H., Kangawa, K., Minamino, N., Matsuo, H., Ueda, M., Hanaoka, M., Hirose, T. and Numa, S. 1989. Primary structure and expression from complementary DNA of skeletal muscle ryanodine receptor. Nature 339: 439-445.

Thomas, R. C. 1969. Membrane current and intracellular sodium changes in a snail neurone during extrusion of injected sodium. J. Physiol. 201: 495-514.

Thomas, R. C. 1972. Intracellular sodium activity and the sodium pump in snail neurones. J. Physiol. 220: 55-71.

Thomas, R. C. 1977. The role of bicarbonate, chloride and sodium ions in the regulation of intracellular pH in snail neurones. J. Physiol. 273: 317-338.

Venosa, R. A. and Horowicz, P. 1981. Density and apparent location of the sodium pump in frog sartorius muscles. J. Memb. Biol. 59: 225-232.

Verveen, A. A. and DeFelice, L. J. 1974. Membrane noise. Prog. Biophys. Mol. Biol. 28: 189-265.

Wei, A., Covarrubias, M., Butler, A., Baker, K., Pak, M. and Salkoff, L. 1990. K^+ current diversity is produced by an extended gene family conserved in Drosophila and mouse. Science 248: 599-603.

Young, J. Z. 1936. The giant nerve fibres and epistellar body of cephalopods. Q. J. Microsc. Sci. 78: 367-386.

Zipser, B. and McKay, R. 1981. Monoclonal antibodies distinguish identifiable neurones in the leech. Nature 289: 549-554.

3. Cellular Neurobiology: Synaptic Transmission

Direct Signal Transmission Occurs at Electrical Synapses

Historical Background

Since neurons generate electrical signals, it is reasonable to assume that they can transmit these signals electrically to other neurons, in a sense across intercellular resistances. This was postulated in the 1950s, mainly by Eccles, as being the dominant mode of transmission in the CNS. However, the pioneering work on neuromuscular synapses by Katz and his coworkers resulted in this concept being completely discarded in favor of chemical synaptic transmission. It is ironic that Eccles, who later contributed significantly to the understanding of chemical synapses, abandoned his original idea of electrical synapses just about the time that Furshpan and Potter, working with Katz, first demonstrated electrical synaptic transmission. Since then electrical synapses have been found alongside the more numerous chemical synapses in almost all nervous systems studied.

An electrical signal can propagate from one neuron to another via current flow

If two neurons are closely apposed then some of the current which causes a potential change in the first cell could reach the second cell and also cause a potential change there. The problem with this type of signal transmission is that without special structural modifications only a fraction of the current crosses over into the second cell (Fig. 3.1a). The current path from the active site in the first cell and across the cell membrane of the second, has a much higher resistance than the current path back to the active site via the extracellular space.

This problem could be alleviated to some extent if the current were to flow between a number of neuronal processes which are very closely apposed to one another. Although this has not yet been demonstrated, it could in principle occur in nerve pathways consisting of many neighboring nonmyelinated axons. Most neurons, however, are separated

by intercellular gaps of 10–20 nm, so this type of transmission cannot be widespread. Another way to enhance current flow between neurons would be via a specialized insulation around the intercellular contact site. This does in fact occur, and is the basis for an inhibitory transmission in the Mauthner neuron system of some lower vertebrates.

A much more effective electrical coupling is achieved by linking two neurons via subcellular junctional elements (Fig. 3.1b). High conductance intercellular bridges, which link the cytoplasm of two cells, allow current to be transferred directly from an active to a neighboring cell, without having to overcome the relatively high resistance of one, or even

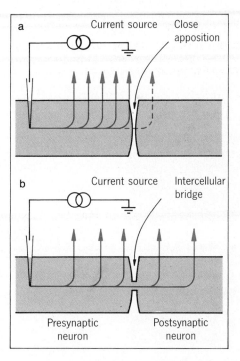

Fig. 3.1 Electrical signal transfer between neurons. **a** Even when two nerve fibers lie close together, only a small amount of current can flow from one fiber to its neighbor. **b** Electrical coupling is much more effective when both fibers are connected by intercellular bridges

both, cell membranes. This greatly facilitates the current that flows from one cell to the other as compared with the current that flows across the cell membrane and through the extracellular space. The majority of electrical synapses consist of groups of junctions like these. At such contact sites, the normal intercellular space between two cells is reduced to about 2 nm.

Connexon molecules form the basis of electrical synapses

Electrical synapses are based on *gap junctions*. These are cell-linking structures that also occur in many nonneuronal epithelial and mesenchyme tissues. Ions with a molecular weight of less than 1 kDa can move from one cell to the next through such contact sites. Gap junctions are characterized by numerous similar macromolecular structures which bridge the intercellular space (Fig. 3.2). Each one of these individual structures is composed of a barrel-shaped assembly of two proteins called *connexons*. A connexon is a transmembrane protein made up of six similar subunits, each about 30 kDa large, which are arranged symmetrically around a central pore of about 2 nm diameter. Each of the subunits has several hydrophobic regions about 20 amino acids long, a structural motif found in many membrane proteins, and indicating helical transmembrane regions.

In order to form a functional intercellular canal, two connexons must join across the intercellular gap. It seems likely that the central canal can be opened or closed by conformational changes in the subunits. This might occur via a rotation in the position of the subunits in the membrane, similar to the closing mechanism of an iris diaphragm.

Signal transmission at electrical synapses is fast

There are almost no signal delays at electrical synapses because the speed of transmission is determined solely by the electrotonic properties of the pre- and postsynaptic membranes. As a consequence of their fast signal transmission, electrical synapses are frequently found in neuronal circuits which are optimized for high speed. This is the case, for example, in circuits which evoke fast escape behavior where milliseconds can mean the difference between life and death.

Most electrical synapses have symmetrical resistance properties, that is, an ionic current encounters the same resistance in both directions. Such *nonrectifying electrical synapses* can, for example, contribute to the synchronization of activity in reciprocally coupled neurons. Other electrical synapses can vary their conductance in a voltage-dependent manner. Electrical synapses which have *rectifying*

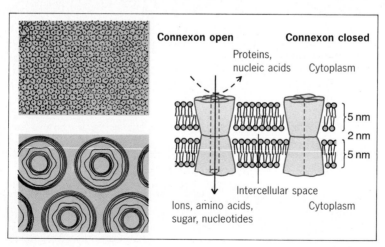

Fig. **3.2**   Molecular organization of electrical synapses. Electrical synapses consist of many molecular aggregates which lie close together, and which are visible in the electron microscope (top left). Information about the molecular organization of such connexon molecules can be obtained by diffraction analysis (bottom left). A model depicts how the subunits of a connexon are arranged around a central canal, and how this canal, which connects two cells, can be opened and closed (right) (after Unwin and Henderson, and Bretscher)

properties belong to this group (Fig. 3.3). These allow a depolarizing current occurring during an action potential, for example, to flow from the presynaptic into the postsynaptic cell, but not vice versa. The transfer properties of many electrical synapses can also be altered by factors such as changes in the intracellular pH value and in intracellular Ca^{2+} concentration. It seems that transmission at electrical synapses can be influenced by everything that switches the connexons back and forth between their open and closed conformations.

A significant drawback of an electrical synapse is that it cannot perform signal amplification. Pre- and postsynaptic nerve processes must therefore be matched to one another.

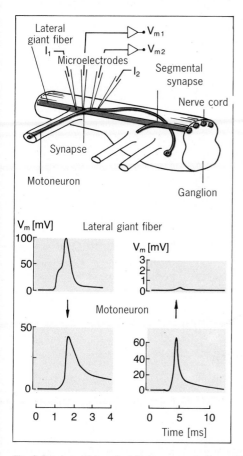

Fig. 3.**3** A rectifying electrical synapse. In the segmental ganglia of the crayfish a depolarizing synaptic current can flow from the lateral giant fiber into a motoneuron without much decrement. However, current flow from the motoneuron back into the giant fiber is more difficult (after Furshpan and Potter)

The current that is produced at a small, 1–2 µm presynaptic ending can barely influence a postsynaptic giant fiber with a diameter of 100 µm. The situation is different in chemical synapses.

The Presynaptic Terminal of a Chemical Synapse Converts Electrical into Chemical Signals

Anatomical basis

Chemical synapses are specialized communication sites between two neurons at which signal transmission occurs via chemical neurotransmitters. It is the role of the presynaptic terminal to convert a change in electrical potential into a secretory process. For this purpose the presynaptic part of the synapse possesses subcellular components common to all secretory cells. A high density of transmitter-filled vesicles, having diameters between 30 and 150 nm, is characteristic. The ultrastructure of different presynaptic terminals is very variable. The best studied are the *directional synapses,* at which transmitter release is restricted to a spatially small region opposite the postsynaptic site (Fig. 3.**4**). In synapses of this kind the synaptic vesicles are concentrated at specialized active zones. These active zones consist of long or round electron-dense structures which are found near the presynaptic membrane and are associated with a series of intramembrane particles (Ca^{2+} channels?). Exocytotic fusion of the vesicles with the presynaptic membrane occurs at these sites. During and shortly after vesicle fusion, empty vesicles appear as pocket-shaped depressions at the active zones. After exocytosis, those regions of the presynaptic membrane which derive from the fused vesicles are recovered out of the membrane, and either recycled for the formation of new vesicles, or degraded. At other, nondirectional, synapses, like those of the postganglionic neurons of the vertebrate autonomic nervous system, there are hardly any specializations at the presynaptic membrane, and vesicle fusion can occur in an nondirected manner all over the presynaptic terminal. The released transmitter can diffuse across several hundred micrometers and so influence an extensive postsynaptic target area. In the "extreme" case of neurosecretion, the transmitter substance is even released into the blood system and so can reach quite distant targets.

Transmitter substances relay signals at chemical synapses

The general concept of synaptic signal transmission via a chemical messenger, a transmitter, has its origins in experiments carried out by Loewi in 1920 on the neural release of acetylcholine from the vagus nerve of the frog heart. Since then, this concept has been continually changing because of the discovery of new transmitters and transmitter mechanisms. In a broader sense, every substance that is released at the synapses of a neuron, and influences another nerve or effector cell in a specific way, can be considered as a transmitter. In order to qualify as a transmitter substance in a more narrow sense, however, a substance must satisfy several strict criteria. The substance should

— be synthesized in the neuron;
— be found in sufficiently high concentration at the presynaptic terminal;
— have the same effect on a target cell when applied externally in physiologically appropriate concentrations;

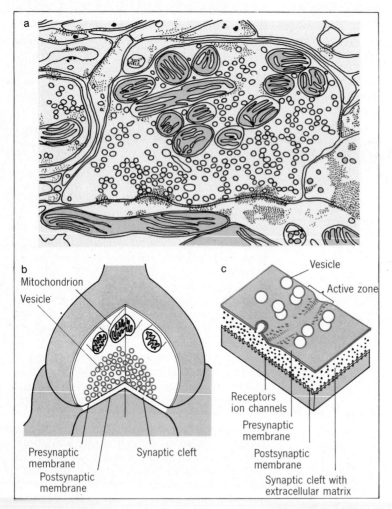

Fig. 3.**4**   Ultrastructure of a chemical synapse. **a** A synaptic terminal as seen in the electron microscope. The presynaptic terminal is filled with vesicles and also contains mitochondria. **b** Schematic representation of a chemical synapse. **c** An enlargement of the presynaptic and postsynaptic membranes at an active zone shows the fusion of several vesicles with the cell membrane (after Stevens and Reese)

— be blocked in its action by the same pharmacological substances as block synaptic transmission;

— be removed in a specific way from the extracellular synaptic space.

A detailed experimental analysis of all these criteria has only been undertaken for a few substances, among them acetylcholine. Despite this, there are good grounds for believing that there are a large number of different transmitter substances.

There are two main groups of transmitters in the nervous system. On the one hand, there are small neuroactive molecules which consist mainly of amines, and are termed classic transmitters; and on the other hand, there are neuroactive *peptides*. Some neurons possess only a single transmitter substance. However, several transmitter substances may coexist in a neuron. Such coexistence of different transmitters often involves a low molecular weight transmitter and a neuropeptide. Several neuropeptides can also occur in one neuron since multiple neuropeptides are often formed by cleavage from a larger polypeptide. Whatever combination of neurotransmitters a neuron uses, it seems to release the same combination at all its synapses.

The classic neurotransmitters are small charged molecules

At the latest count the transmitters include *at least* eight different substances of the small molecule type (Fig. 3.5). All of these small and mostly positively charged molecules are produced in relatively short biosynthetic chain reactions by intermediate metabolism, under the influence of cytoplasmic enzymes. Their synthesis can therefore occur in the cell body as well as in the synaptic terminals. The latter is important because it allows a reconversion of inactivated transmitter substances directly at the synaptic effector site.

The first transmitter substance discovered, and the only low molecular weight transmitter not synthesized directly from an amino acid, is *acetylcholine*. Acetylcholine is produced from acetylcoenzyme A and choline by cholinacetyltransferase. Acetylcholine is the transmitter substance of spinal motoneurons and the postganglionic terminals of the vertebrate parasympathetic nervous system. In addition, acetylcholine occurs as a transmitter in the CNS and in the peripheral nervous system of vertebrates and invertebrates.

The monoamines *dopamine* and norepinephrine *(noradrenaline)* are transmitters

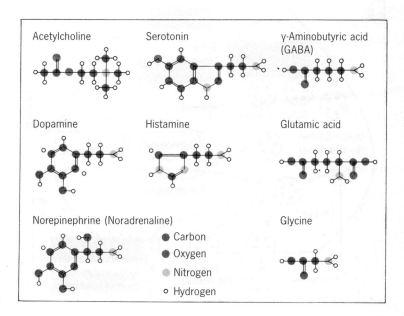

Acetylcholine   Serotonin   γ-Aminobutyric acid (GABA)

Dopamine   Histamine   Glutamic acid

Norepinephrine (Noradrenaline)   Glycine

● Carbon
● Oxygen
● Nitrogen
○ Hydrogen

Fig. 3.5   Structure of some low molecular weight neurotransmitter substances

which belong to the catecholamines as they have a catechol core (a 3,4-dihydroxybenzole ring). They are found, among other places, in many invertebrate neurons, as well as in the central and autonomic nervous systems of vertebrates. Norepinephrine is the most important transmitter in ganglion cells of the sympathetic nervous system. Both transmitters are synthesized from the amino acid tyrosine (Fig. 3.6). Epinephrine *(adrenaline)* is also assumed to play a role as a neurotransmitter, but occurs in the brain in much smaller amounts than norepinephrine. Two substances related to the catecholamines, and which probably also play a role as transmitters, are octopamine and tyramine. Both are found in invertebrate neurons.

Serotonin is an indolamine; it has an indole ring in addition to the catechol. Serotonin is synthesized from the amino acid tryptophane. *Histamine* is an imidazole that is produced from histidine. These transmitter substances are often classed together with the cate-

amino acids *glutamate, γ-aminobutyric acid* (GABA), and *glycine.* Glutamate occurs at many excitatory synapses in the vertebrate CNS, and is an important transmitter at neuromuscular synapses in arthropods. GABA is an amino acid that is widespread in the nervous system, and is the neurotransmitter for many inhibitory synapses. Glycine is found in certain neurons of the vertebrate spinal cord. The amino acid *aspartate* also counts as a possible neurotransmitter. What is special about these transmitter substances is that they are ubiquitous as amino acids in all cells. Since only certain amino acids function as transmitters, it is likely that the neurons that use these amino acid transmitters have special mechanisms and compartments (vesicles?) for their storage and release.

The number and diversity of neuroactive peptides is determined by the genome

The number of putative transmitter systems has risen immensely since the discovery of the neuropeptides. These molecules consist of

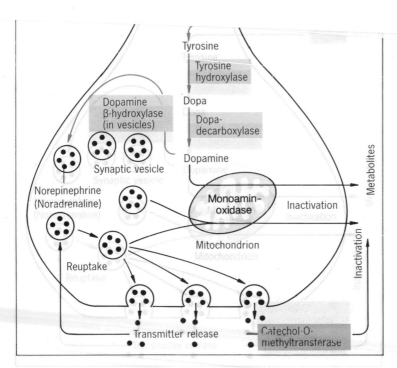

Fig. 3.**6** Simplified depiction of the synthesis, storage, release, and reuptake of the neurotransmitter norepinephrine (noradrenaline) at a synaptic terminal (after Iversen)

Reichert, Introduction to Neurobiology
ISBN 3-13-784701-X (GTV), 0-19-521010-7 (OUP)
Georg Thieme Verlag, Stuttgart · New York 1992

which can act as neuroactive substances are known. Some researchers estimate that there could be thousands. Several of these substances have been known for some time as hormones, for example, ACTH and vasopressin, which are released from the pituitary; gastrin and cholecystokinin, which are intestinal hormones; and somatostatin and LHRII, which are produced in the hypothalamus. It is not very surprising that peptides like these, which can act as hormonal messenger substances over large distances, are also employed as neurotransmitters for synaptic signal transmission over short distances. There are also continuous transitions in the action of a neuroactive peptide as a hormone or as a transmitter. In intermediate cases like this, which defy any exact definition, one speaks of a *neuromodulatory* action. Two neuropeptide groups, the endorphins and the enkephalins, are particularly interesting because they produce analgesic or euphoric effects in humans. They are termed endogenous opiates because they activate the same receptors in the nervous system as do the plant opiates.

Neuropeptides differ from the classic transmitters mainly in the way in which they are produced. Their structure is encoded directly by the genome. Often several neuropeptides are encoded on a single coherent mRNA, and then translated into a large, multifunctional polyprotein (Fig. 3.8a) This translation occurs at the membrane-bound polysomes of the cell body. The secretory precursor protein undergoes molecular processing in the Golgi apparatus, and in the secretory vesicles which derive from the Golgi apparatus (posttranslational modification). This can result in amplification since several copies of the same neuropeptide can occur in one polyprotein. For example, the precursor protein for enkephalin can contain five distinct copies of enkephalin. Neuropeptides with related, synergistic, functions can also occur on the same precursor protein, and so enter the same vesicles. Since the molecular refining processes can vary in different neurons, the same polyprotein can serve to produce different, neuron-specific, neuropeptides. Similar considerations hold for the molecular refinement of the primary transcript

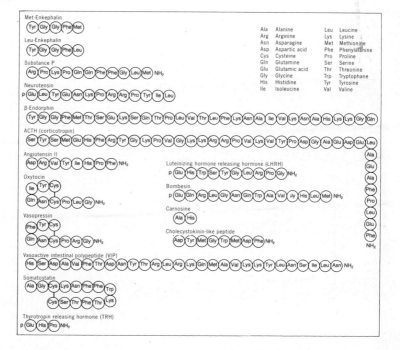

Fig. 3.**7** Amino acid sequences of several neuropeptides (after Iversen)

RNA to mRNA, termed posttranscriptional processing. The calcitonin gene, for example, produces a primary RNA which is the raw material for two different, tissue-specific, mRNAs. Since the encoding of similar precursor proteins can occur through families of related genes, one frequently finds groups of related neuropeptides, that is, groups of different neuropeptides with a high degree of homology in their amino acid sequences (Fig. 3.8b).

Due to their method of synthesis, neuropeptides are formed in the cell body and can probably only be incorporated into vesicles there. These vesicles must therefore be transported from the cell body to the synaptic terminals.

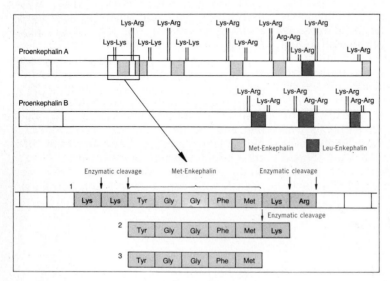

Fig. 3.8a Synthesis of neuropeptides from precursor molecules. Enkephalins (met-enkephalin and leu-enkephalin) are synthesized by enzymatic splitting of two precursor peptides (proenkephalins). Both precursor peptides contain several enkephalin sequences. Enzymatic cleavage sites are characterized by the amino acids lysine and arginine

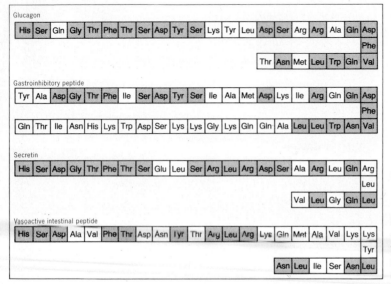

Fig. 3.8b The molecular relatedness of different neuropeptides is revealed in amino acid sequence homology (after Snyder and Bloom)

Depolarization of the presynaptic terminal activates voltage-dependent Ca^{2+} channels

How do potential changes in the presynaptic terminals of chemical synapses lead to the secretion of transmitter substances? In cells which translate an electrical excitation into another form of activation, it generally holds that this translation is regulated by Ca^{2+} currents which are controlled by voltage-dependent Ca^{2+} channels. Inward flowing Ca^{2+} ions function as intracellular messengers which can activate further biochemical processes.

At the squid giant synapse, a particularly favorable preparation, the relationship between the depolarization of the presynaptic terminal and the generation of a postsynaptic potential can be studied quantitatively. It turns out that small presynaptic depolarizations are insufficient to evoke a postsynaptic potential. However, as soon as a threshold level of depolarization, generally between 25 and 40 mV, is exceeded, then a postsynaptic potential is generated. Beyond this threshold value, the amplitude of the postsynaptic potential depends very strongly on the amplitude of the presynaptic depolarization (Fig. 3.**9**). Moreover, it does not seem to matter whether the presynaptic depolarization is evoked by an action potential or an electrotonic potential.

Experiments with pharmacological blockers show that synaptic transmission is not initiated by either an inward Na^+ current or by an outward K^+ current at the presynaptic terminal. Rather, it is an inward Ca^{2+} current into the presynaptic terminal, evoked by depolarization, which elicits the chemical part of the transmission process (Fig. 3.**10**). The larger the inward Ca^{2+} current, the greater the amplitude of the evoked postsynaptic potential. This presynaptic Ca^{2+} current has the following properties:

— It is evoked when the presynaptic depolarization exceeds a threshold value.

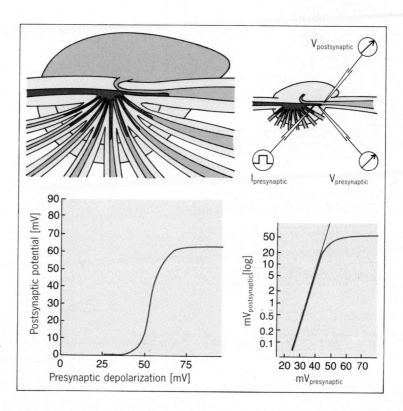

Fig. 3.**9**   Relationship between presynaptic depolarization and postsynaptic potential. At the squid giant synapse, transmission can be studied directly at the synaptic terminal using intracellular electrodes (top). In the suprathreshold region, the amplitude of the postsynaptic potential is strongly dependent on the amplitude of the presynaptic depolarization (bottom) (after Katz and Miledi, and Llinas)

– The current is somewhat delayed and typically begins only toward the end of a presynaptic action potential. This is the main reason for a delay of about 0.5 ms in signal transmission at chemical synapses.
– Above the threshold value, the inward Ca^{2+} current is strongly voltage-dependent.
– The inward Ca^{2+} current is dependent on the duration of the depolarizing phase of an action potential.

The properties of the Ca^{2+} inward current can be accounted for by the molecular properties of voltage-dependent Ca^{2+} channels. When these Ca^{2+} channels are open, then a Ca^{2+} current into the cell results due to the steep slope of the chemical gradient for Ca^{2+} ions (from 1 mmol to 100 nmol), which is directed inward. The voltage-dependent Ca^{2+} channels in the presynaptic membrane seem to be concentrated very near the sites of transmitter release. They have the following properties:

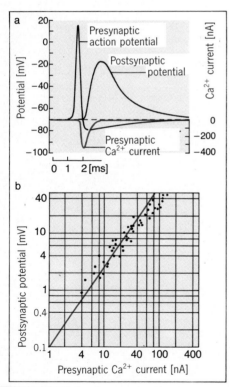

Fig. 3.**10a,b**   The role of Ca^{2+} in synaptic transmission. **a** Presynaptic action potential, presynaptic Ca^{2+} influx and postsynaptic potential at the squid giant synapse. **b** Dependence of the amplitude of the postsynaptic potential on the presynaptic influx of Ca^{2+}

– The Ca^{2+} channels are activated and switch to the open configuration when the cell membrane is sufficiently depolarized.
– The activation time of the Ca^{2+} channels is substantially longer than that of the Na^+ channels.
– The probability of a Ca^{2+} channel opening is voltage-dependent and increases **e**-fold for every 6 mV of suprathreshold depolarization.
– During a continuous depolarization the Ca^{2+} channels inactivate only slowly and incompletely.

The voltage-dependent Ca^{2+} channel has a structure similar to that of the voltage-dependent Na^+ channel (about 60% amino acid sequence homology). The channel protein is thought to be a long polypeptide that consists of four internally homologous transmembrane domains, each of which is able to cross the membrane six times in an α-helical conformation.

An influx of Ca^{2+} ions into the presynaptic terminal leads to a transient increase in the local Ca^{2+} concentration, which is then rapidly reduced by cellular homeostatic mechanisms. It is this transient increase in the free intracellular Ca^{2+} concentration which leads to transmitter release. At the squid giant synapse the influx of Ca^{2+} ions has been quantitatively studied using both fluorescent, Ca^{2+}-sensitive,

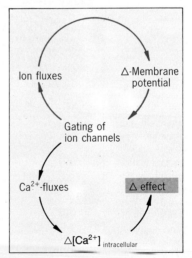

Fig. 3.**10c**   General scheme for the role of Ca^{2+} in the transduction of electrical excitation into another activity form (after Llinas and Hille)

dyes and voltage clamp experiments (Fig. 3.11). Further, injection of Ca²⁺ ions into the presynaptic terminal has provided direct evidence for the action of intracellular Ca^{2+} on transmitter release at this synapse.

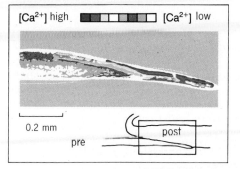

[Ca²⁺] high   [Ca²⁺] low

0.2 mm

pre   post

Fig. 3.11 Localization of the presynaptic (pre) Ca^{2+} inward current at an active squid giant synapse by fluorescent Ca^{2+}-sensitive dyes (post = postsynaptic) (after Smith)

Transmitter release occurs in quanta

The transmitter release evoked by increasing the intracellular Ca^{2+} concentration is not continuous. Transmitter is actually emitted from the presynaptic terminal in small elementary units. These units are termed *quanta*. A quantum of released transmitter leads to the generation of a unitary postsynaptic potential, called a miniature postsynaptic potential (mPSP). The normal postsynaptic potential is made up of many unitary miniature potentials. The quantal nature of transmitter release has been described for all chemical synapses studied to date, and has been most thoroughly analyzed at the vertebrate neuromuscular synapse by Katz.

The starting point of these investigations was the discovery that spontaneous miniature postsynaptic potentials can occur in the absence of presynaptic stimulation (Fig. 3.12a). These miniature potentials, which at the neuro-

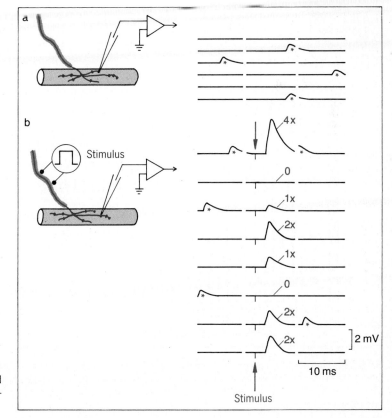

Fig. 3.12 Unitary potentials at the neuromuscular synapse.
a Miniature postsynaptic potentials (*) occur spontaneously.
b Under certain circumstances, small postsynaptic potentials whose amplitude fluctuates in a stepwise manner can be elicited in the muscle fiber by presynaptic activation (after Liley)

muscular synapse of vertebrates are also called miniature end-plate potentials (mEPP), occur at low frequency, and are randomly distributed in time. The amplitude of the spontaneous miniature potentials varies around a mean value of about 0.4 mV under normal conditions.

Small postsynaptic potentials can also be evoked by presynaptic action potentials when the extracellular Ca^{2+} concentration is greatly reduced. The amplitude of these small evoked potentials does not vary in a regular way, but seems to fluctuate in a stepwise manner (Fig. 3.12b). A statistical analysis of the amplitude distribution of these evoked postsynaptic potentials shows that they are composed of multiple integrals of a single unitary potential, and that the amplitude distribution of this unitary potential corresponds to that of the spontaneous miniature potentials (Fig. 3.13).

Two important deductions result from this and similar experiments.

– Transmitter release occurs in multimolecular packets, each of which evokes a small postsynaptic unitary potential. Accordingly, the normal postsynaptic potential, which appears to be continuously graded in amplitude, is in fact composed of a variable number of such unitary potentials.

– The change in the extracellular Ca^{2+} concentration does not change the size of the quanta released, but rather the probability of a given quantum being released. The more Ca^{2+} that flows into the presynaptic terminal, the more quanta of transmitter are released.

At the vertebrate neuromuscular synapse, about 200 quanta are released per presynaptic action potential under normal conditions. Each one of these quanta consists of 5000–10 000 molecules of acetylcholine. In contrast, at most central nervous synapses, but also at the neuromuscular synapses of many invertebrates, the number of quanta released per action potential is much lower, typically between 1 and 10.

Synaptic vesicles fuse with the presynaptic membrane

Quanta of transmitter have a morphological correlate, namely the synaptic vesicles in the presynaptic terminal. It is assumed that each vesicle contains several thousand transmitter molecules, and therefore exactly one quantum. The vesicles can fuse with the presynaptic membrane at special binding sites, and thereby release their contents exocytotically into the

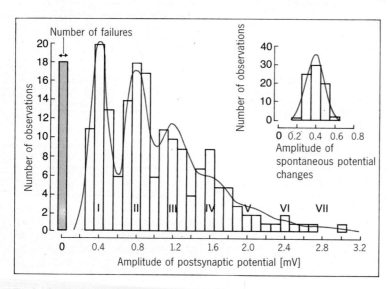

Fig. 3.13   Amplitude histogram of evoked small postsynaptic potentials and spontaneous miniature postsynaptic potentials at the neuromuscular synapse. In the amplitude distribution of the evoked postsynaptic potentials, maxima occur at whole-number multiples (I,II,III,IV,V,VI,VII) of the mean amplitude of the spontaneous miniature postsynaptic potentials (after Boyd and Martin)

synaptic cleft. The various stages of fusion of synaptic vesicles can be "frozen" in time by rapidly cooling synapses at various times following presynaptic stimulation (Fig. 3.14). Analysis of the frog neuromuscular synapse with the electron microscope shows that exactly one vesicle fuses with the presynaptic membrane per quantum released. In addition, these investigations indicate that the individual vesicles fuse independently of one another. The fact that the process of vesicle fusion leads to an increase in membrane capacitance means that this process can, in principle, also be followed in the living cell by electrophysiological measurements of capacitance.

The role of intracellular Ca^{2+} is critical in the process of vesicle fusion. It is namely the increase in the intracellular Ca^{2+} concentration in the synaptic terminal which initiates the binding and fusion of the synaptic vesicles with the presynaptic membrane. Up to now it has not been possible to determine whether vesicle fusion is caused directly by Ca^{2+} ions, or whether Ca^{2+} acts indirectly via Ca^{2+}-binding proteins, like calmodulin for example. A Ca^{2+}/calmodulin complex could lead to adhesion, and finally fusion, of the vesicle membrane with the cell membrane via the phosphoprotein synapsin I, which occurs specifically, and in high concentrations, on the cytoplasmic side of synaptic vesicles.

Transmitter molecules are already packed into vesicular structures during their synthesis. In this way they are protected from enzymatic degradation, are osmotically neutral, and can be transported and stored in high concentration within a neuron. There are specific, active uptake systems for small molecular transmitters in the vesicle membrane, so that the refilling of vesicles can occur in the synaptic terminal. In some presynaptic terminals there is also a certain amount of neurotransmitter free in the cytoplasm. Whether these free transmitter molecules can be released via a nonvesicular method is currently under investigation.

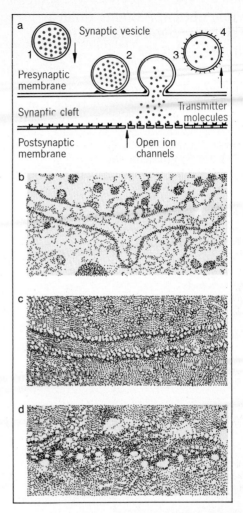

Fig. 3.**14** Fusion of vesicles with the presynaptic membrane. **a** During synaptic transmission, transmitter-filled vesicles approach the presynaptic membrane (1). They then bind to specialized membrane sites (2), after which they fuse with the membrane and empty their contents into the synaptic cleft (3). Vesicle membrane is actively recovered from the presynaptic membrane (4). **b** Electron micrograph of a cross-section through part of a chemical synapse. Vesicles have been "frozen" in the process of fusion at the active synapse. **c** View of the membrane proteins of a presynaptic active zone before the synaptic release of transmitter. **d** Immediately after synaptic activation. At the active zone, vesicles fuse with the presynaptic membrane, leaving behind depressions (after Heuser and Stevens)

Transmembrane Proteins Control Postsynaptic Signal Generation at Chemical Synapses

Principle

The postsynaptic membrane is the receiver element of a chemical synapse. It is the site at which a chemical signal from the presynaptic terminal, is acquired, converted, and made available to interact with other neural signals. This process begins with the fact that on release from the presynaptic terminal, transmitter molecules rapidly diffuse across the synaptic cleft (in approx. 0.2 ms) and interact with specific receptor proteins on the postsynaptic membrane. As a result of this interaction, molecular reactions are evoked in the postsynaptic terminal whose consequence is generally a change in the electrical properties of the postsynaptic membrane. Such changes can develop quickly or slowly. They can have an excitatory or inhibitory effect on the postsynaptic cell. The effects can be short (milliseconds), or long term (potentially days or months).

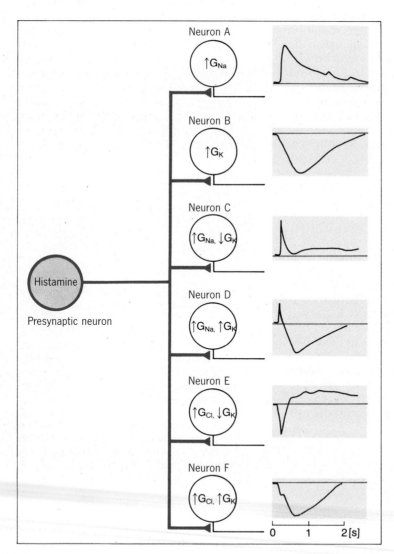

Fig. 3.**15**   The same transmitter can have different postsynaptic effects. A histaminergic neuron in *Aplysia* synapses with several postsynaptic neurons. The postsynaptic potentials evoked by histamine in these neurons have different polarities and time courses. G = conductance (after Kandel)

Neurotransmitters bind to receptors on the postsynaptic membrane

Transmitter molecules can only exert an effect on the postsynaptic cell if they encounter the right receptor molecules on the postsynaptic membrane. These receptor molecules are concentrated on the postsynaptic membrane, and are oriented in such a way that an active binding site for the appropriate transmitter lies free on the extracellular surface. For every neurotransmitter there are receptor molecules which specifically bind the neurotransmitter with a high, enzyme-like affinity. As a result of the transient binding of the appropriate transmitter to its receptor, an allosteric conformational change in the receptor molecule occurs, which leads to further postsynaptic effects being evoked.

The postsynaptic effect of a given transmitter is determined by the nature of the postsynaptic receptor molecules, and not by the nature of the transmitter. Since there can be different receptor types for the same transmitter, one and the same transmitter can have different effects on different postsynaptic cells (Fig. 3.15). The same transmitter can act in an excitatory way on one cell and in an inhibitory way on another. It is, thus, misleading to speak of an "excitatory" or "inhibitory" transmitter without specifying the postsynaptic mode and site of action. Various highly specific neuropharmacological agents and neurotoxins can be used to characterize the different receptor types which bind the same neurotransmitter. For example, one can differentiate pharmacologically between nicotinic and muscarinic acetylcholine receptors in that the former are activated by the alkaloid nicotine and blocked by the snake venom α-bungarotoxin, while the latter are activated by the alkaloid muscarine and blocked by atropine.

There is a large diversity of different receptor types, since there are generally several receptor types for every neurotransmitter. Despite this diversity, it seems that at all chemical synapses studied to date the transient transmitter–receptor binding initiates only two fundamental postsynaptic mechanisms. Depending on the receptor type, there is either a rapid change in the ionic permeability of the postsynaptic membrane, or a change in the biochemical activity of the postsynaptic cell, or both (Fig. 3.16).

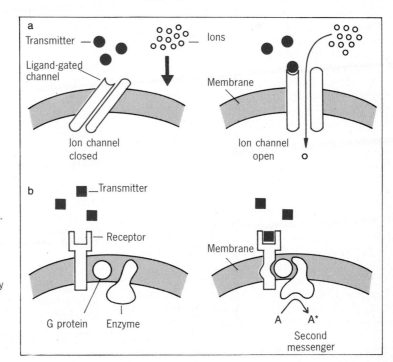

Fig. 3.16   Schematic representation of the two main mechanisms for transmitter–receptor systems at chemical synapses. **a** The transmitter causes a change in the ionic permeability of the postsynaptic cell by acting on the ion channel. **b** The transmitter initiates changes in the biochemical activity of the postsynaptic cell

a
Transmitter
Ligand-gated channel
Ions
Membrane
Ion channel closed
Ion channel open   o

b
Transmitter
Receptor
Membrane
G protein   Enzyme
A   A*
Second messenger

Transmitter-gated ion channels allow the direct conversion of a chemical signal into an electrical signal

Transmitter-dependent ion channels, which are also termed transmitter-gated ion channels, ligand-gated ion channels or simply *receptor channels,* are transmembrane complexes which combine the properties of receptors and ionophores. They have specific binding sites for neurotransmitters, and, as ion channels, can assume different quasi-stable closed and open conformations. They are switched between conformations of different permeability by transmitter action. More precisely, the transition from one conformation to another becomes energetically favorable as a result of binding the correct ligand. The switching or gating of transmitter-dependent ion channels is generally very fast, which leads to the generation of postsynaptic potentials within milliseconds. Transmitter-gated ion channels are characterized by having different ion selectivities. There are transmitter-gated ion channels which preferentially allow only a single ionic species, such as K^+ or Cl^-, to pass. Others, by contrast, allow cations to pass unspecifically, but are largely impermeable to anions. In contrast to the voltage-gated ion channels, many transmitter-gated ion channels are only weakly affected by voltage changes across the membrane. However, there are also important receptor channels which can be activated in both a transmitter- and voltage-dependent manner.

The transmitter-gated ion channel whose properties have been most intensively studied is the *nicotinic acetylcholine receptor channel* of the vertebrate neuromuscular synapse. This receptor channel occurs with a high density (10 000 receptors/μm2) in the postsynaptic membrane, and can be isolated in high concentration from the electroplaques (transformed muscle cells) of certain electric fish. The receptor–ion channel complex is a pentamer consisting of four different polypeptide chains, α, β, γ, and δ, and has the composition $\alpha_2\beta\gamma\delta$ (Fig. 3.17). Each of these polypeptides, whose molecular weight lies between 40 and 65 kDa, is coded by its own gene. All four genes have a high degree of sequence homology, which indicates a divergent evolution from a common original gene. The amino acid chain of each polypeptide subunit crosses the membrane several times in an α-helical conforma-

tion. The hydrophilic N-terminal is glycosylated and lies on the extracellular side of the membrane. The five polypeptide units are arranged in a highly symmetrical ring-shaped manner around a central transmembrane pore. The whole cylinder-shaped complex is embedded in the membrane, and extends about 7 nm out into the extracellular space, and 4 nm into the intracellular space.

The extracellular parts of the two α subunits each have a binding site for acetylcholine. They are, therefore, the actual "receptive" subunits. The conformational changes in both the α subunits are assumed to produce a cooperative restructuring of all the subunits, which results in the central transmembrane channel opening. In its open configuration the nicotinic acetylcholine receptor channel is permeable to cations, but largely impermeable to anions. This cation selectivity might be related to the fact that the polypeptide regions, which are arranged around the extracellular opening of the central channel pore, carry a negative net charge. As a result of such localized net charges, positively charged cations can be pulled into the region of the opening, and thus be available to diffuse from there in high concentration through the channel. The diameter of the channel is about 3 nm on the synaptic side, and narrows further toward the cytoplasmic side. In its open state the channel has a conductance which varies between 30 and 50 pS depending on the animal. Investigations on the permeability of various cations through the open channel show that the diameter of the channel at its narrowest point is about 0.65 nm, and is therefore large enough to allow the passage of hydrated Na^+ and K^+ ions.

Put simply, the gating behavior of the acetylcholine receptor can be represented as a three-phase process:

- Two transmitter molecules bind to the receptor and induce a cooperative conformational change in the receptor–ion channel complex.
- The ion channel opens for a stochastically variable period, which on the average is about 1 ms long.
- The ion channel closes, and both the transmitter molecules can diffuse away from the receptor.

In its details, however, the kinetic gating behavior of the acetylcholine receptor is remarkably complex. The transition from a closed to an open conformation proceeds through several intermediate states, and even in its functionally "open" state, the channel appears to undergo numerous very rapid transitions between open and closed conformations. Further, due to the continued presence of transmitter molecules at the receptor, there is a decline in the total conductance, termed a desensitization. The receptor can pass through a series of "desensitized states" which resemble the inactivated state of the voltage-dependent Na⁺ channel.

In the vertebrate nervous system there are numerous, different, nicotinic acetylcholine receptor types, whose amino acid se-

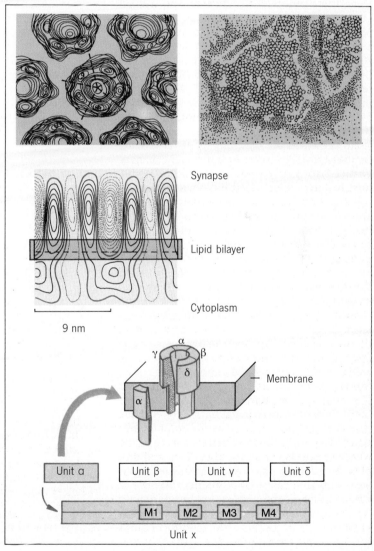

Synapse

Lipid bilayer

Cytoplasm

9 nm

Membrane

Fig. 3.**17**   The nicotinic acetylcholine receptor channel. Diffraction analysis (top left) and electron micrograph (top right) show that the receptor channel is a pentamer consisting of five units arranged around a central canal. A cross-section through the postsynaptic membrane (middle) shows that the receptor channel extends through the membrane, and has structural domains on both the synaptic and cytoplasmic sides. The five polypeptide units of the receptor channel (2 x α, β, γ, and δ) reside together in the membrane to form an ion channel (bottom). Every polypeptide unit is coded by its own gene. All the subunits display a high degree of homology in their amino acid sequences. M = transmembrane region (after Brisson, Unwin and Stevens)

quences are somewhat different from those in the receptor type present in muscle cells. All these receptor types are nevertheless highly homologous, and have a very high level of structural conformity. Further, all the nicotinic acetylcholine receptor types in vertebrates have amino acid sequences which are homologous with those of insects. This demonstrates an evolutionary relationship between the receptor molecules which stretches back over more than 350 million years.

The structure of numerous other transmitter-dependent ion channels seems to be similar to that of the acetylcholine receptor, which points to a family of related ion channel genes that are derived from a common original gene. A $GABA_A$-receptor–ion channel complex, for example, is also thought to consist of several homologous polypeptide subunits. Again, every polypeptide chain spans the membrane several times in an α-helical conformation. The α- and β–subunits of the $GABA_A$-receptor–ion channel complex have about 50% homologous amino acid sequences between them, and about 25% homologous amino acid sequences with the subunits of the acetylcholine receptor. A glycine-receptor–ion channel complex seems to be constructed out of homologous polypeptide subunits in a similar way.

The properties of the glutamate receptor are particularly interesting. There are at least three pharmacologically distinct glutamate receptor channel types. One binds the agonist quisqualate and is called the Q-receptor. Another binds the agonist kainate and is called the K-receptor. The third binds the agonist N-methyl-D-aspartate and is known as the *NMDA-receptor*. Q- and K-receptors are often termed non-NMDA receptors. Activation of the Q- and K-receptors normally leads to the opening of ion channels which are permeable to Na^+ and K^+ ions. This is a similar mode of action to the nicotinic acetylcholine receptor. In the case of the NMDA-receptor, however, there is a further dimension. The NMDA-receptor channel has several conductance states. The prevailing conductance state of the NMDA-receptor channel is determined not only by binding the neurotransmitter glutamate, but also by the membrane potential. If the postsynaptic membrane is at rest or depolarized only slightly, then the ion channel is blocked by Mg^{2+}. In this state, binding of glutamate only makes the receptor channel permeable to a small extent, and then only to Na^+ and K^+ ions. If the membrane is depolarized more strongly, then the Mg^{2+} block is removed. In this state, binding of glutamate makes the receptor channel much more permeable, not only to monovalent cations, but also to Ca^{2+} ions (Fig. 3.18). This process can lead to the formation of regenerative postsynaptic potentials. The state of the NMDA-receptor channel can also be influenced allosterically by glycine. The special type of synaptic signal processing at the NMDA-receptor channel is assumed to have important consequences for activity-dependent processes in the nervous system.

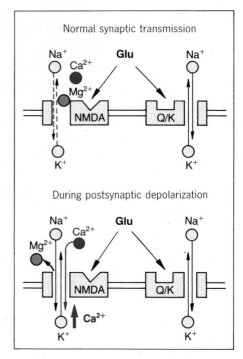

Fig. 3.**18** Properties of glutamate receptors. Activation of Q/K receptors leads to the opening of ion channels which are permeable to Na^+ and K^+. Activation of NMDA receptors at the normal resting potential raises the permeability of cation channels only slightly since these are blocked by Mg^{2+} (top). The Mg^{2+} blockade of the NMDA channel is removed by postsynaptic depolarization which, thus, considerably increases the permeability of the activated ion channel to Na^+, K^+ and Ca^{2+} (bottom). Glu = glutamic acid (after Nicoll et al.)

Synaptic receptors can initiate biochemical changes in the postsynaptic cell

Not all receptors exert a direct effect on the permeability of the postsynaptic membrane. A second class of postsynaptic receptors evokes a set of biochemical reactions in the postsynaptic cell following the binding of transmitter. The end effect of these biochemical reactions can be an allosteric conformational change, or a covalent modification, of an ion channel. In both cases, changes in the electrical properties of the postsynaptic membrane will result. Other processes can also be evoked by the biochemical reaction cascades, even those involved in the regulation of gene activity. These amplifying reaction chains are complex. They can themselves be regulated at several sites, and their molecular program can be modified in different neurons. Characteristic for synapses at which this type of signal processing occurs are slower gating kinetics, and a longer time of action for the induced postsynaptic processes (a time span of seconds, minutes, or longer).

The muscarinic acetylcholine receptors, β-adrenergic receptors and serotonin receptors are all well-known receptor systems which initiate postsynaptic reaction chains. All three receptor types are large transmembrane proteins which have homologous amino acid sequences. The polypeptide chain in each of these proteins is assumed to form seven hydrophobic α-helical regions which can span the cell membrane (Fig. 3.19). However, the muscarinic acetylcholine receptor, β-adrenergic receptor, and serotonin receptor do not function directly as ion channels.

The initiation of the biochemical reaction chains in these and similarly functioning receptor systems begins with the binding of the transmitter to the postsynaptic receptor. This causes a conformational change to occur in the receptor. The transmitter–receptor complex then interacts with a coupling protein in the membrane. This coupling protein is usually one of the heterotrimeric guanosine phosphate-binding proteins called *G proteins*. As a result of this interaction an exchange of GDP for GTP occurs at the G protein. The G protein is thereby activated, and depending on the cell type, can then initiate various other signal-amplifying reactions. In the simplest case these reactions can be the initiation of conformational changes in neighboring ion channels. A lateral diffusion of the activated G protein is assumed to bring about interactions between the G protein and ion channels in the membrane. Intracellular reaction cascades can also be initiated by the activated G protein, and two of these reaction cascades have been intensively studied (Fig. 3.20). In both, intracellularly-acting, low molecular weight messenger substances, termed *second messengers,* are involved.

In the first reaction type the G protein binds to the catalytic subunit of an adenylate cyclase. This is then activated and catalyses in turn the conversion of ATP into *cAMP*. cAMP can then activate cAMP-dependent protein kinases. The protein kinases can finally phosphorylate various protein substrates and thereby change their properties. If these protein substrates are ion channels in the membrane (or are associated with ion channels in the membrane), then a change in membrane conductance can result. In the second reaction type, the activated G protein activates a membrane-bound phosphodiesterase which then carries out the hydrolysis of the membrane lipid phosphatidylinositol 4,5-biphosphate to diacylglycerol (DG) and inositol triphosphate (IP$_3$). DG and IP$_3$ are also second messengers which can activate protein kinase C or initiate the release of Ca^{2+} from intracellular reservoirs. Both can change the signal transfer properties of the postsynaptic cell.

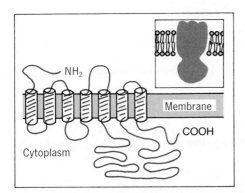

Fig. 3.**19**   Molecular organization of the muscarinic acetylcholine receptor, considerably simplified. The polypeptide chain of the receptor molecule crosses the membrane several times and has a relatively large intracellular region (after Peralta et al.)

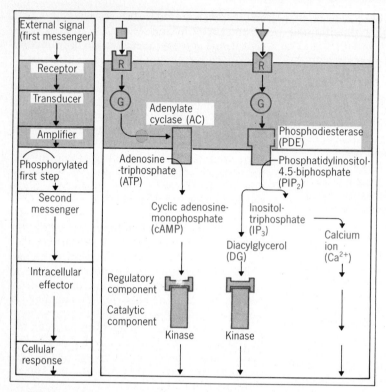

Fig. 3.**20**   Intracellular reaction cascades which can be initiated by transmitter–receptor binding. Activated receptors interact with transducing G proteins (G) which then activate various amplifying enzymes. These evoke internal signals which are transmitted by second messengers. Second messenger molecules can, among other things, bind to the regulatory subunits of protein kinases, whose catalytic subunit is then activated. The catalytic subunit can then act as a cellular effector by phosphorylating specific proteins and thereby evoke various cellular responses (after Berridge)

Transmitter action has time constraints

It is not enough just to control transmitter release during signal transfer at chemical synapses. The released transmitter must also be quickly removed from the synaptic cleft, so that the signal can be temporally delimited, and a subsequent signal generated at the synapse. There are three important mechanisms for the removal of released transmitter:

— *Diffusion* of transmitter out of the synaptic cleft occurs at all synapses. Since the postsynaptic receptors are concentrated at the subsynaptic membrane, diffusion away from the receptor sites limits the transmitter's postsynaptic effects.
— Extracellular enzymatic *degradation* of the transmitter is used, especially in the case of acetylcholine. This molecule is split into choline and acetate by an acetylcholinester-

ase which is located in the extracellular matrix of the synaptic cleft. This results in cessation of the postsynaptic action of the transmitter (acetylcholine), and at the same time makes choline available for presynaptic reuptake and reuse. An inhibition of acetylcholinesterase by certain neurotoxins, nerve gases or insecticides can have disastrous consequences for the organism. An uncontrolled accumulation of acetylcholine at neuromuscular synapses causes a permanent excitation of the postsynaptic muscle cells, and so paralyses important motor systems like the respiratory system.
— The *reuptake* of a transmitter substance by the presynaptic terminal or glia cells is the most common method for functionally inactivating a released transmitter. All biogenic amines are removed from the synaptic cleft by highly specific reuptake mechanisms at

the presynaptic membrane. There are several neuropharmacological substances which block the reuptake mechanisms for neurotransmitters and thereby amplify transmitter action at certain synapses. However, in such cases a persistent and high concentration of neurotransmitter can also cause desensitization phenomena in postsynaptic receptors.

The presence at the presynaptic membrane of binding sites for the released transmitter is important, not only for the reuptake of transmitter from the synaptic cleft. At many presynaptic terminals the released transmitter can selectively react with autoreceptors in order to perform various regulatory functions.

The way in which peptide transmitters are inactivated is not yet totally understood. Extracellularly acting peptidases are likely to play an important role. Peptides are probably only slowly removed from the synaptic extracellular space, which partly explains their persistent effects.

Postsynaptic Potentials

Origin and significance

Presynaptic transmitter release generates postsynaptic potentials at most chemical synapses. Postsynaptic potentials result from conductance changes in the postsynaptic membrane. Like action potentials, they can be thought of as transient disturbances of the resting potential of the cell. However, in contrast to action potentials, synaptic potentials are neither regenerative nor stereotyped in their expression. They are mostly small and can summate with one another as local, passively propagated potentials. Many of the properties of synaptic potentials are determined by the properties of the transmitter–activated postsynaptic ion channels.

The transmitter-gated opening of ion channels in the postsynaptic membrane leads to the formation of local potentials

The opening of a transmitter-gated ion channel leads to an elementary conductance increase in the postsynaptic membrane. An elementary conductance increase can result in a change in the ionic current across the membrane if there is an electromotive force for permeable ions. Such a change in ionic current can be mea-

sured as an elementary ionic current using the *patch clamp* method (Fig. 3.**21a**). Elementary ionic currents have a seemingly rectangular time course, but higher resolution shows that they actually have a fine structure which is characteristic for each channel.

The amplitude of the elementary ionic current i depends on the conductance of the ion channel g_i and the electromotive force EMF, which acts on permeable ions:

$$i = g_i (EMF)$$

The electromotive driving force for an elementary synaptic ionic current is the difference between the membrane potential V_m, and the steady state equilibrium potential for the permeable ions, termed the *reversal potential*, V_{rev}. Therefore

$$i = g_i (V_m - V_{rev})$$

If the ion channel is permeable only to a single ionic species, then the reversal potential is equal to the equilibrium potential for this ionic species. If the ion channel is permeable to several ionic species, then the reversal potential depends on the permeabilities and concentrations of all permeable ion species. In general, the reversal potential can be quantitatively determined from the Goldman equation. For the reversal potential therefore, (analogous to the resting potential): the greater the permeability to an ionic species, the more the reversal potential is determined by the equilibrium potential for this ionic species.

During the postsynaptic potential, the membrane potential is driven toward the reversal potential. This is because the elementary ionic current that flows through an open ion channel evokes a potential change in the postsynaptic membrane which moves the membrane potential towards the reversal potential. In this respect it is important to note that (Fig. 3.**21b**):

— The synaptic elementary current is inward-directed (depolarizing) when the membrane potential is more negative than the reversal potential; and outward-directed (hyperpolarizing) when the membrane potential is more positive than the reversal potential.
— The strength of the synaptic elementary current increases the further the membrane

potential deviates from the reversal potential.
- No net current flows through an ion channel when the membrane potential is equal to the reversal potential.
- The gating behavior, and therefore the unitary conductance, of an ion channel often changes only insignificantly for different values of the membrane potential (most of the transmitter-dependent ion channels have only a small voltage-dependency).

The conductance increase in the postsynaptic membrane that results from the opening of a single ion channel is relatively small (Table 3.1). In the case of the acetylcholine receptor at the frog muscle endplates, for example, this is about 30 pS per channel for a mean open time of about 1.5 ms. In a resting muscle fiber this leads to a maximum elementary ionic current of only 2–3 pA, and produces a postsynaptic potential of less than 1 µV. However, since there are a large number of transmitter-gated ion channels in the postsynaptic membrane, a sizeable total conductance change can result from the simultaneous activation of many ion channels acting in parallel. For a homogeneous population of transmitter-activated postsynaptic ion channels, the total conductance increase ΔG, which results from n activated ion channels with an elementary conductance g_i, is given by

$$\Delta G = n \times g_i$$

As a result of this conductance increase, a transmitter-induced total synaptic current of

$$I = \Delta G \, (V_m - V_{rev})$$

is evoked. At the neuromuscular endplate of vertebrates, acetylcholine can activate more than 200 000 channels within a few milliseconds. This can lead to a maximum total ionic current of almost 0.1 mA, and a postsynaptic potential change of about 60 mV, starting from the resting potential.

The total synaptic current, which is composed of numerous statistically fluctuating elementary synaptic currents, has a continuous time course. The same holds for the postsynaptic potential that is evoked by this current. However, compared with the synaptic current, the postsynaptic potential has a slower time

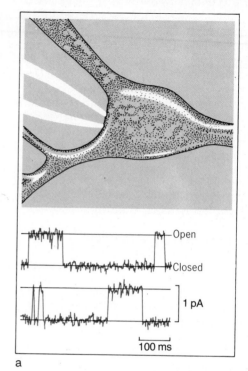

a

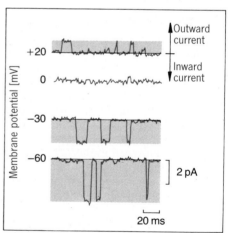

b

Fig. 3.21 Elementary postsynaptic ion currents measured with the patch clamp technique. **a** Ion currents which flow through single transmitter-gated ion channels can be measured after application of the appropriate neurotransmitter via a patch electrode in contact with the cell membrane. The ion channel studied here fluctuates between open and closed states, and in its open state allows a rectangular-shaped ionic current of about 1 pA to flow through. **b** The direction and amplitude of the elementary current through a transmitter-dependent ion channel depend on the value of the membrane potential (after Neher and Sakmann)

Table 3.1   Single-channel conductances

Preparation	Transmitter	g(pS)	Permeable ions
Aplysia neurons	Acetylcholine	8	Cations
Locust muscle cells	Glutamate	130	Cations
Rat myotubes	Acetylcholine	49	Cations
Crayfish muscle cells	GABA	9	Cl⁻
Mouse spinal neurons in cell culture	GABA	18	Cl⁻
Mouse spinal neurons in cell culture	Glycine	30	Cl⁻
Lamprey brainstem neurons	Glycine	73	Cl⁻

course. This is because, as a typical electrotonic potential, it is influenced by the passive electrical properties of the postsynaptic cell membrane. The total ionic current and the "macroscopic" postsynaptic potential have the same dependence on membrane potential and the same reversal potential, as do the elementary currents (Fig. 3.22). The "macroscopic" postsynaptic potential also drives the membrane potential toward the reversal potential.

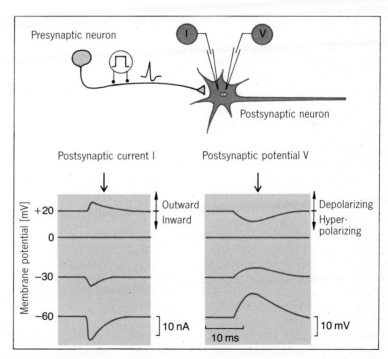

Fig. 3.22   Dependence of a postsynaptic current and a postsynaptic potential on the membrane potential, shown schematically. Polarity and amplitude of the "macroscopic" total postsynaptic current show the same dependence on membrane potential, and have the same reversal potential, as the elementary currents. The same holds for the "macroscopic" postsynaptic potential which is evoked by the total postsynaptic current

Postsynaptic potentials can be excitatory or inhibitory

Voltage-dependent processes in the postsynaptic cell, such as the development of action potentials, or the release of transmitter, can be influenced by postsynaptic potentials. One speaks of an excitatory postsynaptic potential (EPSP) when the postsynaptic potential contributes to the generation of an action potential and/or synaptic transmitter release in the postsynaptic neuron. One speaks of an inhibitory postsynaptic potential (IPSP) when the postsynaptic potential opposes the development of an action potential and/or synaptic transmitter release in the postsynaptic neuron.

The distinction between EPSP and IPSP is clearest when dealing with a postsynaptic neuron which generates action potentials. In this case a postsynaptic potential is an EPSP when its reversal potential is more positive than the threshold for generation of an action potential. Due to the fact that a postsynaptic potential drives the membrane potential toward its reversal potential, an EPSP is depolarizing for all values of the membrane potential that are more negative than its reversal potential. A depolarizing EPSP will therefore contribute to a suprathreshold depolarization of the membrane.

The nicotinic acetylcholine receptor, for example, produces an EPSP. The ion channel of this acetylcholine receptor type is almost equally permeable to Na^+ and K^+. The reversal potential for this EPSP therefore lies approximately in the middle between E_{Na} and E_K, usually between –10 and 0 mV (Fig. 3.23). At the reversal potential the net Na^+ inward current and the net K^+ outward current are equal. For values of membrane potential that are more positive than the reversal potential, the K^+ outward current predominates, and a hyperpolarizing PSP develops. For values of membrane potential more negative than than the reversal potential, the Na^+ inward current predominates, and a depolarizing PSP develops. Since both the resting potential and the threshold for action potential generation are considerably more negative than the reversal potential, a depolarizing EPSP is always evoked over the normal working range of the synapse.

Similar considerations show that a postsynaptic potential is an IPSP when its reversal potential is more negative than the threshold for the generation of an action potential. Because it holds again that a postsynaptic potential drives the membrane potential toward its reversal potential, an IPSP will oppose every depolarization beyond the reversal potential, and therefore a suprathreshold depolarization as well. This occurs in two ways:

– The IPSP is hyperpolarizing at these potential values and thereby opposes a depolarizing EPSP.
– The conductance increases due to the IPSP cause a reduction in the amplitude of simultaneously occurring EPSPs—a sort of "short-circuit" of the membrane. This occurs because, according to Ohm's law, an excitatory ionic current can evoke only relatively smaller EPSPs if the membrane conductance is increased by inhibition.

IPSPs can be evoked by transmitter-dependent K^+ channels, or by transmitter-dependent Cl^- channels. The $GABA_A$-receptor–ion channel complex, for example, is a Cl^- channel and one of the most important inhibitory ion channels in the vertebrate brain. Although both channel types are generally activated independently, they are similar in that their reversal potentials (which in this case correspond to the respective equilibrium potentials) are more negative than the threshold for evoking an action potential. Typical values are –60 mV for Cl^-, and –70 mV for K^+. At Cl^- channels there is a net inflow of Cl^- ions for membrane potential values that are more positive than the reversal potential for Cl^-. For K^+ channels there is a net outward flow of K^+ ions at membrane potential values that are more positive than the reversal potential for K^+. In both cases a hyperpolarizing IPSP is generated which drives the membrane potential away from the threshold for action potential generation (Fig. 3.23). The fact that depolarizing potentials are generated by K^+ and Cl^- channels at membrane potential values which are more negative than the reversal potential does not alter the inhibitory effect of these IPSPs. These channels have an inhibitory effect even at the reversal potential where, by definition, no potential changes are generated. This is because they still oppose every deviation of the membrane potential from this value which lies below the threshold for the development of an action potential.

In cases where the postsynaptic cell does not produce action potentials, a postsynaptic potential has to be considered an EPSP if it favors the release of transmitter from the postsynaptic cell, and as an IPSP if it opposes the release of transmitter from the postsynaptic cell. The same is true when a synapse is formed with another presynaptic terminal. In such cases, the ensuing excitatory or inhibitory processes can become quite complex. A "presynaptic inhibition" of a presynaptic terminal by another inhibitory synapse can occur, for example, either via an inactivation of a synaptic Ca^{2+} channel in the terminal (inhibition of transmitter release by decrease in the presynaptic Ca^{2+} inflow), or via a conductance increase in the presynaptic membrane, so that the amplitude of the action potential in the presynaptic terminal is attenuated (inhibition of transmitter release by a decrease in the presynaptic depolarization).

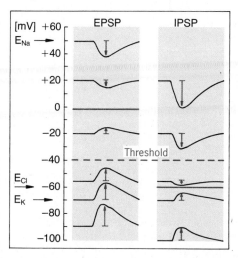

Fig. 3.**23** Dependence of an EPSP and an IPSP on the membrane potential, shown schematically. The reversal potential of the EPSP lies above the threshold for an action potential (here −40 mV). The reversal potential of the IPSP lies below the threshold for an action potential. The EPSP is depolarizing (has an excitatory effect) in the subthreshold range, and in part of the suprathreshold range. The IPSP is hyperpolarizing (has an inhibitory effect) in the suprathreshold range and in part of the subthreshold range

Postsynaptic potentials can result from the transmitter-gated closure of ion channels

Up to now we have only considered mechanisms which evoke postsynaptic potentials via

conductance increases. There are, however, instances where postsynaptic potentials result from the transmitter-gated closure of ion channels, that is, from conductance decreases. In some neurons there are ion channels in the postsynaptic membrane which are open at the resting potential, and thus contribute to the generation of the resting potential, but which can be closed by transmitter action. These include, for example, a particular class of K^+ channels, which can be influenced by the muscarinic acetylcholine receptor (M channels). Since this process is mediated by a diffusible second messenger, the site of transmitter action can even be distant from the site of conductance decrease.

The transmitter-gated closure of such a K^+ channel has excitatory postsynaptic effects. At the resting potential, the closure of a normally open K^+ channel leads to a decrease in the K^+ outward current, and thereby to a depolarization of the membrane. This is because the membrane potential then assumes a new steady-state equilibrium value which lies nearer to E_{Na}. Further, as a result of a decreased conductance of the postsynaptic membrane, the amplitude of all other EPSPs is increased. This follows Ohm's law in that the current flowing at an excitatory synapse will produce a correspondingly greater voltage change if there is a decrease in total membrane conductance.

The effects of synapses which function by conductance decrease are often of long duration (seconds or minutes). The ion channels at these synapses can be modified covalently by transmitter action. Ion channels which can be closed by transmitter action sometimes show a strong voltage-dependence in their gating behavior. They can therefore also be involved in the generation of an action potential in the postsynaptic cell. Since, as open ion channels, they also contribute to the resting potential, they are best considered as "multifunctional ion channels" which defy any strict classification.

The transmission properties of chemical synapses can be modified by repetitive activation

The transmission properties of a chemical synapse can in many cases be modified by its own previous activity. This process is termed homosynaptic plasticity and is at least partly responsible for the experience-dependent functioning of neuron assemblies. In synaptic *depression* the effects of a synapse decrease following prior activation. In synaptic *facilitation* the effects of a synapse increase following prior synaptic activation.

Synaptic depression has been studied in detail in mechanosensory neurons of molluscs and crustaceans (Fig. 3.**24a**). Repeated activation of these sensory neurons, either by mechanical stimuli or electrical stimulation, leads to a decrease in the amplitude of the synaptic potentials which these neurons evoke in postsynaptic cells. The site of action of this type of synaptic depression has been localized to the presynaptic terminal. The synaptic "fatigue" process is based on a decline in the number of transmitter quanta that are released per presynaptic action potential.

Synaptic facilitation has been characterized at the vertebrate neuromuscular synapse. During rapid and repeated stimulation of the presynaptic motor axon, the amplitude of the evoked postsynaptic potential increases (Fig. 3.**24b**). This effect, termed facilitation, decays after a few hundred milliseconds at the neuromuscular synapse. A more persistent effect on synaptic transmission can be evoked by high frequency (50/s) stimulation of the motor axon (Fig. 3.**24c**). After such a "tetanic" stimulation the capacity for synaptic transmission is at first temporarily reduced (posttetanic depression). However, after a few minutes there follows a rapid increase in the synaptic effect

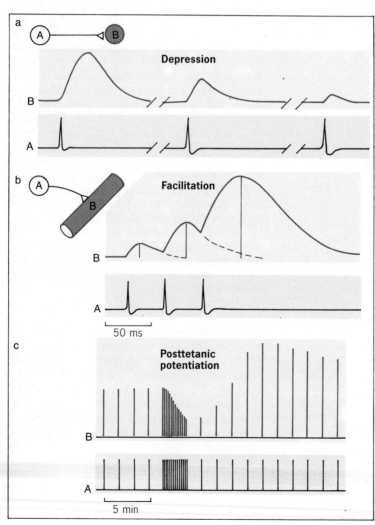

Fig. 3.**24** Synaptic plasticity. **a** Synaptic depression: decrease in the amplitude of the postsynaptic potential during repetitive stimulation. **b** Synaptic facilitation: increase in the amplitude of the postsynaptic potential during repetitive stimulation. **c** Posttetanic potentiation: long-term increase in the postsynaptic potential following high frequency stimulation

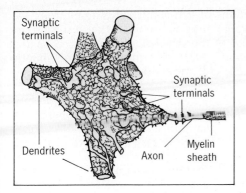

Synaptic
terminals

Synaptic
terminals

Dendrites

Axon

Myelin
sheath

a

Fig. 3.**25**   Synaptic integration. **a** Numerous synaptic terminals
on a spinal motoneuron. **b** The summed postsynaptic potential is
translated into action potentials. In many neurons this occurs at the
axon hillock (after Poritsky and Eckert)

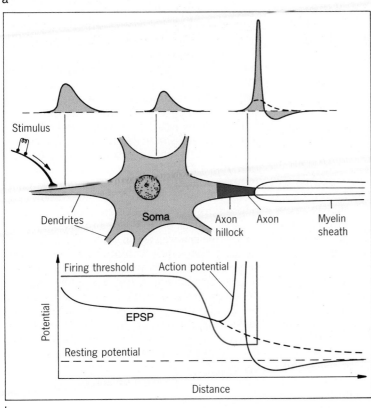

Stimulus

Dendrites   **Soma**   Axon   Axon   Myelin
hillock   sheath

Firing threshold   Action potential

Potential

EPSP

Resting potential

Distance

b

which is termed *posttetanic potentiation* (PTP). As a result, the amplitude of an evoked postsynaptic potential can be double that of a control value. This posttetanic potentiation can last for minutes.

The facilitatory phenomena at the neuromuscular synapse are assumed to result at least partly from an activity-dependent increase in the residual Ca^{2+} concentration in the presynaptic terminal. The Ca^{2+} ions which temporarily remain in the terminal following a prior action potential, summate with those Ca^{2+} ions which enter the terminal during a subsequent action potential. This results in a small increase in the effective Ca^{2+} concentration in the presynaptic terminal. Because of the nonlinear relationship between presynaptic Ca^{2+} concentration and transmitter release, the small amount of additional Ca^{2+} in the presynaptic terminal then leads to a considerable enhancement of evoked transmitter release.

Postsynaptic potentials are integrated and converted into propagated neuronal activity

The postsynaptic potential at the neuromuscular synapse in vertebrate skeletal muscle is evoked by a single presynaptic cell, can reach up to 60 mV, and leads without fail to an action potential under normal conditions. Most neurons, by contrast, receive hundreds or thousands of synaptic contacts from different presynaptic cells (Fig. 3.**25a**). The postsynaptic potentials which are generated at these synapses are small. Typical EPSPs generally amount to less than 1 mV. In order to evoke an action potential in the postsynaptic cell, many such postsynaptic potentials must summate. In addition, besides EPSPs, most neurons also receive numerous IPSPs which can reduce the effectiveness of the summated EPSPs. Different combinations of various presynaptic neurons are active at different times. The resulting response of the cell to the numerous changing synaptic inputs is determined by neuronal integration, that means by spatial and temporal summation of all the postsynaptic potentials. The geometric relationship between excitatory and inhibitory synapses, and the properties of passive signal transmission in the various processes of a neuron play an important role in this process.

The resulting summated postsynaptic potential can itself influence transmission at the neuron's output synapses. However, for this to happen the signal must propagate to the appropriate site of synaptic action. If input and output synapses lie close to one another, this can occur via passive, electrotonic signal conduction. If input and output synapses lie relatively far apart, signal conduction can only occur after the summated postsynaptic potentials have been converted into action potentials. In many neurons this conversion occurs at a special site where the membrane threshold for initiation of action potentials is particularly low (Fig. 3.**25b**). This site, which is termed the impulse initiation zone or axon hillock, often forms the initial segment of the axon. In such neurons a considerable amount of neuronal integration takes place in the impulse initiation zone. This is because the value which the summated postsynaptic potential assumes at this site determines whether or not action potentials are produced. Action potentials are produced then, and only then, when excitation exceeds inhibition at this site by a critical minimal value. If action potentials are indeed generated, then the amplitude and time course of the summated postsynaptic potentials are encoded in the frequency and temporal discharge pattern of the propagated action potentials.

References

General Reviews

Akil, H., Watson, S. J., Young, E., Lewis, M. E., Khachaturian, H., and Walker, J. M. 1984. Endogenous opioids: Biology and function. Annu. Rev. Neurosci. 7: 223-255

Alberts, B. D., Bray, D., Lewis, J., Raff, M., Roberts, K., and Watson, J. D. 1989. Molecular Biology of the Cell, 2nd edition, Garland, New York

Almers, W. and Tse R. W. 1990. Transmitter release from synapses: Does a preassembled fusion pore initiate exocytosis? Neuron 4: 813-818.

Augustine, G. J., Charlton, M. P. and Smith, S. J. 1987. Calcium action in synaptic transmitter release. Annu. Rev. Neurosci. 10: 633-693

Bradford, H. F. 1986. Chemical Neurobiology. Freeman, New York

Cooper, J. R., Bloom, F. E. and Roth, R. H. 1991. The Biochemical Basis of Neuropharmacology, 6th edition, Oxford University Press, New York

Edelman, G. M., Gall, W. E. and Cowan, W. M. (eds.) 1987. Synaptic Function. Wiley, New York

Hall, Z. W. (ed.). 1992. An Introduction to Molecular Neurobiology, Sinauer, Sunderland

Hammond, C. and Tritsch, E. 1990. Neurobiologie Cellulaire. Doin Editeurs, Paris

Hertting, B. and Spatz, H. C. (eds.) 1988. Modulation of Synaptic Transmission and Plasticity in Nervous Systems. Springer, Berlin

Hertzberg, E. L., Lawrence, T. S. and Gilula, N. B. 1988. Gap junctional communication. Annu. Rev. Physiol. 43: 479-491

Kaczmarek, L. K. and Levitan, I. B. (eds.) 1987. Neuromodulation: The Biochemical Control of Neuronal Excitability. Oxford University Press, New York

Kandel, E. R., Schwartz, J. H. and Jessel, T. M. (eds.) 1991. Principles of Neural Science, 3rd edition. Elsevier, New York

Kehoe, J. and Marty, A. 1991. Certain slow synaptic responses: Their properties and possible underlying mechanisms. Annu. Rev. Biophys. Bioeng. 9: 437-465.

Kelly, R. B. 1988. The cell biology of the nerve terminal. Neuron 1: 431-438

Levitan, I. B. 1988. Modulation of ion channels in neurons and other cells. Annu. Rev. Neurosci. 11: 119-136

Loh, Y. P., Brownstein, M. J. and Gainer, H. 1984. Proteolysis in neuropeptide processing and other neural functions. Annu. Rev. Neurosci. 7: 189-222

McCarthy, M. P., Earnest, J. P., Young, E. F., Choe, S. and Stroud, R. M. 1986. The molecular neurobiology of the acetylcholine receptor. Annu. Rev. Neurosci. 9: 383-414

McKelvy, J. F. and Blumberg, S. 1986. Inactivation and metabolism of neuropeptides. Annu. Rev. Neurosci. 9: 415-434

Mountcastle, V. B. 1980. Medical Physiology, 14th edition. Mosby, St. Louis

Nathans, J. 1987. Molecular properties of the muscarinic acetylcholine receptor. Annu. Rev. Neurosci. 10: 195-236

Nestler, E. J. and Greengard, P. 1984. Protein Phosphorylation in the Nervous System. Wiley, New York

Nicoll, R. A., Malenka, R. C. and Kauer, J. A. 1990. Functional comparison of neurotransmitter receptor subtypes in mammalian central nervous system. Physiol. Rev. 70: 513-565

Nicholls, J. G., Martin, A. R. and Wallace, B. 1992. From Neuron to Brain, 3rd edition, Sinauer, Sunderland

O'Dowd, B. F., Lefkowitz, R. J. and Caron, M. G. 1989. Structure of the adrenergic and related receptors. Annu. Rev. Neurosci. 12: 67-84

O'Shea, M. J. and Schaffer, M. 1985. Neuropeptide function: The invertebrate contribution. Annu. Rev. Neurosci. 8: 171-198

Reichardt, L. R. and Kelley, R. B. 1983. A molecular description of nerve terminal function. Annu. Rev. Biochem. 52: 871-926

Sakmann, B. and Neher E. (eds.) 1983. Single-Channel Recording. Plenum, New York

Shepherd, G. M. 1988. Neurobiology, 2nd edition, Oxford University Press, New York

Shepherd, G. M. 1979. The Synaptic Organization of the Brain, 2nd. edition, Oxford University Press, New York

Siegel, G. J., Agranoff, B. W., Albers, R. W. and Molinoff, P. B. (eds.) 1989. Basic Neurochemistry: Molecular, Cellular and Medical Aspects. 4th edition, Raven Press, New York

Snyder, S. H. 1986. Drugs and the Brain. Scientific American Books, New York

Sossin, W. S., Fisher, J. M. and Sheller, R. H. 1989. Cellular and molecular biology of neuropeptide processing and packaging. Neuron 2: 1407-1417.

Sudhoff, T. C. and Jahn, R. 1991. Proteins of synaptic vesicles involved in exocytosis and membrane recycling. Neuron 6: 1-20

Trimble, W. S., Linial, M. and Scheller, R. H. 1991. Cellular and molecular biology of the presynaptic nerve terminal. Annu. Rev. Neurosci. 14: 93-122

Original Publications

Adams, P. R., Brown, D. A. and Constanti, A. 1982. Pharmacological inhibition of the M-current. J. Physiol. 332: 223-262.

Adams, P. R., Brown, D. A. and Constanti, A. 1982b. M-currents and other potassium currents in bullfrog sympathetic neurones. J. Physiol. 330: 537-572.

Adams, W. B. and Levitan, I. B. 1982. Intracellular injection of protein kinase inhibitor blocks the serotonin-induced increase in K⁺ conductance in Aplysia neuron R 15. Proc. Natl. Acad. Sci. USA 79: 3877-3880.

Anderson, C. R. and Stevens, C. F. 1973. Voltage clamp analysis of acetylcholine produced end-plate current fluctuations at frog neuromuscular junction. J. Physiol. 235: 655-691.

Ascher, P. 1972. Inhibitory and excitatory effects of dopamine on Aplysia neurones. J. Physiol. 225: 173-209.

Ascher, P., Marty, A. and Neild, O. 1978. The mode of action of antagonists of the excitatory response to acetylcholine in Aplysia neurones. J. Physiol. 278: 207-235.

Atwood, H. L., Lang, F. and Morin, W. A. 1972. Synaptic vesicles: Selective depletion of crayfish excitatory and inhibitory axons. Science 176: 1353-1355.

Bähler, M. and Greengard, P. 1987. Synapsin I bundles F-actin in a phosphorylation-dependent manner. Nature 326: 704-707.

Ballivet, M., Patrick, J., Lee, J. and Heinemann, S. 1982. Molecular cloning of cDNA coding for the gamma subunit of Torpedo acetylcholine receptor. Proc. Natl. Acad. Sci. USA 79: 4466-4470.

Barnard, E. A., Wieckowski, J. and Chiu, T. H. 1971. Cholinergic receptor molecules and cholinesterase molecules at mouse skeletal muscle junction. Nature 234: 207-209.

Berg, D. K., Kelly, R. B., Sargent, P. B., Williamson, P. and Hall, Z. W. 1972. Binding of α-bungarotoxin to acetylcholine receptors in mammalian muscle. Proc. Natl. Acad. Sci. USA 69: 147-151.

Betz, W. J. and Sakmann, B. 1973. Effects of proteolytic enzyme on function and structure of frog neuromuscular junctions. J. Physiol. 230: 673-688.

Birks, R. I. 1974. The relationship of transmitter release and storage to fine structure in a sympathetic ganglion. J. Neurocytol. 3: 133-160.

Blackman, J. G., Ginsborg, B. L. and Ray, C. 1963. Synaptic transmission in the sympathetic ganglion of frog. J. Physiol. 167: 355-373.

Boistel, J. and Fatt, P. 1958. Membrane permeability change during inhibitory transmitter action in crustacean muscle. J. Physiol. 144: 176-191.

Bowery, N. G., Brown, D. A. and Marsh, S. 1979. γ-Aminobutyric acid efflux from sympathetic glial cells: Effect of "depolarizing" agents. J. Physiol. 293: 75-101.

Brightman, M. W. and Reese, T. S. 1969. Junctions between intimately apposed cell membranes in the vertebrate brain. J. Cell Biol. 40: 668-677.

Brooks, V. B. 1956. An intracellular study of the action of the repetitive nerve volleys and of botulinum toxin on miniature end-plate potentials. J. Physiol. 134: 264-277.

Brown, D. A., Caulfield, M. P. and Kirby, P. J. 1979. Relation between catecholamine-induced cyclic AMP changes and hyperpolarization in isolated rat sympathetic ganglia. J. Physiol. 290: 441-451.

Bullock, T. H. and Hagiwara, S. 1957. Intracellular recording from the giant synapse of the squid. J. Gen. Physiol. 40: 565-577.

Burden, S., Hartzell, H. C. and Yoshikami, D. 1975. Acetylcholine receptors at neuromuscular synapses: Phylogenetic differences detected by snake alphaneurotoxins. Proc. Natl. Acad. Sci. USA 72: 3245-3249.

Bourne, H. R., Sanders, D. A. and McCormick, R. 1990. The GTPase superfamily: A conserved switch for diverse cell functions. Nature 348: 125-132.

Burrows, M. 1979. Synaptic potentials effect the release of transmitter from locust nonspiking interneurons. Science. 204: 81-83.

Burrows, M. and Siegler M. V. S. 1976. Transmission without spikes between locust interneurones and motoneurones. Nature 262: 222-224.

Cantino, D. and Mugnaini, E. 1975. The structural basis for electrotonic coupling in the avian ciliary ganglion: A study with thin sectioning and freezefracturing. J. Neurocytol. 4: 505-536.

Caspar, D. L. D., Goodenough, D. A., Makowski, L. and Phillips, W. C. 1977. Gap junction structures. I. Correlated electron microscopy and x-ray diffraction. J. Cell Biol. 74: 605-628.

Ceccarelli, B., Hurlburt, W. P. and Mauro, A. 1973. Turnover of transmitter and synaptic vesicles at the frog neuromuscular junction. J. Cell Biol. 57: 499-524.

Claudio, T., Ballivet, M., Patrick, J. and Heinemann, S. 1983. Nucleotide and deduced amino acid sequences of Torpedo californica acetylcholine receptor γ subunit. Proc. Natl. Acad. Sci. U.S.A. 80: 1111-1115.

Collier, B. and MacIntosh, F. C. 1969. The source of choline for acetylcholine synthesis in a sympathetic ganglion. Can. J. Physiol. Pharmacol. 47: 127-135.

Colquhoun, D. and Sakmann, B. 1981. Fluctuations in the microsecond time range of the current through single acetylcholine receptor ion channels. Nature 294: 464-466.

Cooke, J. D. and Quastel, D. M. J. 1973. The specific effect of potassium on transmitter release by motor nerve terminals and its inhibition by calcium. J. Physiol. 228: 435-458.

Coombs, J. S., Eccles. J. C. and Fatt, P. 1955. The specific ion conductances and the ionic movements across the motoneuronal membrane that produce the inhibitory post-synaptic potential. J. Physiol. 130: 326-373.

Couteaux, R. and Pécot-Dechavassine, M. 1970. Vésicules synaptiques et poches au niveau des zones actives de la jonction neuromusculaire. C. R. Acad. Sci. (Paris) 271: 2346-2349.

Cull-Candy, S. G., Miledi, R. and Parker, I. 1980. Single glutamate-activated channels recorded from locust muscle fibres with perfused patch-clamp electrodes. J. Physiol. 321: 195210.

Cull-Candy, S. G. and Mildei, R. 1981. Junctional and extra-junctional membrane channels activated by GABA in locust muscle fibres. Proc. R. Soc. Lond. B 211: 527-535.

Curtis, D. R. and Johnston, G. A. R. 1974. Amino acid transmitters in the mammalian central nervous system. Ergeb. Physiol. 69: 97-188.

Dale, H. H., Feldberg, W. and Vogt, M. 1936. Release of acetylcholine at voluntary motor nerve endings. J. Physiol. 86: 353-380.

De Camilli, P. and Jahn, R. 1990. Pathways to regulated exocytosis in neurons. Annu. Rev. Physiol. 52: 624-645

De Groat, W. C. 1972. GABA-depolarization of a sensory ganglion: Antagonism by picrotoxin and bicuculline. Brain Res. 38: 71-88.

del Castillo, J. and Katz, B. 1954. Quantal components of the end-plate potential. J. Physiol. 124: 560-573.

del Castillo, J. and Katz, B. 1954. Statistical factors involved in neuromuscular facilitation and depression. J. Physiol. 124: 574-585.

del Castillo, J. and Katz, B. 1954. Changes in the endplate activity produced by presynaptic polarization. J. Physiol. 124: 586-604.

del Castillo, J. and Katz, B. 1955. On the localization of acetylcholine receptors. J. Physiol. 128: 157-181.

del Castillo, J. and Stark, L. 1952. The effect of calcium ions on the motor endplate potentials. J. Physiol. 116: 507-515.

De Robertis, E. 1967. Ultrastructure and cytochemistry of the synaptic region. Science 156: 907914.

Dickenson-Nelson, A. and Reese, T. S. 1983. Structural changes during transmitter release at synapses in the frog sympathetic ganglion. J. Neurosci. 3: 42-52.

Dodd, J. and Horn, J. P. 1983. Muscarinic inhibition of sympathetic C neurones in the bullfrog. J. Physiol. 334: 271-291.

Dodge, F. A. and Rahamimoff, R. 1967. Cooperative action of calcium ions in transmitter release at the neuromuscular junction. J. Physiol. 193: 419-432.

Dowdall, M. J., Boynes, A. F. and Whittaker, V. P. 1974. Adenosine triphosphate. A constituent of cholinergic synaptic vesicles. Biochem. J. 140: 1-12.

Dwyer, T. M., Adams, D. J. and Hille, B. J. 1980. The permeability of the endplate channel to organic cations in frog muscle. J. Gen. Physiol. 75: 469-472.

Eccles, J. C., Eccles, R. M. and Magni, F. 1961. Central inhibitory action attributable to presynaptic depolarization produced by muscle afferent volleys. J. Physiol. 159: 147-166.

Eccles, J. C., Katz, B. and Kuffler, S. W. 1942. Effect of eserine on neuromuscular transmission. J. Neurophysiol. 5: 211-230.

Eccles, J. C. and O'Connor, W. J. 1939. Responses which nerve impulses evoke in mammalian striated muscles. J. Physiol. 97: 44-102.

Edwards, C. 1982. The selectivity of ion channels in nerve and muscles. Neuroscience 7: 1335-1366.

Elliot, T. R. 1904. On the action of adrenalin. J. Physiol. 31: 20-26.

Erulkar, S. D. and Weight, F. F. 1977. Extracellular potassium and transmitter release at the giant synapse of squid. J. Physiol. 266: 209-218.

Faber, D. S. and Korn, H. 1982. Transmission at a central inhibitory synapse. I. Magnitude of unitary postsynaptic conductance change and kinetics of channel activation. J. Neurophysiol. 48: 654-678.

Fahrenkrug, J. and Emson, P. C. 1982. Vasoactive intestinal polypeptide: Functional aspects. Br. Med. Bull. 38: 265-270.

Falck, B., Hillarp, N.-A., Thieme, G., and Thorp, A. 1962. Fluorescence of catecholamines and related compounds condensed with formaldehyde. J. Histochem. Cytochem. 10: 348-354.

Fambrough, D. M. 1970. Acetylcholine sensitivity of muscle fiber membranes; Mechanism of regulation by motoneurons. Science 168: 372-373.

Fambrough, D. M. 1974. Acetylcholine receptors: Revised estimates of extrajunctional receptor density in denervated rat diaphragm. J. Gen. Physiol. 64: 488-572.

Fatt, P. and Katz, B. 1951. An analysis of the end-plate potential recorded with an intracellular electrode. J. Physiol. 115: 320-370.

Fatt, P. and Katz, B. 1952. Spontaneous subthreshold activity at motor nerve endings. J. Physiol. 117: 109-128.

Fermeau, R. T., Jr., Autelitano, D. J., Blum, M., Wilcox, J. and Roberts, J. L. 1989. Intervening sequencespecific in situ hybridization: Detection of the proopiomelanocortin gene primary transcript in individual neurons. Mol. Brain Res. 6: 197-201.

Fernandez, J. M., Neher, E. and Gomperts, B. D. 1984. Capacitance measurements reveal stepwise fusion events in degranulating mast cells. Nature 312: 453-455.

Fertuck, H. C. and Salpeter, M. M. 1974. Localization of acetylcholine receptor by ^{125}I-labeled alpha-bungarotoxin binding at mouse motor endplates. Proc. Natl. Acad. Sci. USA 71: 1376-1378.

Frank, E. 1973. Matching of facilitation at the neuromuscular junction of the lobster: A possible case for influence of muscle on nerve. J. Physiol. 233: 635-658.

Furshpan, E. J. 1964. "Electrical transmission" at an excitatory synapse in a vertebrate brain. Science 144: 878-880.

Furshpan, E. J. and Potter, D. D. 1959. Transmission at the giant motor synapses of the crayfish. J. Physiol. 145: 289-325.

Gerschenfeld, H. M. and Paupardin-Tritsch, D. 1974. Ionic mechansims and receptor properties underlying the responses of molluscan neurones to 5- hydroxytryptamine. J. Physiol. 243: 427-456.

Glusman, S. and Kravitz, E. A. 1982. The action of serotonin on excitatory nerve terminals in lobster nerve-muscle preparations. J. Physiol. 325: 223-241.

Gold, M. R. 1982. The effects of vasoactive intestinal peptide on neuromuscular transmission in the frog. J. Physiol. 327: 325-335.

Gold, M. R. and Martin, A. R. 1983. Characteristics of inhibitory postsynaptic currents in brainstem neurones of the lamprey. J. Physiol. 342: 85-98.

Gold, M. R. and Martin, A. R. 1983. Analysis of glycine-activated inhibitory post-synaptic channels in brainstem neurones of the lamprey. J. Physiol. 342: 99-117.

Graubard, K., Raper, J. A. and Hartline, D. K. 1980. Graded synaptic transmission between spiking neurons. Proc. Natl. Acad. Sci. USA 77: 3733-3735.

Greengard, P. 1976. Possible role for cyclic nucleotides and phosphorylated membrane proteins in postsynaptic action of neurotransmitters. Nature 260: 101-108.

Grenningloh, G., Rienitz, A., Schmitt, B., Methsfessel, C., Zensen, M., Beyreuther, K., Gundelfinger, E. D. and Betz, H. 1987. The strychnine-binding subunit of the glycine receptor shows homology with nicotinic acetylcholine receptors. Nature 328: 215-220.

Grinnell, A. D. 1970. Electrical interaction between antidromically stimulated frog motoneurones and dorsal root afferents: Enhancement by gallamine and TEA. J. Physiol. 210: 17-43.

Hall, Z. W., Bownds, M. D. and Kravitz, E. A. 1970. The metabolism of gamma aminobutyric acid in the lobster nervous system. J. Cell Biol. 46: 290299.

Hamill, O. P., Bormann, J. and Sakmann, B. 1983. Activation of multiple-conductance state chloride channels in spinal neurones by glycine and GABA. Nature 305: 805-808.

Hamill, O. P. and Sakmann, B. 1981. Multiple conductance states of single acetylcholine receptor channels in embryonic muscle cells. Nature 294: 462-464.

Harris, A. J., Kuffler, S. W. and Dennis, M. J. 1971. Differential chemosensitivity of synaptic and extrasynaptic areas on the neuronal surface membrane in parasympathetic neurons of the frog, tested by microapplication of acetylcholine. Proc. R. Soc. Lond. B 177: 541-553.

Hartzell, H. C., Kuffler, S. W. and Yoshikami, D. 1975. Postsynaptic potentiation: Interaction between quanta of acetylcholine at the skeletal neuromuscular synapse. J. Physiol. 251: 427463.

Hartzell, H. C., Kuffler, S. W., Stickgold, R. and Yoshikami, D. 1977. Synaptic excitation and inhibition resulting from direct action of acetylcholine on two types of chemoreceptors on individual amphibian parasympathetic neurones. J. Physiol. 271: 817-846.

Heuser, J. E. and Reese, T. S. 1973. Evidence for recycling of synaptic vesicle membrane during transmitter release at the frog neuromuscular junction. J. Cell Biol. 57: 315-344.

Heuser, J. E., Reese, T. S. and Landis, D. M. D. 1974. Functional changes in frog neuromuscular junctions studied with freeze-fracture. J. Neurocytol. 3: 109-131.

Heuser, J. E., Reese, T. S., Dennis, M. J., Jan, Y., Jan, L. and Evans, L. 1979. Synaptic vesicle exocytosis captured by quick freezing and correlated with quantal transmitter release. J. Cell Biol. 81: 275-300.

Heuser, J. E. and Reese, T. S. 1981. Structural changes after transmitter release at the frog neuromuscular junction. J. Cell Biol. 88: 564580.

Hökfelt, T., Johansson, O., Ljungdahl, A, Lundberg, J. M. and Schultzberg, M. 1980. Peptidergic neurones. Nature 284: 515-521.

Hollmann, M., O'Shea-Greenfield, A., Rogers, S. W. and Heinemann, S. 1989. Cloning by functional expression of a member of the glutamate receptor family. Nature 342: 643-648.

Hughes, J., Beaumont, A., Fuentes, J. A., Malfroy, B. and Unsworth, C. 1981. Opioid peptides: Aspects of their origin, release and metabolism. J. Exp. Biol. 89: 239-255.

Hughes, J., Smith, T. W., Kosterlitz, H. W., Fothergill, L. A., Morgan, B. A. and Morris, H. R. 1975. Identification of two related pentapeptides from the brain with potent opiate agonist activity. Nature 258: 577-579.

Iversen, L. L., Lee, C. M., Gilbert, R. F., Hunt, S. and Emson, P. C. 1980. Regulation of neuropeptide release. Proc. R. Soc. Lond. B 210: 91-111.

Jackson, M. B., Lecar, H., Mathers, D. A. and Barker, J. L. 1982. Single channel currents activated by γ-aminobutyric acid, muscimol, and (-)-pentobarbital in cultured mouse spinal neurons. J. Neurosci. 2: 889-894.

Jan, Y. N., Jan, L. Y. and Kuffler, S. W. 1979. A peptide as a possible transmitter in sympathetic ganglia of the frog. Proc. Natl. Acad. Sci. USA 76: 1501-1505.

Jan, Y. N., Jan, L. Y. and Kuffler, S. W. 1980. Further evidence for peptidergic transmission in sympathetic ganglia. Proc. Natl. Acad. Sci. USA 77: 5008-5012.

Jessell, T. M. and Iversen, L. L. 1977. Opiate analgesics inhibit substance P release from rat nucleus. Nature 268: 549-551.

Johnson, E. W. and Wernig, A. 1971. The binomial nature of transmitter release at the crayfish neuromuscular junction. J. Physiol. 218: 757-767.

Katz, B. and Miledi, R. 1964. The development of acetylcholine sensitivity in nerve-free segments of skeletal muscle. J. Physiol. 170: 389-396.

Katz, B. and Miledi, R. 1965. The measurement of synaptic delay, and the time course of acetylcholine release at the neuromuscular junction. Proc. R. Soc. Lond. B 161: 483-495.

Katz, B. and Miledi, R. 1967. The release of acetylcholine from nerve endings by graded electrical pulses. Proc. R. Soc. Lond. B 167: 23-38.

Katz, B. and Miledi, R. 1967. The timing of calcium action during neuromuscular transmission. J. Physiol. 189: 535-544.

Katz, B. and Miledi, R. 1967. A study of synaptic transmission in the absence of nerve impulses. J. Physiol. 192: 407-436.

Katz, B. and Miledi, R. 1968. The role of calcium in neuromuscular facilitation. J. Physiol. 195: 481492.

Katz, B. and Miledi, R. 1972. The statistical nature of the acetylcholine potential and its molecular components. J. Physiol. 224: 665-699.

Katz, B. and Miledi, R. 1973. The effect of atropine on acetylcholine action at the neuromuscular junction. Proc. R. Soc. Lond. B 184: 221-226.

Katz, B. and Miledi, R. 1977. Transmitter leakage from motor nerve endings. Proc. R. Soc. Lond. B 196: 59-72.

Kawagoe, R., Onodera, K. and Takeuchi, A. 1981. Release of glutamate from the crayfish neuromuscular junction. J. Physiol. 312: 225-236.

Kehoe, J. 1972. Ionic mechanisms of a two-component cholinergic inhibition in Aplysia neurones. J. Physiol. 225: 85-114.

Kehoe, J. 1972. The physiological role of three acetylcholine receptors in synaptic transmission in Aplysia. J. Physiol. 225: 147-172.

Kennedy, D., Calabrese, R. and Wine, J. J. 1974. Presynaptic inhibition: primary afferent depolarization in crayfish neurons. Science 186: 451-454.

Kistler, J., Stroud, R. M., Klymkowsky, M. W., Lalancett, R. A. and Fairclough, R. H. 1980. Structure and function of an acetylcholine receptor. Biophys. J. 37: 371-383.

Klein, M., Shapiro, E. and Kandel, E. R. 1980. Synaptic plasticity and the modulation of the Ca^{++} current. J. Exp. Biol. 89: 117-157.

Kravitz, E. A., Kuffler, S. W., Potter, D. D. and van Gelder, N. M. 1963. Gamma-aminobutyric acid and other blocking compounds in crustacea. II. Peripheral nervous system. J. Neurophysiol. 26: 729-738.

Kravitz, E. A., Kuffler, S. W. and Potter, D. D. 1963. Gamma-aminobutyric acid and other blocking compounds in crustacea. III. Their relative concentrations in separated motor and inhibitory axons. J. Neurophysiol. 26: 739-751.

Kriebel, M. E. and Gross, C. E. 1974. Multimodal distribution of frog miniature end-plate potentials in adult, denervated and tadpole leg muscle. J. Gen. Physiol. 64: 85-103.

Kuffler, S. W. and Sejnowski, T. J. 1983. Peptidergic and muscarinic excitation at amphibian sympathetic synapses. J. Physiol. 341: 257-278.

Kuffler, S. W. and Yoshikami, D. 1975. The distribution of acetylcholine sensitivity at the post-synaptic membrane of vertebrate skeletal twitch muscles: Iontophoretic mapping in the micron range. J. Physiol. 244: 703-730.

Kuffler, S. W. and Yoshikami, D. 1975. The number of transmitter molecules in a quantum: An estimate from iontophoretic application of acetylcholine at the neuromuscular junction. J. Physiol. 251: 465-482.

Kuno, M. 1964. Quantal components of excitatory synaptic potentials in spinal motoneurones. J. Physiol. 175: 81-99.

Kuno, M. 1964. Mechanism of facilitation and depression of the excitatory synaptic potential in spinal motoneurones. J. Physiol. 175: 100-112.

Kuno, M. and Rudomin, P. 1966. The release of acetylcholine from the spinal cord of the cat by antidromic stimulation of motor nerves. J. Physiol. 187: 177-193.

Kuno, M. and Weakly, J. N. 1972. Quantal components of the inhibitory synaptic potentials in spinal motoneurones of the cat. J. Physiol. 224: 287-303.

Kuo, J. F. and Greengard, P. 1969. Cyclic nucleotide-dependent protein kinases, IV. Widespread occurrence of adenosine 3, 5-monophosphate-dependent protein kinase in various tissues and phyla of the animal kingdom. Proc. Natl. Acad. Sci. USA 64: 1349-1355.

Lassignal, N. and Martin, A. R. 1977. Effect of acetylcholine on postjunctional membrane permeability in eel electroplaque. J. Gen. Physiol. 70: 23-36.

Lev-Tov, A. and Rahamimoff, R. 1980. A study of tetanic and post-tetanic potentiation of miniature end-plate potentials at the frog neuromuscular junction. J. Phyiol. 309: 247-273.

Linder, T. M. and Quastel, D. M. J. 1978. A voltage-clamp study of the permeability change induced by quanta of transmitter at the mouse endplate. J. Physiol. 281: 535-556.

Loewi, O. 1921. Über humorale Übertragbarkeit der Herznervenwirkung. Pflügers Arch. 189: 239-242.

Lømo, T. and Rosenthal, J. 1972. Control of ACh sensitivity by muscle activity in the rat. J. Physiol. 221: 493-513.

Madison, D. V. and Nicoll, R. A. 1986. Cyclic adenosine 3', 5'-monophosphate mediates β-receptor actions of noradrenaline in rat hippocampal pyramidal cells. J. Physiol. 372: 245-259.

Magleby, K. L. and Miller, D. C. 1981. Is the quantum of transmitter release composed of subunits? A critical analysis in the mouse and frog. J. Physiol. 311: 267-287.

Magleby, K. L. and Stevens, C. F. 1972. The effect of voltage on the time course of end-plate currents. J. Physiol. 223: 151-171.

Magleby, K. L. and Stevens, C. F. 1972. A quantitative description of endplate currents. J. Physiol. 223: 173-197.

Magleby, K. L. and Zengel, J. E. 1982. A quantitative description of stimulation-induced changes in transmitter release at the frog neuromuscular junction. J. Gen. Physiol. 80: 613-638.

Martin, A. R. and Pilar, G. 1963. Dual mode of synaptic transmission in the avian ciliary ganglion. J. Physiol. 168: 443-463.

Martin, A. R. and Pilar, G. 1964. Quantal components of the synaptic potential in the ciliary ganglion of the chick. J. Physiol. 175: 1-16.

Matsuda, T., Wu, J.-Y., and Roberts, E., 1973. Immunochemical studies on glutamic acid decarboxylase (EC 4.1.1.15) from mouse brain. J. Neurochem. 21: 159-166.

Matsuda, T., Wu, J. Y., and Roberts, E. 1973. Electrophoresis of glutamic acid decarboxylase (EC 4.1.1.15) from mouse brain in sodium dodecyl sulphate polyacrylamide gels. J. Neurochem. 21: 167-172.

Matthews, G. and Wickelgren, W. O. 1979. Glycine, GABA and synaptic inhibition of reticulospinal neurones of the lamprey. J. Physiol. 293: 393-415.

McAfee, D. A. and Greengard, P. 1972. Adenosine 3', 5'-monophosphate: Electrophysiological evidence for a role in synaptic transmission. Science 178: 310-312.

Miledi, R., Parker, I. and Sumikawa, K. 1982. Synthesis of chick brain GABA receptors by frog oocytes. Proc. R. Soc. Lond. B 216: 509-515.

Miledi, R. and Sumikawa, K. 1982. Synthesis of cat muscle acetylcholine receptors by Xenopus oocytes. Biomed. Res. 3: 390-399.

Minchin, M. C. W. and Iversen, L. L. 1974. Release of [³H]-gamma-aminobutyric acid from glial cells in rat dorsal root ganglia. J. Neurochem. 23: 533-540.

Muller, K. J. and Nicholls, J. G. 1974. Different properties of synapses between a single sensory neurone and two different motor cells in the leech CNS. J Physiol. 238: 357-369.

Muller, K. J. and Scott, S. A. 1981. Transmission at a "direct", electrical connexion mediated by an interneurone in the leech. J. Physiol. 311: 565-583.

Nakajima, Y. and Reese, T. S. 1983. Inhibitory and excitatory synapses in crayfish stretch receptor organs studied with direct rapid-freezing and freeze-substitution. J. Comp. Neurol. 213: 66-73.

Nakajima, Y., Tisdale, A. D. and Henkart, M. P. 1973. Presynaptic inhibiton at inhibitory nerve terminals: A new synapse in the crayfish stretch receptor. Proc. Natl. Acad. Sci. USA 70: 2462-2466.

Nastuk, W. L. 1953. Membrane potential changes at a single muscle end-plate produced by transitory application of acetylcholine with an electrically controlled microjet. Fed. Proc. 12: 102.

Neher, E. and Steinbach, J. H. 1978. Local anaesthetics transiently block currents through single acetylcholine-receptor channels. J. Physiol. 277: 153-176.

Neyton, J. and Trautmann, A. 1985. Single-channel currents of an intercellular junction. Nature 317: 331-335.

Nicholls, J. G. and Purves, D. 1972. A comparison of chemical and electrical synaptic transmission between single sensory cells and a motoneurone in the central nervous system of the leech. J. Physiol. 225: 637-656.

Nicholls, J. G. and Wallace, B. G. 1978. Modulation of transmission at an inhibitory synapse in the central nervous system of the leech. J. Physiol. 281: 157-170.

Noda, M., Takahashi, H., Tanabe, T., Toyosato, M., Furutani, Y., Hirose, T., Asai, M., Inayam, S., Miyata, T. and Numa, S. 1982. Primary structure of alpha-subunit precursor of Torpedo californica a-cetylcholine receptor deduced from cDHA sequence. Nature 299: 793-797.

Noda, M., Takahashi, H., Tanabe, T., Toyosato, M., Furutani, Y., Hirose, T., Asai, M., Takashima, H., Inayam, S., Miyata, T. and Numa, S. 1983. Primary structure of beta- and gamma-unit precursor of Torpedo californica acetylcholine receptor deduced from cDNA sequence. Nature 301: 251-255.

Noda, M., Takahashi, H., Tanabe, T., Toyosato, M., Kikyotani, S., Furutani, Y., Hirose, T., Takashima, H., Inayama, S., Miyata, T. and Numa, S. 1983. Structural homology of Torpedo californica acetylcholine receptor subunits. Nature 305: 528-532.

Onodera, K. and Takeuchi, A. 1980. Distribution and pharmacological properties of synaptic and extrasynaptic glutamate receptors on crayfish muscle. J. Physiol. 306: 233-249.

Orkand, P. M. and Kravitz, E. A. 1971. Localization of the sites of γ-aminobutyric acid (GABA) uptake in lobster nerve-muscle preparations. J. Cell Biol. 49: 75-89.

Otsuka, M., Iversen, L. L., Hall, Z. W. and Kravitz, E. A. 1966. Release of gamma-aminobutyric acid from inhibitory nerves of lobster. Proc. Natl. Acad. Sci. USA 56: 1110-1115.

Otsuka, M., Kravitz, E. A. and Potter, D. D. 1967. Physiological and chemical architecture of a lobster ganglion with particular reference to γ-amino-butyrate and glutamate. J. Neurophysiol. 30: 725-752.

Otsuka, M., Obata, K., Miyata, Y. and Tanaka, Y. 1971. Measurement of γ-aminobutyric acid in isolated nerve cells of cat central nervous system. J. Neurochem. 18: 287-295.

Parnas, H., Dudel, J. and Parnas, I. 1982. Neurotransmitter release and its facilitation in crayfish. Pflügers Arch. 393: 1-14.

Parnas, I., Dudel, J. and Grossman, Y. 1982. Chronic removal of inhibitory axon alters excitatory transmission in a crustacean muscle fiber. J. Neurophysiol. 47: 1-10.

Parnas, I., Pamas, H. and Dudel, J. 1982. Neurotransmitter release and its facilitation in crayfish. II. Duration of facilitation and removal processes of calcium from the terminal. Pflügers Arch. 393: 232-236.

Parnas, I. and Strumwasser, F. 1974. Mechanisms of long-lasting inhibition of a bursting pacemaker neuron. J. Neurophysiol. 37: 609-620.

Patlak, J. B., Gration, K. A. F. and Usherwood, P. N. R. 1979. Single glutamate-activated channels in locust muscle. Nature 278: 643-645.

Peper, K., Dreyer, F., Sandri, C., Akert, K. and Moor, H. 1974. Structure and ultrastructure of the frog motor end-plate: A freeze-etching study. Cell Tissue Res. 149: 437-455.

Pert, C. B. and Snyder, S. H. 1973. Opiate receptor: Demonstration in nervous tissue. Science 179: 1011-1014.

Porter, C. W. and Barnard, E. A. 1975. The density of cholinergic receptors at the endplate postsynaptic membrane: Ultrastructural studies in two mammalian species. J. Membr. Biol. 20: 31-49.

Pritchett, D. B., Sonthoimer, H., Shivers, B. D. Ymer, S., Kettenmann, H., Schofield, P. R. and Seeburg, P. H. 1989. Importance of a novel GABA_A receptor subunit for benzodiazepine pharmacology. Nature 338: 582-585.

Rehm, H., Wiedenmann, B. and Betz, H. 1986. Molecular characterization of synaptophysin, a major calcium-binding protein of the synaptic vesicle membrane. EMBO J. 5: 535-541.

Rudomin, P., Engberg, I. and Jiménez, I. 1981. Mechanisms involved in presynaptic depolarization of group I and rubrospinal fibers in cat spinal cord. J. Neurophysiol. 46: 532-548.

Sargent, P. B., Yau, K.-W. and Nicholls, J. G. 1977. Synthesis of acetylcholine by excitatory motoneurons in central nervous system of the leech. J. Neurophysiol. 40: 453-460.

Schultzberg, M., Hökfelt, T. and Lundberg, J. M. 1982. Coexistence of classical neurotransmitters and peptides in the central and peripheral nervous systems. British Med. Bull. 38: 309-313.

Shapovalov, A. I. and Shiriaev, B. I. 1980. Dual mode of junctional transmission at synapses between single primary afferent fibres and motoneurones in the amphibian. J. Physiol. 306: 1-15.

Shkolnik, L. J. and Schwartz, J. H. 1980. Genesis and maturation of serotonergic vesicles in identified giant cerebral neuron of Aplysia. J. Neurophysiol. 43: 945-967.

Sotelo, C., Llinás, R., and Baker, R. 1974. Structural study of inferior olivary nucleus of the cat: Morphological correlates of electrotonic coupling. J. Neurophysiol. 37: 541-559.

Sotelo, C. and Taxi, J. 1970. Ultrastructural aspects of electrotonic junctions in the spinal cord of the frog. Brain Res. 17: 137-141.

Südhof, T. C., Czernik, A. J., Kao, H.-T., Takei, K., Johnston, P. A., Horiuchi, A., Kanazir, S. D., Wagner, M. A., Perin, M. S., De Camilli, P. and Greengard, P. 1989. Synapsins: Mosaics of shared and individual domains in a family of synaptic vesicle phosphoproteins. Science 245: 1474-1480.

Takeuchi, A. and Takeuchi, N. 1960. On the permeability of the end-plate membrane during the action of transmitter. J. Physiol. 154: 52-67.

Takeuchi, A. and Takeuchi, N. 1965. Localized action of gamma-aminobutyric acid on the crayfish muscle. J. Physiol. 177: 225-238.

Takeuchi, A. and Takeuchi, N. 1966. On the permeability of the presynaptic terminal of the crayfish neuromuscular junction during synaptic inhibition and the action of γ-aminobutyric acid. J. Physiol. 183: 433-449.

Takeuchi, A. and Takeuchi, N. 1967. Anion permeability of the inhibitory postsynaptic membrane of the crayfish neuromuscular junction. J. Physiol. 191: 575-590.

Takeuchi, A. and Takeuchi, N. 1969. A study of the action of picrotoxin on the inhibitory neuromuscular junction of the crayfish. J. Physiol. 205: 377-391.

Toyoshima, C. and Unwin, N. 1988. Ion channel of acetylcholine receptor reconstructed from images of postsynaptic membranes. Nature 336: 247-250.

Unwin, P. N. T. and Zampighi, G. 1980. Structure of the junction between communicating cells. Nature 283: 545-549.

Vizi, S. E. and Vyskocil, F. 1979. Changes in total and quantal release of acetylcholine in the mouse diaphragm during activation and inhibition of membrane ATPase. J. Physiol. 286: 1-14.

Wachtel, H. and Kandel, E. R. 1971. Conversion of synaptic excitation to inhibition at a dual chemical synapse. J. Neurophysiol. 34: 56-68.

Weight, F. and Votava, J. 1970. Slow synaptic excitation in sympathetic ganglion cells: Evidence for synaptic inactivation of potassium conductance. Science 170: 755-758.

Wernig, A. 1972. Changes in statistical parameters during facilitation at the crayfish neuromuscular junction. J. Physiol. 226: 751-759.

Whittaker, V. B., Essman, W. B. and Dowe, G. H. C. 1972. The isolation of pure cholinergic synaptic vesicles from the electric organs of elasmobranch fish of the family Torpedinidae. Biochem. J. 128: 833-846.

Wiersma, C. A. G. 1947. Giant nerve fiber system of the crayfish. A contribution to comparative physiology of synapse. J. Neurophysiol. 10: 23-38.

Zimmerman, H. 1979. Vesicle recycling and transmitter release. Neuroscience 4: 1773-1804.

Zucker, R. S. 1973. Changes in the statistics of transmitter release during facilitation. J. Physiol. 229: 787-810.

4. Sensory Systems

Information Is Acquired by Receptor Cells

The principle of transduction and the sensitivity of receptor cells

To survive, animals must be able to detect and evaluate information about the world around them. They must also obtain information about their own body state. For this to happen, energy from external and internal environmental stimuli must be transformed into changes in electrical potential that can be transmitted and integrated by the nervous system. This process of signal transformation, or sensory *transduction,* normally occurs in specialized cells. It is based on special molecular mechanisms which take place on particular membrane regions of the sensory cells. Sensory cells, also called *receptor cells,* are all specialized to transduce a particular form of stimulus energy. The sensitivity of many receptor cells to their corresponding stimulus is amazing. In many cases it is limited only by the physical properties of the stimulus energy itself, and extends down to the lowest levels of sensitivity that are theoretically possible. Many photoreceptors can be stimulated by single quanta of light. Chemoreceptors in certain insects can respond with potential changes to single molecules of the appropriate type. The ensemble of mechanoreceptors in the human ear can detect oscillations which are an order of magnitude smaller than the diameter of a hydrogen atom.

Specific types of receptors detect specific sorts of stimuli

A given receptor cell is adapted to detect a particular stimulus modality in a highly selective way. Depending on the modality of the corresponding stimulus to which the receptor cell is most sensitive, the various receptor cells can be classified as *chemoreceptors, mechanoreceptors, photoreceptors, thermoreceptors,* or *electroreceptors.* However, the stimulus specificity of a sensory cell is never absolute. For example, nearly

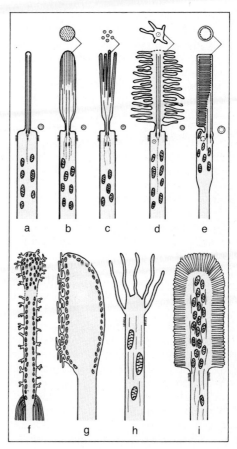

Fig. 4.**1**   Diversity in sensory receptor cells. Outer segments of sense cells specialized for the reception of various stimuli. **a** Sensory cell, flatworm. **b** Mechanoreceptor, insect. **c** Chemoreceptor, insect. **d** Photoreceptor, jellyfish. **e** Photoreceptor, vertebrate. **f** Mechanoreceptor, mammal. **g** Mechanoreceptor, crab. **h** Chemoreceptor, reptile. **i** Photoreceptor, flatworm (after Thurm)

all receptor cells can be excited by electrical current.

Along with their functional diversity, the various receptor cells display an amazing variety of structural specializations (Fig. 4.**1**). In most cases particular regions of the receptor cell are specialized for signal transduction.

Often this involves modified microvilli (arthropod photoreceptors), or modified cilia (vertebrate photoreceptors). However, in some cases the whole cell can participate in stimulus transduction. Some receptor cells have a compact, rounded shape and do not possess any neurite-like processes (mammalian taste receptors). They have a stimulus transduction zone at their apical end, and form synapses with interneurons at the proximal end opposite, without an axon in between. By contrast, other sensory cells (such as insect gustatory sense cells) have a transduction zone near the cell body and a long axon which extends from the periphery to the brain, where it forms synapses. Receptor cells display no less structural diversity than the neurons of the CNS.

Sensory cells can occur individually or in special aggregates. The simplest examples are individual nerve cells whose stimulus-receiving dendrites occur as "free nerve endings" in the tissue, like the thermosensors in vertebrates. In the taste sensilla of insects, several receptor cells are found congregated into a small group within a common cuticular structure. In by far the most complex situation, that of the vertebrate eye, millions of photoreceptors are precisely arranged into a complex sense organ.

Sensory cells are often associated with specialized accessory structures. These are stimulus-conducting structures which often play a role in the selectivity of the receptor cells they are associated with. The pressure- and vibration-sensitive Pacinian corpuscles are found in many mammalian tissues and consist of single mechanosensory neurites which are enveloped by concentrically arranged lamellae of connective tissue. The fact that the Pacinian corpuscle normally responds only to pressure changes rather than to continuous pressure is largely due to the stimulus transmission properties of the lamellar cup. Different accessory structures allow the same receptor type to detect different stimulus parameters. Depending on the type of accessory structure they are associated with, the mechanosensory "hair cells" of vertebrates can detect sound waves, angular velocities, gravitation, or water currents. Accessory structures of amazing sophistication are found in complex sense organs. The human auditory organ, the cochlea, possesses not only 16 000 highly sensitive mechanoreceptors, but also consists of more than a million different movable parts, and is therefore the most complex mechanical apparatus in the body.

The cellular organization of receptor cells and their associated structures is almost always adapted to the reception of a particular type of stimulus. Nevertheless, the primary reason for the stimulus specificity of a receptor cell is not the fine structure of the cell, nor the properties of the accessory structures. It is based on the molecular properties of the transduction process itself.

Transduction processes convert stimulus energy into neuronal activity

Sensory transduction processes generate potential changes across the membrane of the sensory cell. It is therefore not surprising that most receptor cells have molecular mechanisms which act, directly or indirectly, on ion channels to modulate ionic flux across the membrane, and so evoke electrical signals. In many cases the details of how these molecular mechanisms function are still unclear. The actual transduction zones of most receptor cells are generally quite small, and the specialized ion channels which play a role in stimulus transformation are not easily accessible to experimentation. Apart from phototransduction, no complete molecular causal chain for stimulus transformation is known. However, what is clear, is that there is no single mechanism for stimulus transformation. Intermediate steps of varying complexity can be intercalated between stimulus and potential change.

The simplest process, and one that apparently occurs without specialized signal-transforming ion channels, is "transduction" in electroreceptors. These sense cells, which are found in the skin of some fish, detect very weak electric currents, produced either by the fish itself, or emitted by other animals. This process does not involve a true transformation of energy, since one electrical signal is simply transformed into another. The basis of this signal transformation lies in the asymmetric structure of the electroreceptor cell membrane. The cellular surface facing the aqueous external medium has a very low electrical resistance, while that of the opposite basal side is very high. Electric currents which flow through the cell lead therefore to the formation of a potential across the high resistance of the basal cell membrane. Small changes in this potential (in the microvolt range) can then be analyzed by the nervous system.

The transduction processes which occur in mechanoreceptors are somewhat more complicated. Here, special ion channels transform the energy from mechanical stimuli into electrical signals. A well-studied mechanoreceptor is the "hair cell," which occurs in the acoustic, vestibular, and related systems of vertebrates (Fig. 4.2). This cell type is characterized by having stereocilia, which are actually microvilli-like structures of the cell membrane stabilized by actin filaments. The stereocilia lie in a bundle on the apical side of the hair cell. Mechanical deformation of the stereocilia leads to a potential change in the hair cells. The mechanosensitive ion channels are assumed to lie near the tip of each stereocilium. Although the molecular gating mechanism of these channels is not yet known, it is likely that mechanical deformation of the stereocilia directly influences the gating process. The latency between stimulus and conductance change in the receptor membrane is in the region of only a few microseconds and is therefore too short to allow any intervening biochemical steps to occur. The process apparently involves ion channels which are activated by mechanical energy rather than electrical. The ion channels have a conductance of about 20 pS in their open state, and allow most smaller cations to pass relatively nonselectively. Deformation of the stereocilia in one direction seems to preferentially drive these channels into an open state, while deformation in the opposite direction drives them preferentially into a closed state. This gives the hair cell a directional specificity.

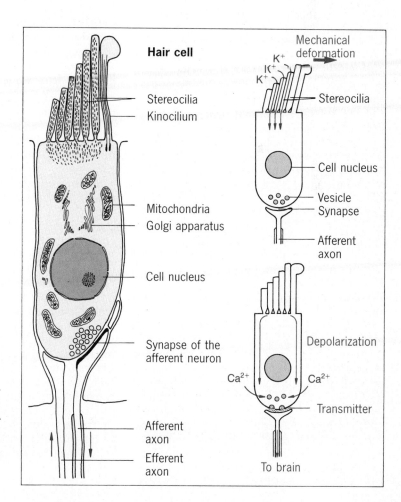

Fig. 4.2   Vertebrate mechano-receptor ("hair cell") from the sacculus of the inner ear (left). Mechanical deformation of the stereocilia leads to a receptor potential in the cell and to the release of transmitter (right) (after Hudspeth)

Further complexity is found in chemosensory stimulus transduction in the sensory cells for taste and smell, where the molecular processes are also not completely understood. In chemosensors, transduction involves at least two stages:

— Stimulus molecules must first bind with suitable receptor molecules on the membrane of the sensory cell. There are probably a multitude of different receptor molecules (or receptor molecule subunits) for the various stimulus molecules.
— After the binding process, ion channels in the cell membrane must switch from a closed to an open state.

It is assumed that the receptor molecules and the ion channels are different macromolecules. It is also assumed that there are further biochemical reaction steps between activation of receptor molecules and the opening of ion channels. It seems likely that a *second messenger* (cAMP, cGMP)-dependent enzyme cascade system is incorporated as a connecting link. Olfactory receptor cells have been shown to possess an olfactory stimulus-dependent adenylate cyclase, as well as ion channels which can be activated by cyclic nucleotides. Indeed, it would not be surprising if comparable molecular processes occur during transduction in chemosensory receptor cells, and during signal transformation at the postsynaptic membrane of a chemical synapse. The capacity to translate information about the chemical state of the environment into an intracellular signal is probably part of the functional repertoire of most cells. In view of the numerous mechanisms employed by "chemosensory" neurons in the CNS for generating postsynaptic signals, several different transduction mechanisms may well exist among the various chemosensory receptors.

In the case of phototransduction, it is clear that similar processes occur during transduction in sensory cells and during synaptic transmission in neurons. In light-sensitive cells, single photons are absorbed by pigment molecules called rhodopsins. This produces conformational changes in the rhodopsin, which initiate subsequent biochemical reactions, and finally lead to a change in the gating behavior of ion channels in the cell membrane. In the photoreceptors of most invertebrates, this involves a conductance increase to Na^+ ions; the cells depolarize in response to light. In the photoreceptors of vertebrates there is a conductance decrease to Na^+ ions; the cells hyperpolarize in response to light. In both cases the respective rhodopsin molecules show a high degree of sequence homology with a certain class of synaptic receptor molecules, namely with the muscarinic acetylcholine receptor and the β-adrenergic receptor. It has been further shown that the reaction chain in vertebrate photoreceptors proceeds via a G-protein activated *second messenger* system that is very similar to the postsynaptic effector mechanism in the muscarinic–cholinergic synapse (p. 69). In invertebrate photoreceptors, biochemical reaction cascades are also interposed between rhodopsin activation and conductance change at the membrane. However, they are not yet completely understood at the molecular level.

Considerable amplification of the sensory signal can occur during transduction

Apart from their high degree of selectivity, receptor cells have the capacity to produce a potential change which contains far more energy than the initiating stimulus. This amplifying function arises partly from the fact that the stimulus-dependent initiation of permeability changes in the cell membrane provides access to the energy stored in the resting potential. A comparable amplification occurs during the generation and conduction of an action potential after a suprathreshold depolarization.

Signal amplification also occurs via biochemical reaction chains. A single activated receptor molecule can influence the gating behavior of numerous ion channels via reaction cascades, and so produce a relatively large transmembrane current. During signal transformation in the photoreceptors of the horseshoe crab *Limulus,* a single absorbed photon can lead to the transient opening of 1000 ion channels in the cell membrane, since signal amplifying second messenger systems are involved in the transduction process. However, signal amplification via biochemical reaction cascades can only occur at the expense of temporal resolution. In the *Limulus* photoreceptor this is apparent in a mean latency of about 200 ms between stimulus and potential change at the most sensitive setting of the transduction apparatus.

Sensory cells also contain a range of mechanisms which lead to increased sensitivity rather than to direct signal amplification. Mechanoreceptive sensory cells, for example, can be equipped with various ion channels in such a way that they begin to oscillate electrically when activated by a particular stimulus. The hair cells in the auditory system of some vertebrates show a well-defined electrical resonance in response to mechanical oscillations. Moreover, they are able to generate a temporal mean of the stimulus intensity since such a sensory cell always encounters many cycles of a sound or vibratory stimulus. This process improves the signal-to-noise relationship during transduction. In many receptors the threshold for stimulus detection can be lowered by enlarging the surface area of transducing membrane, and increasing the density of receptor molecules in the membrane. Sensitivity-increasing mechanisms are, however, not limited to the transduction process but are characteristic of almost all levels of sensory information processing.

Stimulus intensity and time course are encoded in the receptor potential

All transduction processes have one thing in common–they influence the ionic currents which flow across the membrane. This is largely based on opening or closing ion channels in the cell membrane. As a result of sensory transduction, a potential change, called the *receptor potential* or generator potential, is established across the membrane. As the intensity of the stimulus increases, a greater number of channels respond. This produces an increased conductance across the membrane, and results in an increase in the receptor potential. The mechanism that generates this potential is generally similar to that for the synaptic potential.

The time course of the receptor potential can be complex if, in addition to the signal-transducing transmembrane processes, voltage-dependent ion channels are also involved in receptor potential generation. However, in the most simple case for most receptor cells the amplitude of the receptor potential is proportional to the logarithm of the stimulus intensity (Fig. 4.3). This results from the Goldman equation which states that the membrane potential varies with the logarithm of the ionic permeabilities. It follows from this logarithmic relationship that the amplifying action of the

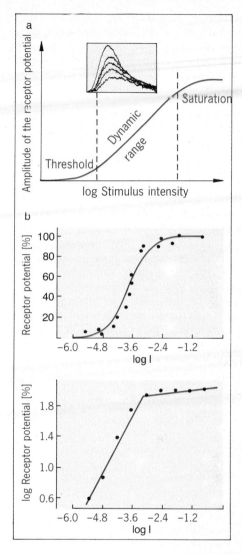

Fig. 4.**3**   Properties of the receptor potential. **a** Within the dynamic range of the receptor cell the amplitude of the stimulus is encoded in the amplitude of the receptor potential. The inset shows the course of a receptor potential for various stimulus intensities. **b** Simplifying, for many receptor cells the amplitude of the receptor potential is proportional to the logarithm of the stimulus intensity over a wide range (after Uttal)

receptor cell becomes progressively weaker with increasing stimulus energy. It also follows that for a given percentage change in stimulus intensity, the receptor potential increases by the same amount over a wide intensity range.

Saturation of the receptor potential is finally reached at very high stimulus intensities, either because the receptor potential approaches its limiting reversal potential, or because all available ion channels are involved in signal transduction. Below the saturation level, in its *dynamic range,* the receptor cell is able to encode the time and amplitude course of a sensory stimulus in the time and amplitude course of its receptor potential.

The receptor potential is a typical electrotonic potential. Its amplitude is continuously variable, and it spreads passively from its site of origin in the receptor cell. In many sensory cells, mainly those which are small and have no axon, the receptor potential directly influences synaptic transmitter release. A depolarizing receptor potential contributes to an increase in transmitter release, a hyperpolarizing receptor potential to a decrease. As at other chemical synapses, the molecular mechanism involves potential changes modulating the Ca^{2+}-dependent exocytosis of transmitter-filled presynaptic vesicles. Some receptor cells have a resting potential that is more negative than the threshold for transmitter release. In these cells the receptor potential first has to reach this threshold level before sensory information can be transmitted to the rest of the nervous sys-

tem. Other receptor cells already release transmitter when "at rest," in the absence of stimuli. This has the advantage that even small changes in the receptor potential can influence transmitter release; the transmission of sensory signals becomes more sensitive as a result. As in some *non–spiking* neurons, this "threshold-free" form of synaptic transmission also allows an additional bidirectional modulation of transmitter release by the receptor potential. Thus, both stimulus increase and stimulus decrease can be signaled with equal sensitivity relative to the value of the resting state.

Electrotonic signal conduction is not sufficient in receptor cells which have a long axon. Here, the information which is contained in the receptor potential must be recoded in the form of action potentials for signal transmission. The way this happens is similar to the transformation of summated postsynaptic potentials into action potentials. This process has been studied in detail in the stretch receptor of the crayfish (Fig. 4.4). Normally the transduction sites and the impulse initiating zone of these receptor cells are spatially separated. The receptor potential must therefore be conducted electrotonically to the impulse initiating zone before action potentials can be generated there. In the transition from a graded re-

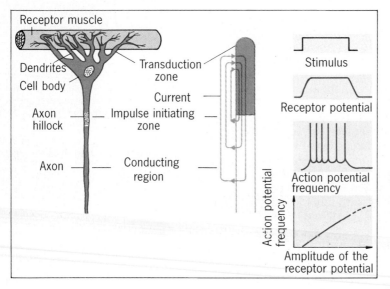

Fig. 4.**4**   Transformation of a receptor potential into an action potential. Stretch receptor of the crayfish, schematic. The stretch receptor can be functionally subdivided into a transduction region, an impulse initiating zone, and a conducting region (left). The strength of the stimulus is first encoded as the amplitude of the receptor potential, and then for propagation as the frequency of the action potentials (right)

ceptor potential to the all-or-nothing excitation of action potentials, the amplitude of the receptor potential is represented by the intervals between successive action potentials. Little information is lost in this recoding since these intervals, and therefore the frequency of the action potentials, can vary almost continually. The action potentials propagate without decrement to the presynaptic terminals of the receptor cells in the CNS, where they effect transmitter release.

Receptor cells adapt

It is a well-known phenomenon that the subjectively perceived stimulus strength decreases with time, even when the intensity of the stimulus remains constant. This reflects the properties of many receptor cells which respond preferentially to changes in the stimulus intensity, and respond with decreasing excitation to constant stimulus strengths. The temporal decrease in receptor response during maintained stimulation is called *adaptation*. Almost all receptor cells adapt. However, different receptor cell types vary with respect to how fast their responses to a constant stimulus decline. Slow adapting, *tonic* receptor cells change their response behavior to maintained stimulation only very little. Our muscle stretch receptor cells belong to this class. They form the basis of our ability to hold the contraction state of our muscles constant over long periods. The mechanoreceptive Pacinian corpuscles belong to the fast-adapting, *phasic* receptor cells which preferentially signal stimulus changes. This explains to some extent the rapid decline in our perception of a maintained pressure stimulus. A phasic and a tonic receptor cell always occur together in the crustacean stretch receptor organs mentioned above (Fig. 4.5).

The adaptation of receptor cells can have different origins. These include, among others:

— *Fatigue of part of the transduction apparatus.* In vertebrate photoreceptors, for example, light absorption causes bleaching of rhodopsin.
— *Changes in membrane conductance.* In some receptor cells there is an increase in the intracellular Ca^{2+} concentration during maintained depolarization which leads to an activation of Ca^{2+}-dependent K^+ channels, and a repolarization of the membrane potential.
— *Time-dependent changes in accessory structures.* A contraction of the pupil of the eye, for example, can reduce the effective light intensity acting on the photoreceptors.

Whatever the mechanism responsible, adaptation plays an important role in extending the dynamic range of the sensory cell. Adaptation contributes to the fact that most receptor cells are sensitive to changes in stimulus intensity across several orders of magnitude. This is important because detecting changes in a given situation is much more relevant to an animal's survival than precisely determining the absolute energy level of a stimulus.

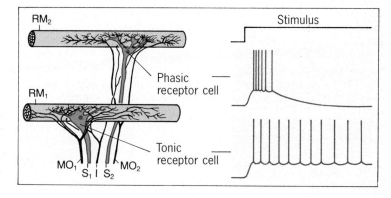

Fig. 4.**5** Slow and fast adapting receptor cells. Morphology (left) and response behavior (right) of the phasic and tonic stretch receptor cells of the crayfish. S_1 = tonic receptor cell, S_2 = phasic receptor cell, RM_1 = muscle bundle of the tonic receptor cell, RM_2 = muscle bundle of the phasic receptor cell, MO_1 = motor fiber for RM_1, MO_2 = motor fiber for RM_2, I = inhibitory fiber (after Burkhardt)

Stimulus modality is encoded by the destination of receptor information

Stimulus intensity is initially represented by the amplitude of the receptor potential. In order to transmit this information to the CNS it is recoded as frequency–modulated action potentials. This method of transmitting stimulus intensities is the same for all sensory messages. The temporal sequence of action potentials with which stimulus intensity is transmitted to the CNS does not indicate whether the sensory message contains information about light, sound, touch, or pain. How is the brain informed about the modality, the sensory quality, of the perceived stimulus? The answer is that this does not come from the transmitted signal itself, but from the connectivity of the neurons in the sensory systems. Messages which come from photoreceptors are interpreted as information about light intensity because they are transmitted to visual brain centers by visual interneurons, and are separate from messages about other sensory modalities. If, for example, these messages were sent in error to acoustic brain centers because of the development of aberrant sensory pathways, then they would be interpreted as acoustic information. A light stimulus would lead to an auditory percept instead of a visual one. For every sensory modality there are individually reserved transmission channels, each of which has a defined, private address in the brain.

Information Processing Begins in the Sense Organs

The complexity of information processing

An enormous amount of sensory information is taken up by all the sensory cells. This abundance of information must subsequently be neuronally processed. The first thing that has to be established is whether a stimulus has occurred or not. If yes, then the strength and quality of the stimuli must be analyzed. The spatial and temporal properties of the stimulus configuration must be determined. Finally, significant features, patterns or arrangements must be extracted from the multitude of stimuli. The complexity of the mechanisms involved in this sensory information processing is far greater than those occurring during reception of primary stimuli. In cases where many sensory cells are aggregated into complex sense organs,

an important component of information processing can already occur peripherally, in the sense organ.

Sensory multichannel systems are often arranged topographically in sense organs

According to information theory the aggregation of many receptors into a sense organ corresponds to the formation of a sensory multichannel system. Clearly, more information can be transmitted in this way than by a single channel system. But beyond simple multiplication, the functional grouping of several single channels also increases the possibilities for a comparative, recombinant form of information processing.

When several independent sensory channels transmit information about the same stimulus, averaging can be carried out, which leads to increased sensitivity. In this way weak signals can be detected with greater certainty against a noisy background. The signal-to-noise ratio of a single channel can be improved $\sqrt{n}$ times in a system which consists of n different, independent, channels. With a single channel, averaging can be achieved only with longer duration stimuli and at the expense of increased response latency.

The information transmitting properties of a sensory multichannel system can also be improved if the individual receptor units differ quantitatively or qualitatively in their sensitivity. Such a division of the response range among various receptor cells leads to an increase in the sensitivity of the whole sense organ. Each receptor cell can then concentrate, as a specialist, on accurately registering a specific, often narrowly defined stimulus range (Fig. 4.6). If the receptor cell had to deal with the whole intensity range, then a lowering of its sensitivity would be unavoidable, despite capacity for adaptation. Examples of receptor cell types with such a fractionation of the response range are

- the photoreceptor cells of vertebrates and higher invertebrates (different systems for dim and intense light, receptors with different spectral sensitivity)
- the mechanoreceptive sense cells of the Golgi organs of vertebrates (specialized for narrow angular ranges of limb position), and
- the antennal olfactory receptor cells of many insects (different response spectra of single cells in response to different odors).

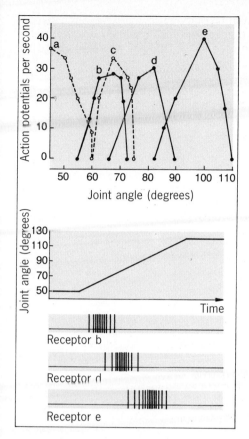

Fig. 4.**6**   Division of the response range of different receptor cells. Relationship between the action potential frequency and position of the knee joint in different joint receptors (a–e) of the cat (above). Different receptors are activated sequentially during constantly increasing stretching of the knee (bottom) (after Skoglund)

A decisive advantage of a sensory multichannel system is the opportunity to encode the location or direction of a stimulus. This is possible if the many receptors are arranged in a spatially structured, quasi-epithelial way in the sense organ. An example of this is the retina of an image-forming eye. Stimuli from the external visual world are imaged onto the structured array of photoreceptor cells in the retina, and represented by them as a spatially structured pattern of neural excitation. In this type of topographic representation stimulus signals from neighboring regions of the external world are imaged onto neighboring parts of the retina. A topographic representation of visual information is maintained in the interneuronal networks of the retina, and in many visual centers in the brain.

Convergence, divergence and lateral inhibition are organizational principles in sensory networks

The formation of spatially ordered, multichannel sensory systems allows neighboring groups of neurons to process correlated sensory inputs locally. This occurs through various types of connections which are formed either at the level of the sensory receptors, or include the postsynaptic sensory interneurons. *Divergence* occurs when a single neuron synapses with several subsequent neurons. In this way an individual neuron can influence a considerable number of postsynaptic neurons. *Convergence* occurs when different neurons all synapse with the same target neuron. This allows the activity of whole groups of sensory cells to be integrated. Convergence is widespread in sense organs since the number of receptor cells considerably exceeds the number of interneurons there. In the cat retina for example, about 1500 photoreceptor cells converge onto about 100 bipolar cells, and these converge via further intercalated interneurons onto a single ganglion cell which then projects to the brain (Fig. 4.7). However, in the cat retina we also find connections in which the output signal of a single photoreceptor diverges onto at least two bipolar cells, from there onto 5 amacrine cells, and is distributed via further intercalated interneurons to 2 ganglion cells. As this example shows, convergence and divergence frequently occur in the same neuronal network.

Another widespread form of local processing in multichannel sensory systems is *lateral inhibition*. This was first discovered in the retina of the horseshoe crab *Limulus* (Fig. 4.8). In the compound eye of this animal the excitation of one ommatidium by incident light is attenuated when neighboring ommatidia are illuminated as well. The reason for this are reciprocal inhibitory connections which are formed between the individual ommatidia. The inhibitory connections are strongest between immediate neighbors and decrease with interommatidial distance in the retina. Lateral inhibition can have several functional consequences, such as:

— *Contrast enhancement* (Fig. 4.**9**). The reception of a spatial or temporal contrast causes neighboring sensory channels to receive different levels of excitatory input. This contrast can be enhanced by lateral inhibition.

Assume that one sensory channel receives a stronger stimulus signal than another, neighboring sensory channel. As a result of lateral inhibition, the first sensory channel will inhibit the second more strongly than the other way around. The output of the second channel will therefore be overly attenuated with respect to that of the first. This then

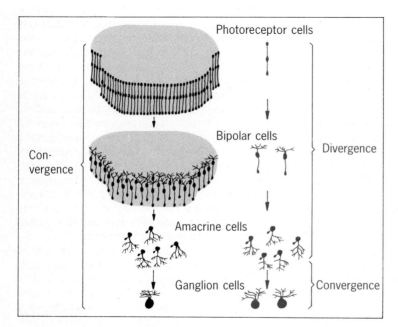

Fig. 4.**7**   Convergence and divergence in the cat retina. Convergence (left) and divergence (right) occur in the same cellular network (after Sterling, Freed and Smith)

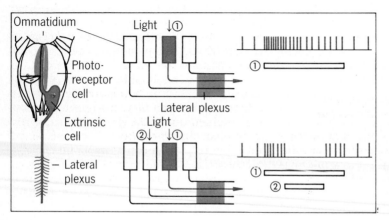

Fig. 4.**8**   Lateral inhibition in the retina of the horseshoe crab (Limulus). Structure of an ommatidium (left). The excitation of the extrinsic cell on illumination of an ommatidium (1) is attenuated by the additional illumination of neighboring ommatidia (2) (after Ratliff and Hartline)

means that an enhanced input contrast will be propagated.

— *Regulation of sensitivity.* The sensitivity of a sensory system can be attenuated during strong stimulation by high threshold lateral inhibition. Such a type of lateral inhibition can therefore contribute to adaptation.

— *Movement detection* If laterally inhibiting connections are formed asymmetrically in a topographically organized sensory system, then the system can detect stimulus movement. The outputs of the system will be different depending on the direction of movement of the stimulus with respect to the orientation of the inhibitory connections.

— *Sharpening of the input range.* If the input ranges of neighboring receptor channels partly overlap, then lateral inihibition can result in a reduction in this overlap.

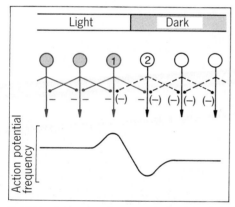

Fig. 4.**9** Contrast enhancement by lateral inhibition, greatly simplified. The differential excitation resulting from presentation of a contrast is amplified by lateral inhibition. The firing rate of receptor 1 in the light is higher than that of neighboring receptors in the light. The firing rate of receptor 2 in the dark is lower than that of neighboring receptors in the dark. – = strong inhibition (–) = weak inhibition

Sense organs are under the efferent control of the central nervous system

Sensory information does not only flow centrally from the periphery. As a result of centrifugal connections, *feedback* of sensory information is also possible. This means that signals in an initial layer of the sense organ can be influenced by signals in downstream elements of the same sense organ. Moreover, the brain itself plays an important role in the control of sensory information flow from the periphery. The CNS is not only a passive receiver of information from the sense organs, but also influences the uptake of this information. The sensitivity of a sensory system can be raised or lowered by the CNS. This control is usually exercised by efferent neuronal connections, which can intervene at various sites in the sensory system.

The efferent control of sensory information can occur at the level of the accessory structures. The sensitivity of the stretch receptor organs in crustacea, and of the muscle spindles in vertebrates, is influenced by the central control of the intrinsic muscle fibers in these sensory structures (Fig. 4.**5**). Since the mechanoreceptive sensory cells are embedded in these muscle fibers, the sensory discharge is influenced by the initial tension of the muscle. By setting the muscle tension appropriately, the CNS can optimally match the sensitivity of the sensory apparatus to various stimulus conditions. Other examples for the efferent control of accessory structures by the brain include the pigment cells in arthropod eyes, the iris muscles in the vertebrate eye, and the tympanal muscles in the vertebrate ear.

The CNS can exert a direct efferent control over receptor cells. In the crustacean stretch receptor organs, both the phasic and tonic receptor cells are innervated by several inhibitory efferent fibers which can change the sensitivity of the receptor cells (Fig. 4.**10**). The receptor cells can even be completely shut down. During maximum inhibition, the receptor potential of these sensory cells does not reach the threshold for action potentials, even on strong stretch stimulation. Comparable cases of efferent inhibition at the level of sense cells are found in the auditory systems of amphibia, reptiles and mammals. In the lateral line system of fish, inhibitory as well as excitatory efferent control mechanisms are present. Efferent control can also act on peripheral sensory interneurons. In the visual system of birds, there is an efferent control over certain retinal amacrine cells from the isthmooptic nucleus. All these cases demonstrate that the brain actively participates in determining the content of inflowing information.

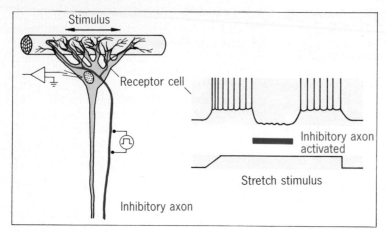

Fig. 4.**10** Efferent control of the stretch receptor in the crayfish by inhibitory innervation. Structure of the stretch receptor with efferent innervation by an inhibitory axon (left). The response of the receptor to a stretch stimulus is inhibited by the activation of the efferent axon (right) (after Kuffler and Eyzaguirre)

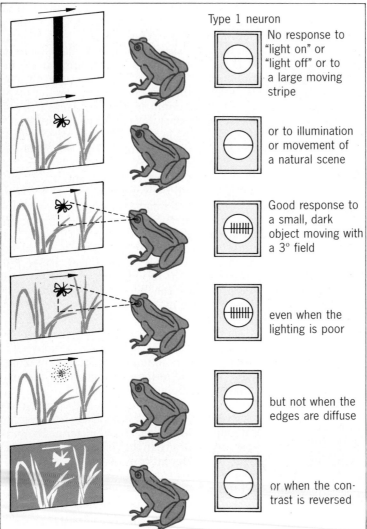

Fig. 4.**11** Sensory filtering in the retina of the frog. Response behavior of a ganglion cell (after Bullock and Horridge)

Abstraction of information by sensory filters begins in the peripheral ganglia

To extract relevant information from the abundance of received stimuli requires the capacity for neuronal abstraction. This is the job of neuronal circuits which are termed *sensory filters*. Sensory filtering in peripheral sense organs is made possible by the numerous neuronal interactions which take place in sensory networks.

A classic example of sensory filtering has been demonstrated in the retina of the frog. Recordings were made from retinal ganglion cells which "ignore" the majority of visual stimuli and react only to very specific features in the visual field. For example, one particular ganglion cell type is only excited when a small dark object, about the size of a fly, moves in front of a light background somewhere in the visual field (Fig. 4.**11**). The neuron does not respond to a light being switched on or off, nor does it respond to large moving objects. There is no response when the small object is stationary with respect to the background, or when the whole scene moves. In short, the neuron seems to be specialized to detect flying insects.

Central Processing of Sensory Information

The function of projection centers

Most afferent sensory neurons run from the periphery to discrete central nervous regions termed sensory *projection centers,* and form synaptic connections with follower interneurons there. The interneurons in every projection center carry out some of the sensory information processing, integrate this with other types of information, and then transmit the processed information to subsequent centers. In many cases sensory information is initially separated according to modality and then processed further. The central visual system of arthropods is a perfect example of such a "specific" system. The three sequentially arranged and anatomically distinct optic ganglia, the lamina, medulla, and lobula, process almost exclusively visual information (Fig. 4.**12**). In other cases sensory information already receives a multimodal character in the initial stages of central processing. Sensory systems which, by divergence of the input pathways and convergence with other inputs, are specialized from the beginning to transmit "unspecific" information play important integrative roles affecting the whole organism.

Neighboring groups of neurons process sensory inputs which have common information content

Sensory projection centers often have special modular *fine structures.* In some cases these fine structures can be directly observed histologically. In the olfactory system of insects, the axons of the primary sense cells project to about 100 spherically-shaped neuronal aggregates in the antennal lobe of the deutocerebrum. Synaptic interactions between afferent sense cells, intrinsic interneurons, and projection interneurons occur in these centers, termed glomeruli (Fig. 4.**13**). In the males of some insects, one glomerulus is even specialized for processing pheromone signals emitted by the female. In the somatosensory cortex of rodents there are groups of neurons which are assembled into column-like structures called "barrels." Each "barrel" is concerned with the processing of sensory information from one of the vibrissae on the animal's snout (Fig. 4.**14**.).

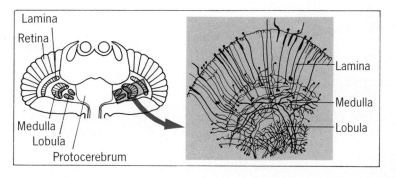
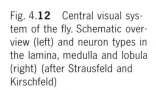

Fig. 4.**12**   Central visual system of the fly. Schematic overview (left) and neuron types in the lamina, medulla and lobula (right) (after Strausfeld and Kirschfeld)

Lamina
Retina
Medulla
Lobula
Protocerebrum

Lamina
Medulla
Lobula

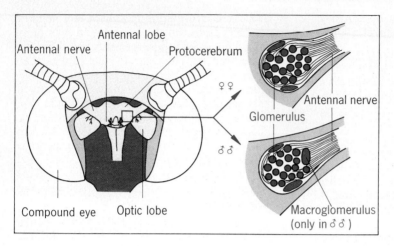

Antennal lobe

Antennal nerve   Protocerebrum

♀♀

♂♂

Glomerulus

Antennal nerve

Compound eye   Optic lobe

Macroglomerulus
(only in ♂♂)

Fig. 4.**13**   Olfactory compartment in the antennal lobe of a moth. Schematic overview (left). Olfactory information is processed in the partially sex-specific glomeruli, and relayed from there to other brain regions (right) (after Hildebrand)

In other cases, like the visual or somatosensory system of mammals, the compartmentalization of the projection centers can only be demonstrated using a combination of anatomical and physiological or biochemical techniques. It turns out that the spatial organization of these aggregates is often column- or band-shaped. In the somatosensory cortex, for example, all the neurons in a given band-like compartment appear to respond to the same submodality. There are aggregates whose many neurons respond either to limb position, to cutaneous contact, or to stimulation of hair fields. The neurons in a band-like compart-ment also obtain their sensory information mostly from the same peripheral body region.

In general, the particular region of the sensory epithelium which on stimulation leads to an excitation or inhibition of a sensory neuron, is termed the *receptive field* of the neuron. Such receptive fields can have different sizes, and a functional fine structure with excitatory and inhibitory regions. The fact that the neurons in a given sensory compartment often have the same receptive field points to an important organizational principle of sensory systems with a modular format.

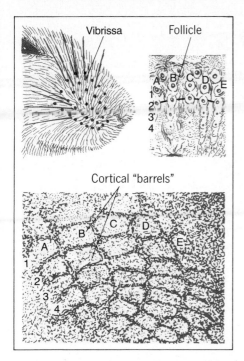

Fig. 4.**14**   Mechanosensory compartment in the somato-sensory cortex of the mouse. The snout of the mouse has an ordered group of long mechanosensory vibrissae (top). The information from each vibrissa is processed by a neuronal aggregate (barrel) in the cortex (bottom) (after Van der Loos et al.)

Position-coded information is transmitted topographically to sequential neural layers

In many sensory systems stimulus properties are represented by the spatial pattern of sensory cell activation. In the vertebrate auditory system, the frequency of a sound stimulus is encoded by the location of the stimulated cochlear hair cells along the basilar membrane. In an image-forming visual system, the position of a light stimulus in the visual field is represented by the position of the stimulated photoreceptor cells in the retina. In the mechanosensory system of the body integument, the location of the stimulus is given by the position of the stimulated sensory cells on the body surface. In these cases the spatial relationships among neighbors, represented as the pattern of activated receptor cells, are partially maintained during the CNS processing of the sensory information.

A classic example of this type of representation is the mammalian mechanosensory system. Here the information from the body surface is relayed topographically via spinal interneurons to nuclei in the brain stem, and from there topographically again to centers in the thalamus, and somatosensory cortex. In this *somatotopic* type of projection, a spatially ordered representation of the body surface is maintained at every level of processing. An impressive illustration of this organization is the somatosensory "homunculus," which represents a projection of the body surface onto the human cortex (Fig. 1.**9**). The characteristic distortions of this type of projection, in particular the large areas used for representing the face and hands, reproduce the high sensitivity and spatial resolution of these body regions to mechanical stimuli.

A comparable situation occurs in the auditory system of mammals. Here the auditory sensory cells project to the central auditory nuclei; from there projections run to the inferior colliculus, then to the medial geniculate, and finally to the auditory cortex. All these processing centers are at least partially *tonotopically* organized. In each of these structures there is a spatially ordered sequence of neuron groups, each of which is involved with auditory signals of similar frequency. These "frequency bands" are arranged so that there is an ordered sequence of sound frequencies being processed from one neuron group to the next (Fig. 4.**15**). In this way the tonotopic organization of the primary sense cells in the cochlea is repeated at all the central levels. Interestingly, characteristic topographic distortions appear in animals which recognize signals on the basis of a particular frequency band. In bats, which during echolocation must detect small deviations from a particular, relatively constant, sound frequency (locating frequency), a large part of the auditory cortex is specialized for processing sound stimuli in this frequency range (Fig. 4.**16**).

The retention of topographically ordered sensory projections in numerous, sequential, processing centers, also helps in the processing of correlated inputs. Common information content, coded positionally in the periphery, can in this way be registered and integrated. However, how are different aspects of the information provided by the same inputs processed?

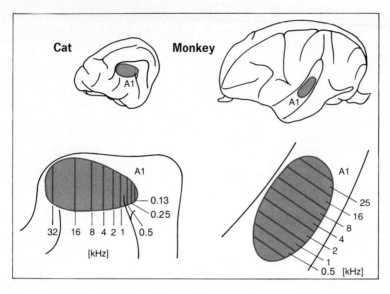

Fig. 4.**15** Tonotopic arrangement of the central auditory area in mammals. Neurons are grouped into frequency bands in the A1 region of the auditory cortex. There is a regular sequence in the sound frequency processed between one neuron group and the next (after Woolsey, Merzenich et al., Ottoson)

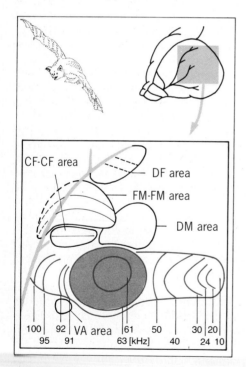

Fig. 4.**16** Tonotopicity in the bat. A large part of the auditory cortex is specialized for processing sound stimuli within a narrow frequency range (echo-locating frequency range) (after Suga)

Parallel and serial information processing occur simultaneously

An analysis of topographic sensory projections shows clearly that there is not only a serial sequence of projection centers, but also that numerous comparable representations of the sensory world can be built up side by side in the central nervous system. Central sensory systems generally consist of subsystems operating in parallel. In every single subsystem, different parameters of a stimulus configuration can be processed simultaneously.

In the central auditory system of mammals, the afferents which leave the organ of Corti arborize in the cochlear nucleus of the brain stem, and tonotopically innervate a number of spatially separate, postsynaptic, neuron groups. In this way several separate topographic representations of the auditory sense organ occur in each of the two cochlear nuclei. A parallel organization is maintained over several projection centers up to the auditory cortex, and is responsible for the fact that several separate tonotopic representations of the frequency spectrum are found there. Various aspects of an auditory stimulus (for example, commencement and duration of stimulus, binaural delay, spatial position of sound sources) can be processed in more or less exclusive transmission channels within these different parallel projection systems.

The somatosensory system of vertebrates is organized in basically the same way. There, multiple sensory representations are also found in the thalamus and somatosensory cortical regions. In the "SI region" of the somatosensory cortex alone there are at least four largely independent and complete topographic representations of the body. In the adjacent SII region there is (at least) one more. Each of these regions seems to process stimuli of mainly one particular somatosensory submodality.

Hierarchically organized higher-order neurons can detect more complex features of the environment

A key element of the functional organization of central sensory systems is the increasingly complex responses of neurons in hierarchically organized higher-order neural centers. There are many examples of this.

— There are neurons in the visual system of insects which respond to specific movement stimuli. These are found not in the retina or lamina, but in the subsequent ganglia of the medulla and lobula. Multimodal neurons which integrate visual and mechanosensory inputs in order to detect particular movements of the animal with respect to its surroundings, occur postsynaptically to the lobula neurons in the brain itself.
— There are neurons in the somatosensory system of primates which respond to tactile stimuli moving across the skin in a directionally specific way, and which are first encountered in higher-order cortical centers. By contrast, precursor neurons do not react to movement, and respond mainly to the presence of tactile stimuli.
— The temporal "association cortex" of primates is a cortical region in which preprocessed sensory information from other primary cortical areas is integrated. In this region there are populations of neurons which respond strongly to complex visual stimuli, stimuli which to some extent have a clear semantic meaning, like faces for example.

Neurons with similarly complex response characteristics, and which may be involved in the perception of complex, naturally occurring stimulus configurations, can be considered as *feature detectors*.

The central nervous system carries out behaviorally relevant recombinations of sensory information

Sensory information can lead, in a more or less complex way, to motor activity, to behavior. However, it is not possible to identify a general watershed between sensory and motor systems. Sensory input can lead via reflex arcs to the direct monosynaptic activation of motoneurons. The same input, however, can also activate motoneurons polysynaptically, via intercalated local interneurons. Finally, as a result of extended ascending and descending connecting loops, sensory input can transit numerous projection centers in the brain before it is used for motor control, and only then following complex integrative processes. The division of central neuronal circuits into sensory and motor systems is to some extent artificial, as can be demonstrated at the level of single neurons. In many cases, single neurons have been described which have sensory receptive properties, as well as motor command functions.

The close interaction between sensory and motor systems, as well as their relationship to behavior, can be seen at many levels in the CNS. The combination of information which is found in multimodal sensory units can often be related to particular behavioral contexts. In the brain of the grasshopper, for example, there are interneurons which integrate visual, aerodynamic and proprioceptive information in order to detect course deviations during flight. In the brain of the barn owl there are neurons which are specialized to integrate auditory input with information about head position, in order to localize sound sources better. In the parietal cortex of monkeys, visual information about the position of a stimulus on the retina is integrated with information about the position of the eyes with respect to the head, in order to localize objects in space with respect to the position of the head. Even in largely unimodal systems, the relationship between sensory information processing and behavior can be clearly demonstrated. In the auditory cortex of the bat, there are topographically organized groups of neurons which employ preprocessed auditory information to encode the velocity and distance of prey, or the position of prey in space with respect to the bat.

The relationship between sensory information processing and behavior is not surprising; it is a product of evolution. The nervous system is a communications and processing machine whose main function is to recognize, decide, command and respond, in a behaviorally relevant way. In Shepherd's words: "Nothing in neurobiology makes sense except in the light of behavior."

The Vertebrate Visual System Exemplifies the Organizational Principles of Sensory Systems

Anatomical foundations and functions

The organization and functioning of a complex sensory system can be illustrated most clearly using a system which has been thoroughly studied from many aspects, namely the visual system of vertebrates. As humans, our perception is strongly visually oriented, so a detailed examination of the organizational principles involved in the reception and processing of visual information by higher vertebrates should be especially relevant.

In our eye, light stimuli from different parts of the environment are imaged in an orderly way onto an array of neural elements onto the retina. The retina has two important functions. The first is that of photoreception and involves two types of photoreceptor cells: first the *cones,* which are important for form and color vision during daylight; and second, ten times as many *rods,* which mediate vision at low light levels. The second important function involves processing the incoming visual information. For this purpose the retina has a complex network of interneurons in addition to the receptor cells. The vertebrate retina is part of the CNS not only because of its embryological mode of development. It can also be considered as part of the brain on the basis of its complexity.

Photoreceptor cells

The transduction of light energy into electrical signals is carried out in the photoreceptor cells. In the dark both the rods and the cones are de-

polarized by a steady Na^+ inward current. In the light these cells are hyperpolarized because the effect of light is to shut down this *dark current* (Fig. 4.17). Structurally, both cell types have an inner and an outer segment. The inner segment contains the cell's synthesis machinery, nucleus, and many mitochondria. The outer segment contains the photopigment and is the actual site of phototransduction. It consists of numerous folded lamellae which serve to increase the membrane surface area exposed to light, and which are continually manufactured at the base of the outer segment. In the rods, these membrane lamellae become dissociated from the cell membrane, and then lie stacked as closed "disks" in the cell. In rods and cones these membranes are packed with the visual pigment molecule *rhodopsin.* This consists of a complex transmembrane protein, opsin, and a covalently bound chromophor, retinal. The retinal is the part of the molecule which absorbs photons. Rhodopsin is an extraordinary molecule. In the dark it has a half-life of over 400 years. Despite this, the energy derived from the absorption of a single photon by a rhodopsin molecule is sufficient to initiate a complex chain of reactions, which can lead to a current of about one picoampere across the cell membrane for about 1 s. This corresponds to energy conversion with a gain of 100 000.

This amplification is carried out by an *enzyme* cascade initiated by rhodopsin, and which involves *second messengers* (Fig. 4.18). Follow-

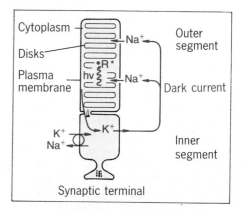

Fig. 4.17   Vertebrate photoreceptor cell. Greatly simplified schematic of a rod. The absorption of a photon (hv) by rhodopsin (R) initiates a reaction chain which leads to a decrease in the dark current (after Lamb)

ing absorption of a photon, rhodopsin is transformed into activated rhodopsin in a series of very fast intermediate steps. This occurs as a result of conformational changes in the protein component of rhodopsin. The conformational change is evoked by the actual lightdependent reaction, which is a stereoisomerization of the retinal. The part of the activated rhodopsin, which lies on the cytoplasmic side of the membrane, can now activate a second type of molecule. This is a G protein, also called transducin. As in many neurotransmitter systems, the activated G protein acts on a target enzyme, in this case a cGMP–phosphodiesterase. This step leads to the hydrolysis of cytoplasmic cGMP. By virtue of this molecular cascade, a single rhodopsin molecule can effect the hydrolysis of millions of cGMP molecules. As a result of the hydrolysis of cytoplasmic cGMP, a reduction in the transmembrane current occurs. This is because cGMP directly holds the cell's Na^+ channels in an open state, probably due to the binding of several cGMP molecules to a single transmembrane channel. If the concentration of cGMP in the cell is lowered by activated phosphodiesterase, cGMP molecules diffuse away from the Na^+ channels, and these close. This in turn results in a reduction of the

inflow of Na^+ ions into the cell, and the cell becomes hyperpolarized. Hyperpolarization then represents the response of the receptor cell to a light stimulus.

Both photoreceptor cell types, rods and cones, have essentially the same transduction mechanism. Despite this, there are some important differences. The rods have a higher gain than the cones. They are more sensitive, but their response is slower. All rods have the same spectral sensitivity. The cones, by contrast, can usually be divided into several groups, each having a different spectral sensitivity. The reason for this are the slightly different types of rhodopsin which occur in the various cones. The pattern of connections with the interneurons in the retina also differs. The rod system is strongly convergent, with many rods projecting onto the same postsynaptic cell. The cones, by contrast, feed into more individualized postsynaptic neuronal channels.

Retinal interneurons

In addition to the photoreceptors, the retina consists of a complex network of interneurons (Fig. 4.19). Each of these interneurons receives and processes information from a particular re-

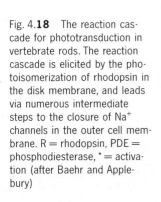

Fig. 4.**18** The reaction cascade for phototransduction in vertebrate rods. The reaction cascade is elicited by the photoisomerization of rhodopsin in the disk membrane, and leads via numerous intermediate steps to the closure of Na^+ channels in the outer cell membrane. R = rhodopsin, PDE = phosphodiesterase, * = activation (after Baehr and Applebury)

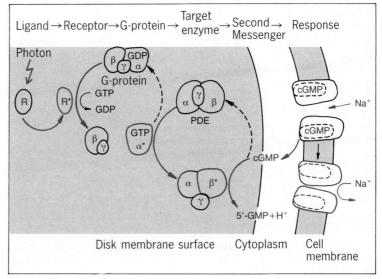

gion of the visual field. Accordingly, each neuron responds to illumination of a very specific region of the retina—the *receptive field* of the respective neuron. A photoreceptor has a very simple and homogeneous receptive field. By contrast, many other neurons in the retina have complex receptive fields with a distinct fine structure. The transformation in the complexity of the receptive fields occurs as a result of processing of visual information in the retinal interneurons. The properties of these inter-

neurons, and the nature of their connections, are diverse, and also show species-specific differences. Despite this, the interneurons can be divided into four classes: the *bipolar cells* and *horizontal cells* of the outer retinal layer, and the *ganglion cells* and *amacrine cells* of the inner retinal layer. Closer examination shows that there are several subclasses even within one type of interneuron. In the retina of the cat, over 70 different types of neurons have already been described.

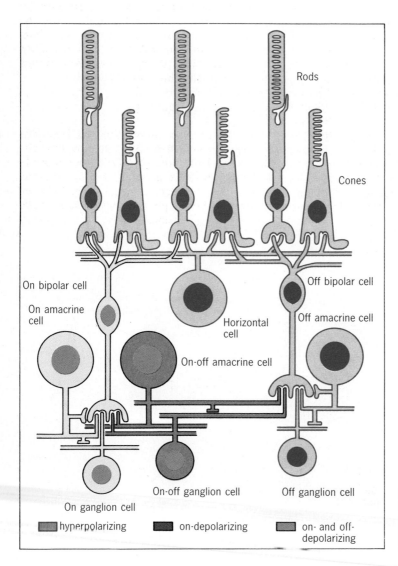

Fig. 4.**19**   Schematic representation of the photoreceptors and interneurons of an amphibian retina (after Miller and Slaughter)

How are the photoreceptor signals transmitted to the interneurons of the retina? A receptor cell forms synapses with bipolar and horizontal cells at the proximal region of its inner segment. Transmitter is continuously released in the dark at these synapses. The photoreceptor cells are continuously depolarized in the dark, and a depolarizing receptor potential leads to transmitter release. This transmitter release is inhibited by the light-dependent hyperpolarization of the photoreceptor cells. In this way a light stimulus is translated into an inhibitory modulation of transmitter output. This modulation of transmitter release by the receptor potential is passive and electrotonic, without action potentials being generated. The modulation is highly sensitive since the transmitter output can varied in a graded manner, without first having to reach a threshold for release.

The released transmitter, probably an amino acid or amino acid derivative, acts on two types of bipolar cells, the *on* and *off* bipolar cells. The synapse from the photoreceptor onto the on bipolar cell is sign inverting, while the synapse onto the *off* bipolar cell is sign conserving (Fig 4 20). The on bipolar cells are inhibited by transmitter. Illumination of the presynaptic photoreceptor cell (reduction in transmitter output) is translated in this cell type into a disinhibition, that is, an excitation. The *off* bipolar cells are excited by transmitter. An illumination of the presynaptic photoreceptor cell (reduction in transmitter output) is translated in this cell type into an inhibition. The retina emphasizes once again that the same transmitter substance can evoke different effects depending on the type of postsynaptic cell.

The synapses between the photoreceptor cells and the bipolar cells are formed in an outer synaptic layer (the outer plexiform layer) of the retina. The bipolar cells for their part form synapses with ganglion cells in an inner synaptic layer (the inner plexiform layer). The responses of the two types of bipolar cells are conducted in parallel across sign-conserving synapses, to the postsynaptic ganglion cells. These are correspondingly divided into *on*-ganglion cells and *off*-ganglion cells. In addition, there are also *on*-*off*-ganglion cells, where the same ganglion cell receives synapses from both types of bipolar cells. Action potentials are generated in the ganglion cells, whose axons project to the brain. Most of the rest of the information processing in the retina takes place electrotonically and passively, without action potentials.

Apart from these direct connections (photoreceptor cell–bipolar cell–ganglion cell), there are also important *lateral connections*. In the outer synaptic layer there are horizontal cells which can mediate interactions between many neighboring photoreceptors. The bipolar cells are affected in two ways as a result of these lateral interactions.

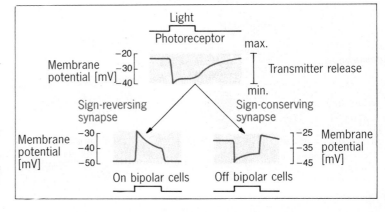

Fig. 4.**20** Synaptic transmission between photoreceptors and bipolar cells. The synapse between photoreceptors and on bipolar cells is sign-inverting in its action, while the synapse between photoreceptors and off bipolar cells is sign-conserving (after Levick and Dvorak)

- A given bipolar cell responds not only to illumination of "its" photoreceptor cells, that is, those presynaptic cells that project directly onto it, but also to illumination of neighboring photoreceptor cells via the intercalated horizontal cells. The receptive field of a bipolar cell, that region of the retina which can influence the cell, can in certain circumstances, be quite wide and extensive.

- Due to the polarity of the lateral interactions through the horizontal cells, an *antagonistic surround* is formed in the bipolar cells. A bipolar cell responds oppositely according to whether light stimuli fall on "its," or on neighboring, photoreceptor cells. Illumination of the center, or of the surround, of the receptive field of a bipolar cell has opposite effects. Thus an *on* bipolar cell which, by definition, is excited by illumination of the center of its receptive field, is inhibited by illumination of the antagonistic surround. An *off* bipolar cell, which is inhibited by illumination of the center of its receptive field, is excited by illumination of the antagonistic surround. Center and surround both belong to the receptive field of a cell; but they have functionally opposite, antagonistic, effects on the cell.

The largely concentric antagonistic surround of the bipolar cells is relayed to the postsynaptic ganglion cells. Ganglion cells therefore also often have functionally structured receptive fields with a center-surround antagonism. *On*-center ganglion cells have an inhibitory surround. *Off*-center ganglion cells have an excitatory surround.

The properties of the ganglion cells are further modified by lateral interactions mediated by the laterally branched amacrine cells

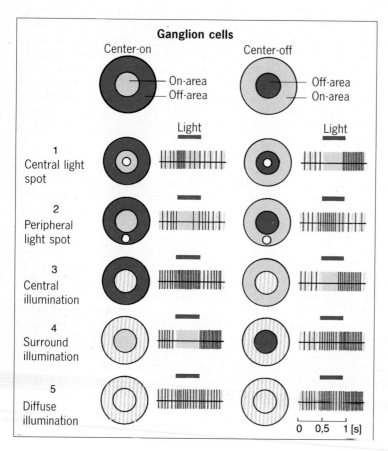

Fig. 4.21 Specialization of retinal ganglion cells for the detection of structured contrast. Response of on and off ganglion cells to variable illumination of their receptive fields. Both ganglion cell types display a concentric antagonistic surround (after Kuffler)

of the inner synaptic layer. Accordingly, several different subclasses of ganglion cells can be distinguished, some of which are motion sensitive. In the retina of many higher mammals for example, there are X/β, Y/α, and W ganglion cells. The X/β cells have cell bodies of medium size, with a highly branched dendritic arbor. They have relatively small receptive fields, respond to stationary illumination, and generate responses which contain both transient and tonic components. The brain uses their information for vision requiring high spatial resolution. The Y/α cells are large cells with little dendritic branching. They have large receptive fields, respond partially to movements in their receptive fields, and generate only transient responses to stationary illumination. They provide information required for coarse target recognition and form analysis. The W cells are small cells. Their information is used for the coordination of head and eye movements. The most common retinal ganglion cell is the X/β cell, comprising about 80% of all ganglion cells. The size of its receptive field varies depending on the region of the retina. The ganglion cells with the smallest receptive fields are in the fovea, which is the region with the highest visual acuity in the retina. The X/β ganglion cells are especially dense in the fovea.

It is important to recognize that there is not only a transfer of information from one cell layer of the retina to the next, but that processing of information already occurs. This involves *convergence,* for example from many rods onto one bipolar cell; *divergence,* for example from one horizontal cell to many cones (feedback) and bipolar cells; and *lateral inhibition,* for example from amacrine cells onto ganglion cells. This information processing begins with the photoreceptor cells, where illumination with light at appropriate wavelengths is an effective stimulus. It ends with the ganglion cells in the retina, where an effective stimulus already involves a complex and structured visual pattern. For an *on* ganglion cell the optimal stimulus is a bright circular light spot, bounded by a dark ring-shaped surround. For an *off* ganglion cell, the opposite luminance relationship holds. These cells barely respond to uniform illumination. Ganglion cells, like the bipolar cells to some extent, are optimized for the *detection of structured contrast* (Fig. 4.21).

The result of all these interactions is a diversity of ganglion cells, all of which have different physiological properties, even though they transmit information about one and the same region of the visual field. In this way, preprocessed information about a given region of the visual field is conducted to the brain via many *parallel channels.*

The projection areas of the retinal ganglion cells

All the visual information which the brain receives about the environment is provided by the retinal ganglion cells. The different ganglion cell types conduct this environmental information in parallel to the various parts of the brain. Various aspects of this information are then processed further in spatially separated neural centers. However, this further processing is is not carried out in one step, but rather as a progressive integration and abstraction of visual information in each of several successively connected neural structures. Parallel and serial information processing therefore characterize the central visual system. An additional common feature of this information processing is the maintenance of an ordered representation of the visual environment. Neighboring cells in all visual centers process information from neighboring regions of the visual field. The projections are *topographic.* In order to understand how this comes about, we first have to understand the basic functional anatomy of the visual system.

A more or less large region of the visual field, the binocular visual field, is viewed by both eyes. This means that to some extent both retinas receive information about the same part of the visual field, and relay this to the brain. The morphological basis on which this relay occurs is organized differently in different vertebrates. For this reason we will only consider the situation in higher mammals. In these animals the following simple projection rules hold for each retina. The ganglion cells in the temporal half of the retina project to the ipsilateral half of the brain, those in the nasal half project to the contralateral side of the brain (Fig. 4.22). The orderly subdivision of the ganglion cell axons from each retina occurs at the optic chiasm—at the point where the optic nerve enters the brain. This simple projection rule has a functional consequence which is just a simple, and is a product of the optics of the eye: that infomation from the right half of the visual field is processed by the left half of the brain, and information from the left half of the visual field by the right half of the brain. This is because the ipsilateral half of the binocular visual field is projected onto the nasal half of the ipsilateral retina, and onto the temporal half of the contralateral retina. This means that the ipsilateral visual field is neurally projected onto the contralateral half of the brain by ganglion cells from both retinas. The processing of visual information then occurs in two symmetrical cellular pathways in the two halves of the brain.

The axons of the retinal ganglion cells which originate from neighboring parts of the retina do not have just one target region in the brain. Some ganglion cells, above all the W cells, but also a few Y cells, project to the superior colliculus. This is a region of the midbrain which is important for the control of eye movements. In the superior colliculus, somatosensory and auditory information are integrated with this visual information and used for the coordination of head and eye movements. Other ganglion cell axons terminate in the pretectal region which is important for the regulation of pupil reflexes.

The majority of the ganglion cells, the X cells from the foveal region of the retina, as well as many Y cells, send their axons into the

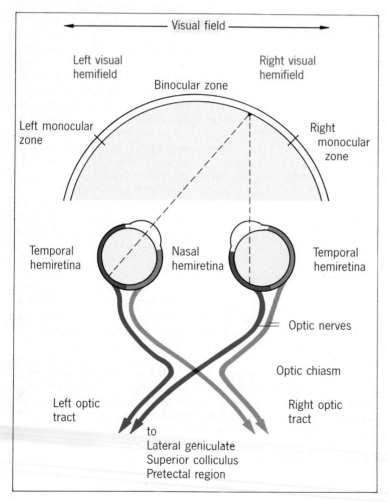

Fig. 4.**22**   Schematic representation of the imaging relationships in the human visual system (after Kelley)

lateral geniculate, which is a part of the thalamus (Fig. **4.23**). The lateral geniculate is built up in layers. The retinal ganglion cell projections to the lateral geniculate are structured in such a way that every layer receives an orderly representation of the contralateral visual field. However, a given layer receives this input only from the ipsilateral, or only from the contralateral, retina. Information about the same region of the visual field is monocularly segregated here. Since an exceedingly high proportion of ganglion cells convey information from the central part of the visual field, this means that the greater part of the lateral geniculate is also concerned with the representation of this region. The physiological properties of the neurons in the lateral geniculate are very similar to those of the retinal ganglion cells, particularly with respect to the structure of their receptive fields with *on* and *off* centers. However, the antagonistic surround is somewhat more strongly expressed in the neurons of the lateral geniculate.

The product of the parallel processing of the visual information in all the layers of the lateral geniculate is relayed by its projection neurons to a particularly important structure in the brain—namely the *visual cortex.* However this is not a one-way street. There are also projections from the visual cortex back to the lateral geniculate. This retrograde projection mediates the cortical control of visual information flow, and in fact involves more axons than the actual forward visual projection.

The visual cortex

In the visual cortex various stimulus parameters from discrete small areas of the visual field are registered and processed in defined microanatomical structures. Neurons are found here which are specialized for object features like orientation, form or color. The way this remarkable structure is organized was worked out by Hubel and Wiesel in a series of elegant experiments on the primary visual cortex.

The primary visual cortex, also called V1 or area 17, receives its input from the lateral geniculate via an extensive optic radiation. The projection of the lateral geniculate neurons onto the cortical neurons is once again topographic. Neighboring neurons receive information about neighboring regions of the visual field. Like the lateral geniculate, the primary visual cortex is composed of numerous layers. In primates one can distinguish six layers (Fig. **4.24**). The majority of the axons from the lateral geniculate terminate in layer IV. Neurons in this layer receive their input monocularly, from either one eye or the other. From layer IV the visual information reaches layers II, III, V, and VI. These projections are also topographically and retinotopically organized. However, in contrast to the monocularly driven neurons in layer IV, most other cortical neurons receive information about a given region of the visual field from both eyes. In most cases the input from one eye dominates somewhat, so that an *ocular dominance* exists for these neurons. The most important exceptions are the neurons which receive information about that peripheral region of the visual field which is only registered monocularly anyway.

Thus, visual information undergoes a transformation in the visual cortex, a conversion from monocularity to binocularity. There

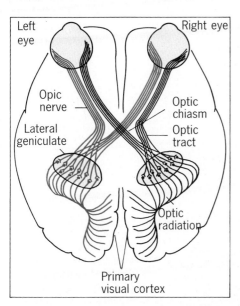

Fig. 4.**23**   Simplified schema of the human visual pathway. The axons of the retinal ganglion cells reach the lateral geniculate via the optic nerve and optic tract. The axons of the projection neurons from the lateral geniculate reach the primary visual cortex via the optic radiation (after Hubel and Wiesel)

are, however, other more important aspects to the visual information processing. One has to do with the complex structure of the receptive field of cortical neurons. The simple, concentric center–surround organization of the receptive field in the cells of the lateral geniculate is no longer found in the majority of cortical neurons. The "simplest" response properties of cortical neurons are those which appear as a sensitivity to a line, stripe or edge having a very specific orientation in a particular part of the visual field (Fig. 4.**25**). The response properties of these *simple cells* of the visual cortex are therefore really quite complicated. These cells have the properties of visual detectors. This detector property becomes even clearer in other neurons of the visual cortex which also respond to lines or edges having a particular orientation, but independently of the position of these objects in the visual field (Fig. 4.**26**). In this case the neurons display an amazing capacity for abstraction. Orientation of the object is important, but not its position in the receptive field. Other *complex cells* of this type respond specifically in a position-independent way to quite complex, geometrically-defined structures, which can even have a particular direction of movement. It is still unclear how the response properties of the simple and complex cells in the visual cortex come about. One hypothesis

is that the properties of the simple cells result from the convergent connections of projection neurons of the lateral geniculate, while for their part, the properties of the complex cells are achieved by the convergent connections of simple cells. The neurons from a given level in this hierarchy "recognize" more than the neurons from a lower level, and also have a greater capacity for abstraction.

Regardless of how the response properties of the cortical neurons arise, they are formed on the basis of a regular, orderly, functional microarchitecture. Every layer in the visual cortex can be divided into multiple aggregates of neurons. The individual aggregates are similar to one another in their morphological dimension, but differ from one another in the functional properties of their neurons. These functional units are called modules. Such functionally differentiated neuron aggregates are arranged microanatomically as columns or ribbons in the cortical layers. They can be demonstrated anatomically with activity-dependent or voltage selective staining methods (Fig. 4.**27**). On the one hand the *module concept* applies to ocular dominance. Neurons which have the same ocular dominance, and receive input from the same region of the visual field, are grouped together microanatomically into columns or ribbons. Ordered rib-

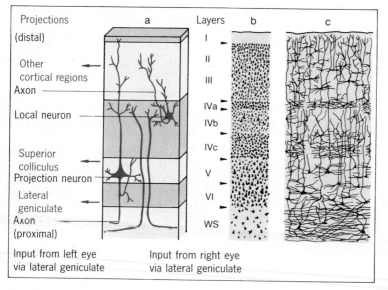

Fig. 4.**24**   Layer-like arrangement of the primary visual cortex of primates. **a** Schematic of the afferent and efferent connections for the different layers of the primary visual cortex. **b** Representation of the laminar cytoarchitecture of the visual cortex (Nissl staining). **c** Representation of some individual neurons in the primary visual cortex (Golgi staining) (after Kelley, and LeVay et al.)

bons of neurons which receive a stronger input from the left eye alternate with those which receive a stronger input from the right eye. On the other hand the module concept applies to orientation specificity. Neurons which respond to bars or edges with a given orientation, in a particular region of the visual field, are again grouped together microanatomically into a column or band. Neurons in a neighboring orientation band receive their input from the same region of the visual field, but respond to an orientation of the bar or edge which has been rotated by a few degrees. The orientation specificity shifts in a discrete and regular way from one orientation band to the next.

Orientation bands and ocular dominance bands are superimposed in an orderly way. Within one ocular dominance band, the

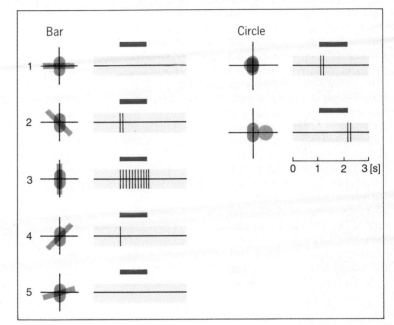

Fig. 4.**25a**   Response properties of a simple cell in the primary visual cortex. The cell responds best to a vertically oriented bar of light in the center of its visual field

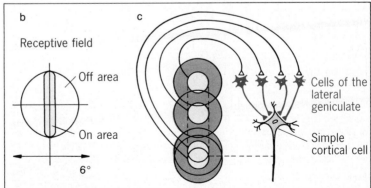

Fig. 4.**25b**   Functional structure of the receptive field of the cell. **c** Hypothetical circuit to explain the response properties of the cell. Numerous presynaptic cells with partly overlapping, concentric receptive fields are assumed to synapse onto the simple cell (after Hubel and Wiesel)

way. Within one ocular dominance band, the orientation sensitivity of groups of neurons changes in a stepwise manner. Likewise, groups of neurons which have an ocular dominance of the left eye alternate with those which have an ocular dominance of the right eye. If we now consider all the orientation bands and ocular dominance bands which are concerned with the same part of the visual field, then we can see that they are once again spatially grouped together in a modular way. In these hyper-

modules, which are also termed *hypercolumns,* all orientations as well as both ocular dominance types are represented by corresponding neuronal bands (Fig. 4.28). In addition there are further neuronal aggregates in the hypercolumn which are not orientation-specific, but are concerned with the processing of color information. In this way every hypercolumn represents a type of cortical computational unit. It contains the neuronal machinery necessary to analyze a given small region of the visual field.

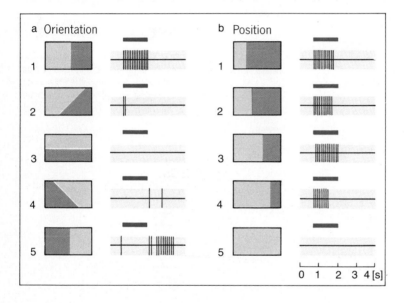

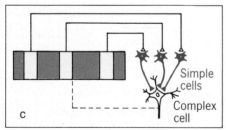

Fig. 4.**26** Response properties of a complex cell in the primary visual cortex. **a** The cell responds best to a vertically oriented edge of light. To excite the cell, the right side of the vertical edge must be illuminated; illumination of the left side produces an inhibition. **b** The cell responds equally well to a vertical edge irrespective of where in the cell's receptive field the edge is presented. **c** Hypothetical circuit to explain the response properties of the cell. Numerous presynaptic cells with partly overlapping, vertical, bar-like receptive fields are assumed to synapse onto the complex cell (after Hubel and Wiesel)

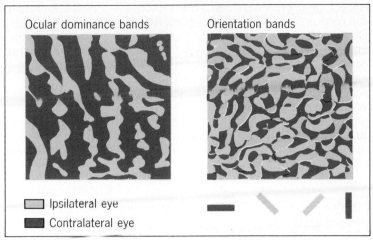

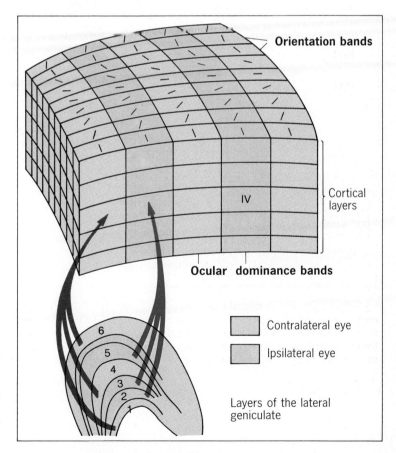

Fig. **4.27** Anatomical representation of functionally differentiated neuron aggregates. Partial view of the cortical surface. The effect of monocular stimulation (left) or differently oriented bars of light (right) on the electrical activity of cortical neuron aggregates can be illustrated following application of voltage-sensitive dyes. In this way the band-shaped arrangement of neurons with the same ocular dominance or the same orientational specificity can be represented *in vivo* (after Blasdel and Salama)

Fig. **4.28** Schematic representation of visual hypercolumns. Ocular dominance bands and orientation bands are illustrated in a simplified way as lying orthogonally to one another (after Kuffler and Nicholls)

Apart from the primary visual cortex, there are still further topographic representations of the visual field in other cortical regions. In primates there are no less than a dozen further representations of the visual field. These other, higher cortical fields receive their visual input partly from layers II and III of the primary visual cortex, partly from extracortical structures like the lateral geniculate or the superior colliculus. All these representations differ from one another in the details of their retinotopic projections, as well as in the stimulus parameters which are preferentially processed there. The neurons in some of these areas are concerned with the movement of objects in three-dimensional space; the neurons in others are primarily concerned with the further processing of form and color information (Fig. 4.29). It therefore seems to be a unifying organizational principle of the sensory cortex to establish numerous parallel representations of the environment, in order to then process different informational parameters in each of these representations.

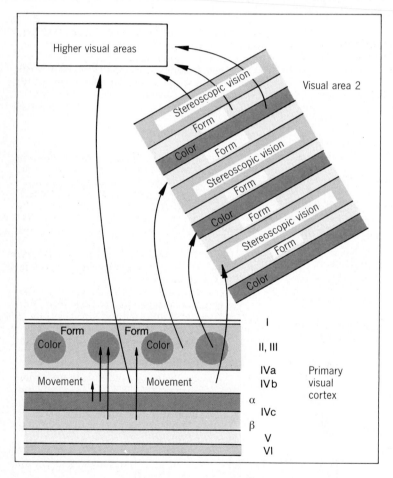

Fig. 4.**29** Schematic diagram showing the functional segregation of visual information in the visual central nervous system of primates (after Livingstone and Hubel)

References

General Reviews

Ali, M. A. (ed.) 1984. Photoreception and Vision in Invertebrates. Plenum, New York

Borselino, A. and Cervetto, L. (eds.) 1984. Photoreceptors. Plenum, New York

Bray, D. 1990. Intracellular signalling as a parallel distributed procress. J. Theor. Biol. 143: 215-231

Camhi, J. M. 1984. Neuroethology. Sinauer, Sunderland

Correia, J. J. and Prachio, A. A. (eds.) 1985. Contemporary Sensory Neurobiology. Liss, New York

Daw, N. W., Brunken, W. J. and Parkinson, D. 1989. The function of synaptic transmitters in the retina. Annu. Rev. Neurosci. 12: 205-226

Dowling, J. E. 1987. The Retina: An Approachable Part of the Brain. Belknap Press, Cambridge

Edelman, G. M., Gall, W. E. and Cowan, W. M. (eds.) 1988. Auditory Function: Neurobiological Bases of Hearing. Wiley, New York

Gilbert, C. D. 1983. Microcircuitry of the visual cortex. Annu. Rev. Neurosci. 6: 217:247

Helmholtz, H. 1889. Popular Scientific Lectures. Longmans, London.

Hubel. D. H. 1982. Cortical neurobiology: A slanted historical perspective. Annu. Rev. Neurosci. 5: 363-370

Hubel, D. H. 1988. Eye, Brain and Vision. Scientific American Library, New York

Hudspeth, A. J. 1985. The cellular basis of hearing: The biophysics of hair cells. Science 230: 745-752.

Kaissling, K. E. 1986. Chemo-electrical transduction in insect olfactory receptors. Annu. Rev. Neurosci. 9: 121-146

Knudsen, E. I., du Lac, S. and Easterly, S. D. 1987. Computational maps in the brain. Annu. Rev. Neurosci. 10: 41-66

Lancet, D. 1986. Vertebrate olfactory reception. Annu. Rev. Neurosci. 9 329-355

Lund, J. S. 1988. Anatomical organization of macaque monkey striate visual cortex. Annu. Rev. Neurosci. 11: 253-288

Lund, J. S. (ed.) 1988. Sensory Processing in the Mammalian Brain: Neural Substrates and Experimental Strategies. Oxford University Press, New York

Marr, D. 1982. Vision. Freeman, San Francisco

Nathans, J. 1987. Molecular biology of visual pigments. Annu. Rev. Neurosci. 10: 163-194

Nicholls, J. G., Martin, A. R. and Wallace, B. 1992. From Neuron to Brain, 3rd edition, Sinauer, Sunderland

Ottoson, D. 1983. Physiology of the Nervous System. Macmillan, London

Roper, S. D. 1989. The cell biology of vertebrate taste receptors. Annu. Rev. Neurosci. 12 329-354

Schwartz, E. A. 1985. Phototransduction in vertebrate rods. Annu. Rev. Neurosci. 8: 339-368

Shapley, R. and Lennie, P. 1985. Spatial frequency analysis in the visual system. Annu. Rev. Neurosci. 8: 547-584

Shepherd, G. M. 1988. Neurobiology, 2nd edition, Oxford University Press, New York

Stavenga, D. G., Hardie, R. C. (eds.) 1989. Facets of Vision. Springer, Berlin

Sterling, P. 1983. Microcircuitry of the cat retina. Annu. Rev. Neurosci. 6: 149-185

Stryer, L. 1986. Cyclic GMP cascade of vision. Annu. Rev. Neurosci. 9: 87-120

Travers, J. B., Travers. S. P. and Norgren, R. 1987. Gustatory neural processing in the hindbrain. Annu. Rev. Neurosci. 10: 595-632

Wall, P. D. and Melzack, R. (eds.) 1989. Textbook of Pain. 2nd edition, Churchill Livingstone, Edinburgh

Yau, K. W. and Baylor, D. A. 1989. Cyclic GMP-activated conductance of retinal photoreceptor cells. Annu. Rev. Neurosci. 12: 289-328

Zeki, S. 1990. Colour vision and functional specialisation in the visual cortex. Discuss. Neurosci. 6: 1-64

Original Publications

Alexandrowicz, J. S. 1951. Muscle receptor organs in the abdomen of Homarus vulgaris and Parlinurus vulgaris. Q. J. Microsc. Sci. 92: 163-199.

Art, J. J., Crawford, A. C., Fettiplace, R. and Fuchs, P. A. 1982. Efferent regulation of hair cells in the turtle cochlea. Proc. R. Soc. Lond. B 216: 377-384.

Barlow, H. B. 1953. Summation and inhibition in the frog's retina. J. Physiol. 119: 69-88.

Barlow, H. B., Blakemore, C. and Pettigrew, J. D. 1967. The neural mechanism of binocular depth discrimination. J. Physiol. 193: 327-342.

Barlow, H. B., Hill, R. M. and Levick, W. R. 1964. Retinal ganglion cells responding selectively to direction and speed of image motion in the rabbit. J. Physiol. 173: 377-407.

Barlow, H. B. and Levick, W. R. 1965. The mechanism of directionally selective units in rabbit's retina. J. Physiol. 178: 477-504.

Baylor, D. A. and Fettiplace, R. 1977. Transmission from photoreceptors to ganglion cells in turtle retina. J. Physiol. 271: 391-424.

Baylor, D. A. and Fettiplace, R. 1977. Kinetics of synaptic transfer from receptors to ganglion cells in turtle retina. J. Physiol. 271: 425-448.

Baylor, D. A., Fuortes, M. G. F. and O'Bryan, P. M. 1971. Receptive fields of cones in the retina of the turtle. J. Physiol. 214: 265-294.

Baylor, D. A. and Hodgkin, A. L. 1973. Detection and resolution of visual stimuli by turtle photoreceptors. J. Physiol. 234: 163-198.

Baylor, D. A., Lamb, T. D. and Yau, K.-W. 1979. The membrane current of single rod outer segments. J. Physiol. 288: 589-611

Baylor D. A., Nunn, B. J. and Schnapf, J. L. 1987. Spectral sensitivity of cones of the monkey Macaca fascicularis. J. Physiol. 390: 145-160.

Berlucchi, G. and Rizzolatti, G. 1968. Binocularly driven neurons in visual cortex of split-chiasm cats. Science 159: 308-310.

Bishop, P. O., Coombs, J. S. and Henry, G. H. 1971. Responses to visual contours: Spatio-temporal aspects of excitation in the receptive fields of simple striate neurones. J. Physiol. 219: 625-657.

Bishop, P. O. and Pettigrew, J. D. 1986. Neural mechanisms of binocular vision. Vision Res. 26: 1587-1600.

Blasdel, G. G. and Lund, J. S. 1983. Termination of afferent axons in macaque striate cortex. J. Neurosci. 3: 1389-1413.

Bowling, D. B. and Michael, C. R. 1980. Projection patterns of single physiologically characterized optic tract fibres in cat. Nature 286: 899-902.

Brown, H. M., Ottoson, D. and Rydqvist, B. 1978. Crayfish stretch receptor: An investigation with voltage-clamp and ion-sensitive electrodes. J. Physiol. 284: 155-179.

Boycott, B. B. and Wässle, H. 1974. The morphological types of ganglion cells of the domestic cat's retina. J. Physiol. 240: 397-419.

Breer, H., Boekhoff, I. and Tareilus, E. 1990. Rapid kinetics of second messenger formation in olfactory transduction. Nature 345: 65-68.

Buck, L. and Axel, R. 1991. A novel multigene family may encode odorant receptors: A molecular basis for odorant recognition. Cell 65: 175-187.

Caldwell, J. H. and Daw, N. W. 1978. Effects of picrotoxin and strychnine on rabbit retinal ganglion cells. Changes in centre surround receptive fields. J. Physiol. 276: 299-310.

Christensen, B. N. and Perl, E. R. 1970. Spinal neurons specifically excited by noxious or thermal stimuli: Marginal zone of the dorsal horn. J. Neurophysiol. 33: 293-307.

Cleland, B. G., Levick, W. R. and Wässle, H. 1975. Physiological identification of a morphological class of cat retinal ganglion cells. J. Physiol. 248: 151-171.

Corey, D. P. and Hudspeth, A. J. 1979. Ionic basis of the receptor potential in a vertebrate hair cell. Nature 281: 675-677.

Costanzo, R. M. and Gardner, E. P. 1980. A quantitative analysis of responses of direction-sensitive neurons in somatosensory cortex of awake monkeys. J. Neurophysiol. 43: 1319-1341.

Cowan, W. M. and Powell, T. P. S. 1963. Centrifugal fibres in the avian visual system. Proc. R. Soc. Lond. B 158: 232-252.

Crawford, A. C. and Fettiplace, R. 1981. An electrical tuning mechanism in turtle cochlear hair cells. J. Physiol. 312: 377-412.

Daniel, P. M. and Whitteridge, D. 1961. The representation of the visual field on the cerebral cortex in monkeys. J. Physiol. 159: 203-221.

Dennis, M. J., Harris, A. J. and Kuffler, S. W. 1971. Synaptic transmission and its duplication by focally applied acetylcholine in parasympathetic neurones in the heart of the frog. Proc. R. Soc. Lond. B 177: 509-539.

Dhallan, R. S., Yau, K.-W., Schrader, K. A. and Reed R. R. 1990. Primary structure and functional expression of a cyclic nucleotide-activated channel from olfactory neurons. Nature 347: 184-187.

Dowling, J. E. and Boycott, B. B. 1966. Organization of the primate retina: Electron microscopy. Proc. R. Soc. Lond. B 166: 80-111.

Dowling, J. E., Lasater, E. M., Van Buskirk, R. and Watling, K. J. 1983. Pharmacological properties of isolated fish horizontal cells. Vision Res. 23: 421-432.

Dowling, J. E. and Werblin, F. S. 1971. Synaptic organization of the vertebrate retina. Vision Res. 3: 1-15.

Dräger, U. C. 1981. Observations on the organization of the visual cortex in the reeler mouse. J. Comp. Neurol. 201: 555-570.

Drujan, B. D. and Svaetichin, G. 1972. Characterization of different classes of isolated retinal cells. Vision Res. 12: 1777-1784.

Dubin, M. W. and Cleland, B. G. 1977. Organization of visual inputs to interneurons of the lateral geniculate nucleus of the cat. J. Neurophysiol. 40: 410-427.

Edwards, C. and Ottoson, D. 1958. The site of impulse initiation in a nerve cell of a crustacean stretch receptor. J. Physiol. 143: 138-148.

Enroth-Cugell, C. and Robson, J. G. 1966. The contrast sensitivity of retinal ganglion cells of the cat. J. Physiol. 787: 517-552.

Eyzaguirre, C. and Kuffler, S. W. 1955. Processes of excitation in the dendrites and in the soma of single isolated sensory nerve cells of the lobster and crayfish. J. Gen. Physiol. 39: 87-119.

Fahrenbach, W. H. 1985. Anatomical circuitry of lateral inhibition in the eye of the horseshoe crab, Limulus polyphemus. Proc. R. Soc. Lond. B 225: 219-249.

Famiglietti, E. V. Jr., Kaneko, A. and Tachibana, M. 1977. Neuronal architecture of on and off pathways to ganglion cells in carp retina. Science 198: 1267-1269.

Ferster, D. 1981. A comparison of binocular depth mechanisms in areas 17 and 18 of the cat visual cortex. J. Physiol. 311: 623-655.

Ferster, D. and LeVay, S. 1978. The axonal arborizations of lateral geniculate neurons in the striate cortex of the cat. J. Comp. Neurol. 182: 923-944.

Ferster, D. and Lindström, S. 1983. An intracellular analysis of geniculocortical connectivity in area 17 of the cat. J. Physiol. 342: 181-215.

Fischer, B. and Poggio, G. F. 1979. Depth sensitivity of binocular cortical neurones of behaving monkeys. Proc. R. Soc. Lond. B 204: 409-414.

Flock, A. and Russell, J. J. 1973. The post-synaptic action of efferent fibres in the lateral line organ of the burbot Lota lota. J. Physiol. 235: 591-605.

Friedlander, M. J., Lin. C.-S., Stanford, L. R. and Sherman, S. M. 1981. Morphology of functionally identified neurons in lateral geniculate nucleus of the cat. J. Neurophysiol. 46: 80-129.

Fuortes, M. G. F. and Poggio, G. F. 1963. Transient responses to sudden illumination in cells of the eye of Limulus. J. Gen. Physiol. 46: 435-452.

Gilbert, C. D. 1977. Laminar differences in receptive field properties of cells in cat primary visual cortex. J. Physiol. 268: 391-421.

Gilbert, C. D. and Wiesel, T. N. 1979. Morphology and intracortical projections of functionally characterised neurones in the cat visual cortex. Nature 280: 120-125.

Gilbert, C. D. and Wiesel, T. N. 1983. Clustered intrinsic connections in cat visual cortex. J. Neurosci. 3: 1116-1133.

Gilbert, C. D. and Wiesel, T. N. 1989. Columnar specificity of intrinisic horizontal and corticocortical connections in cat visual cortex. J. Neurosci. 9: 2432-2442.

Gray, C. M. and Singer, W. 1989. Stimulus-specific neuronal oscillations in orientation columns of cat visual cortex. Proc. Natl. Acad. Sci. USA. 86: 1698-1702.

Guillery, R. W. 1970. The laminar distribution of retinal fibers in the dorsal lateral geniculate nucleus of the cat: A new interpretation. J. Comp. Neurol. 138: 339-368.

Guillery, R. W. and Kaas, J. H. 1971. A study of normal and congenitally abnormal retinogeniculate projections in cats. J. Comp. Neurol. 143: 73-100.

Hagins, W. A., Penn, R. D. and Yoshikami, S. 1970. Dark current and photocurrent in retinal rods. Biophys. J. 10: 380-412.

Hagiwara, S., Kusano, K. and Saito, S. 1960. Membrane changes in crayfish stretch receptor neuron during synaptic inhibition and under action of gammaaminobutyric acid. J. Neurophysiol. 23: 505-515.

Hartline, H. K. 1940. The receptive fields of optic nerve fibers. Am. J. Physiol. 130: 690-699.

Hartline, H. K. 1940. The nerve messages in the fibers of the visual pathway. J. Opt. Soc. Am. 30: 239-247.

Hecht, S., Shlaer, S. and Pirenne, M. H. 1942. Energy, quanta and vision. J. Gen Physiol. 25: 819-840.

Hendrickson, A. E., Ogren, M. P., Vaughn, J. E., Barber, R. P., and Wu, J.-Y. 1983. Light and electron microscope immunocytochemical localization of glutamic acid decarboxylase in monkey geniculate complex: Evidence for GABAergic neurons and synapses. J. Neurosci. 3: 1245-1262.

Hendrickson, A. E., Wilson, J. R. and Ogren, M. P. 1978. The neuroanatomical organizations of pathways between dorsal lateral geniculate nucleus and visual cortex in old and new world primates. J. Comp. Neurol. 182: 123-136.

Hubel, D. H. and Wiesel, T. N. 1959. Receptive fields of single neurones in the cat's striate cortex. J. Physiol. 148: 574-591.

Hubel, D. H. and Wiesel, T. N. 1961. Integrative action in the cat's lateral geniculate body. J. Physiol. 755: 385-398.

Hubel, D. H. and Wiesel, T. N. 1962. Receptive fields, binocular interaction and functional architecture in the cat's visual cortex. J. Physiol. 160: 106-154.

Hubel, D. H. and Wiesel, T. N. 1963. Shape and arrangement of columns in cat's striate cortex. J. Physiol. 165: 559-568.

Hubel, D. H. and Wiesel, T. N. 1965. Receptive fields and functional architecture in two non-striate visual areas (18 and 19) of the cat. J. Neurophysiol. 28: 229-289.

Hubel, D. H. and Wiesel, T. N. 1967. Cortical and callosal connections concerned with the vertical meridian of visual field in the cat. J. Neurophysiol. 30: 1561-1573.

Hubel, D. H. and Wiesel, T. N. 1968. Receptive fields and functional architecture of monkey striate cortex. J. Physiol. 195: 215-243.

Hubel, D. H. and Wiesel, T. N. 1972. Laminar and columnar distribution of geniculo-cortical fibers in the macaque monkey. J. Comp. Neurol. 146: 421-450.

Hubel, D. H. and Wiesel, T. N. 1974. Sequence regularity and geometry of orientation columns in the monkey striate cortex. J. Comp. Neurol. 158: 267-294.

Hubel, D. H., Wiesel, T. N. and Stryker, M. P. 1978. Anatomical demonstration of orientation columns in Macaque monkey. J. Comp. Neurol. 177: 361-380.

Hudspeth, A. J., Poo, M. M. and Stuart, A. E. 1077. Passive signal propagation and membrane properties in median photoreceptors of the giant barnacle. J. Physiol. 272: 25-43.

Humphrey, A. L. and Hendrickson, A. E. 1983. Background and stimulus-induced patterns of high metabolic activity in the visual cortex (area 17) of the squirrel and macaque monkey. J. Neurosci. 3: 345-358.

Humphrey, A. L., Skeen, L. C. and Norton, T. T. 1980. Topographic organization of the orientation column system in the striate cortex of the tree shrew (Tupaia glis). II. Deoxyglucose mapping. J. Comp. Neurol. 192: 549-566.

Hunt, C. C., Wilkinson, R. S. and Fukami, Y. 1978. Ionic basis of the receptor potential in primary endings of mammalian muscle spindles. J. Gen. Physiol. 77: 683-698.

Hyvärinen, J. and Poranen, A. 1978. Movement-sensitive and direction and orientation-selective cutaneous receptive fields in the hand area of the postcentral gyrus in monkeys. J. Physiol. 283: 523-537.

Jansen, J. K. S., Njå. A., Ormstad, K. and Walloe, L. 1971. On the innervation of the slowly adapting stretch receptor of the crayfish abdomen: An electrophysiological approach. Acta Physiol. Scand. 81: 273-285.

Kaneko, A. 1970. Physiological and morphological identification of horizontal, bipolar and amacrine cells in goldfish. J. Physiol. 207: 623-633.

Kaneko, A. 1971. Electrical connexions between horizontal cells in the dogfish retina. J. Physiol. 213: 95-105.

Kaneko, A. and Tachibana, M. 1983. Double color-opponent receptive fields of carp bipolar cells. Vision Res. 23: 381-388.

Kaplan, E. and Shapley, R. M. 1982. X and Y cells in the lateral geniculate nucleus of macaque monkeys. J. Physiol. 330: 125-143.

Kaupp, U. B., Niidome, T., Tanabe, T., Terada, S., Bönigk, W., Stühmer, W., Cook, N. J., Kangawa, K., Matsuo, H. Hirose, T., Miyata, T. and Kelly, J. P. and Van Essen, D. C. 1974. Cell structure and function in the visual cortex of the cat. J. Physiol. 238: 515-547.

Khanna, S. M. and Leonard, D. B. B. 1982. Basilar membrane tuning in the cat cochlea. Science 215: 305-306.

Knudsen, E. I. and Konishi, M. 1978. A neural map of auditory space in the owl. Science 200: 795-797.

Kruger, L., Perl, E. R. and Sedivec, M. J. 1981. Fine structure of myelinated mechanical nociceptor endings in cat hairy skin. J. Comp. Neurol. 198: 137-154.

Kuffler, S. W. 1953. Discharge patterns and functional organization of the mammalian retina. J. Neurophysiol. 16: 37-68.

Kuffler, S. W. 1954. Mechanisms of activation and motor control of stretch receptors in lobster and crayfish. J. Neurophysiol. 17: 558-574.

Kuffler, S. W. and Eyzaguirre, C. 1955. Synaptic inhibition in an isolated nerve cell. J. Gen. Physiol. 39: 155-184.

Lam, D. M.-K. and Ayoub, G. S. 1983. Biochemical and biophysical studies of isolated horizontal cells from the teleost retina. Vision Res. 23: 433-444.

La Vail, J. H. and La Vail, M. M. 1974. The retrograde intraaxonal transport of horseradish peroxidase in the chick visual system: A light and electron microscopic study. J. Comp. Neurol. 157: 303-358.

LeVay, S., Hubel, D. H. and Wiesel, T. N. 1975. The pattern of ocular dominance columns in macaque visual cortex revealed by a reduced silver stain. J. Comp. Neurol. 159: 559-576.

LeVay, S. and McConnell, S. K. 1982. On and off layers in the lateral geniculate nucleus of the mink. Nature 300: 350-351.

Livingstone, M. S. and Hubel, D. H. 1982. Thalamic inputs to cytochrome oxidase-rich regions in monkey visual cortex. Proc. Natl. Acad. Sci. USA 79: 6098-6101.

Livingstone, M. S. and Hubel, D. H. 1983. Specificity of cortico-cortical connections in monkey visual system. Nature 304: 531-534.

Livingstone, M. S. and Hubel, D. H. 1984. Anatomy and physiology of a color system in the primate visual cortex. J. Neurosci. 4: 309-356.

Livingstone, M. S. and Hubel, D. H. 1984. Specificity of intrinsic connections in primate primary visual cortex. J. Neurosci. 4: 2830-2835.

Livingstone, M. S. and Hubel, D. 1988. Segregation of form, color, movement and depth: Anatomy, physiology and perception. Science 240: 740-749.

Lloyd, D. P. D. 1943. Conduction and synaptic transmission of the reflex response to stretch in spinal cats. J. Neurophysiol. 6: 317-326.

Loewenstein, W. R. and Mendelson, M. 1965. Components of receptor adaptation in a Pacinian corpuscle. J. Physiol. 177: 377-397.

Luskin, M. B. and Price, J. L. 1983. The topographic organization of associational fibers of the olfactory system in the rat, including centrifugal fibers to the olfactory bulb. J. Comp. Neurol. 216: 264-291.

Malpeli, J. G. 1983. Activity of cells in area 17 of the cat in absence of input from layer A of lateral geniculate nucleus. J. Neurophysiol. 49: 595-610.

Malpeli, J. G., Schiller, P. H. and Colby, C. L. 1981. Response properties of single cells in monkey striate cortex during reversible inactivation of individual lateral geniculate laminae. J. Neurophysiol. 46: 1102-1119.

Marchiafava, P. L. and Weiler, R. 1982. The photoresponses of structurally identified amacrine cells in the turtle retina. Proc. R. Soc. Lond. B 214: 403-415.

Matsumoto, S. G. and Hildebrand, J. G. 1981. Olfactory mechanisms in the moth Manduca sexta: response characteristics and morphology of central neurons in the antennal lobes. Proc. R. Soc. Lond. B 213: 249-277.

Maturana, H. R., Lettvin, J. Y., McCulloch, W. S. and Pitts, W. H. 1960. Anatomy and physiology of vision in the frog (Rana pipiens). J. Gen. Physiol. 43: 129-175.

McGuire, B. A., Hornung, J.-P., Gilbert, C. D. and Wiesel, T. 1984. Patterns of synaptic input to layer 4 of cat striate cortex. J. Neurosci. 4:3021-3033.

Merzenich, M. M., Kaas, J. H., Sur, M. and Lin, C.-S. 1978. Double representation of the body surface within cytoarchitectonic areas 3b and 1 in "S-1," in the owl monkey (Aotus trivigatus). J. Comp. Neurol. 181: 41-74.

Merzenich, M. M. and Reid, M. D. 1974. Representation of the cochlea within the inferior colliculus of the cat. Brain Res. 77: 397-415.

Michael, C. R. 1981. Columnar organization of color cells in monkey's striate cortex. J. Neurophysiol. 46: 587-604.

Middlebrooks, J. C., Dykes, R. W. and Merzenich, M. M. 1980. Binaural response-specific bands in primary auditory cortex (A1) of the cat: Topographical organization orthogonal to isofrequency contours. Brain Res. 181: 31-48.

Miller, R. F., Frumkes, T. E., Slaughter, M. and Dacheux, R. F. 1981. Physiological and pharmacological basis of GABA and glycine action on neurons of mudpuppy retina. II. Amacrine and ganglion cells. J. Neurophysiol. 45: 764-782.

Mountcastle, V. B. 1957. Modality and topographic properties of single neurons of cat's somatic sensory cortex. J. Neurophysiol. 20: 408-434.

Movshon, J. A., Thompson, I. D. and Tolhurst, D. J. 1978. Spatial summation in the receptive fields of simple cells in the cat's striate cortex. J. Physiol. 283: 53-77.

Movshon, J. A., Thompson, I. D. and Tolhurst, D. J. 1978. Spatial and temporal contrast sensitivity of neurones in areas 17 and 18 of the cat's visual cortex. J. Physiol. 283: 101-120.

Nakajima, S. and Onodera, K. 1969. Membrane properties of the stretch receptor neurones of crayfish with particular reference to mechanisms of sensory adaptation. J. Physiol. 200: 161-185.

Nakajima, S. and Onodera, K. 1969. Adaptation of the geneator potential in the crayfish stretch receptors under constant length and constant tension. J. Physiol. 200: 187-204.

Nakamura, T. and Gold, G. H. 1987. A cyclic nucleotide-gated conductance in olfactory receptor cilia. Nature 325: 442-444.

Nakatani, K. and Yau, K.-W. 1988. Calcium and light adaptation in retinal rods and cones. Nature 334: 69-71.

Nelson, R., Famiglietti, E. V. Jr. and Kolb, H. 1978. Intracellular staining reveals different levels of stratification for on- and off-center ganglion cells in cat retina. J. Neurophysiol. 41: 472-483.

Nicholls, J. G. and Baylor, D. A. 1968. Specific modalities and receptive fields of sensory neurons in the CNS of the leech. J. Neurophysiol. 31: 740-756.

Nunn, B. J. and Baylor, D. A. 1982. Visual transduction in retinal rods of the monkey Macaca fascicularis. Nature 299: 726-728.

Orbach, H. S., Cohen, L. B. and Grinvald, A. 1985. Optical mapping of electrical activity in rat somatosensory and visual cortex. J. Neurosci. 5: 1886-1895.

Palmer, L. A. and Rosenquist, A. C. 1974. Visual receptive fields of single striate cortical units projecting to the superior colliculus in the cat. Brain Res. 67: 27-42.

Pearlman, A. L. and Hughes, C. P. 1976. Functional role of efferents to the avian retina. I. Analysis of retinal ganglion cell receptive fields. J. Comp. Neurol. 166: 111-122.

Pearlman, A. L. and Hughes, C. P. 1976. Functional role of efferents to the avian retina. II. Effects of reversible cooling of the isthmo-optic nucleus. J. Comp. Neurol. 166: 123-132.

Piccolino, M. and Gerschenfeld, H. M. 1980. Characteristics and ionic processes involved in feedback spikes of turtle cones. Proc. R. Soc. Lond. B 206: 439-463.

Poggio, G. F. and Mountcastle, V. B. 1960. A study of the functional contributions of the lemniscal and spinothalamic systems to somatic sensibility. Bull. Johns Hopkins Hosp. 106: 266-316.

Roberts, A. and Bush, B. M. H. 1971. Coxal muscle receptors in the crab: The receptor current and some properties of the receptor nerve fibres. J. Exp. Biol 54: 515-524.

Rolls, E. T. 1989. Information processing in the taste system of primates. J. Exp. Biol. 146: 141-164.

Schiller, P. H. and Malpeli, J. G. 1977. Properties and tectal projections of monkey retinal ganglion cells. J. Neurophysiol. 40: 428-445.

Schiller, P. H. and Malpeli, J. G. 1978. Functional specificity of lateral geniculate nucleus laminae of the rhesus monkey. J. Neurophysiol. 41: 788-797.

Schiller, P. H., Sandell, J. H. and Maunsell, J. H. R. 1986. Functions of the on and off channels of the visual system. Nature 322: 824-825.

Shatz, C. J. 1977. Anatomy of interhemispheric connections in the visual system of Boston Siamese and ordinary cats. J. Comp. Neurol. 173: 497-518.

Shatz, C. J., Lindström, S. and Wiesel, T. N. 1977. The distribution of afferents representing the right and left eyes in the cat's visual cortex. Brain Res. 131: 103-116.

Sillito, A. M. 1979. Inhibitory mechanisms influencing complex cell orientation selectivity and their modification at high resting discharge levels. J. Physiol. 289: 33-53.

Simons, D. J. and Woolsey, T. A. 1979. Functional organization in mouse barrel cortex. Brain Res. 165: 327-332.

Specht, S. and Grafstein, B. 1973. Accumulation of radioactive protein in mouse cerebral cortex after injection of ^{3}H-fucose into the eye. Exp. Neurol. 41: 705-722.

Suga, N., O'Neill, W. E. and Manabe, T. 1978. Cortical neurones sensitive to combinations of information-bearing elements of bisonar signals in the mustache bat. Science 200: 778-781.

Talbot, S. A. and Marshall, W. H. 1941. Physiological studies on neural mechanisms of visual localization and discrimination. Am. J. Ophthalmol. 24: 1255-1264.

Tao Cheng, J.-H., Hirosawa, K. and Nakajima, Y. 1981. Ultrastructure of the crayfish stretch receptor in relation to its function. J. Comp. Neurol. 200: 1-21.

Trotier, D. and MacLeod, P. 1983. Intracellular recordings from salamander olfactory receptor cells. Brain Res. 268: 225-237.

Ts'o, D. Y., Frostig, R. D., Lieke, E. E. and Grinvald, A. 1990. Functional organization of primate visual cortex revealed by high resolution optical imaging. Science 249: 417-420.

Van der Loos, H. and Woolsey, T. A. 1973. Somatosensory cortex: Structural alterations following early injury to sense organs. Science 179: 395-398.

Van Essen, D. C. and Zeki, S. M. 1978. The topographic organization of rhesus monkey prestriate cortex. J. Physiol. 277: 193-226.

Wässle, H., Peichl, L. and Boycott, B. B. 1981. Morphology and topography of on- and off-alpha cells in the cat retina. Proc. R. Soc. Lond. B 272: 157-175.

Welker, C. 1976. Microelectrode delineation of fine grain somatotopic organization of Sm1 cerebral neocortex in albino rat. J. Comp. Neurol. 166: 173-190.

Woolsey, T. A. and van der Loos, H. 1970. The structural organization of layer IV in the somatosensory region (SI) of mouse cerebral cortex. The description of a cortical field composed of discrete cytoarchitectonic units. Brain Res. 17: 205-242.

Yau, K.-W. 1976. Receptive fields, geometry and conduction block of sensory neurones in the central nervous system of the leech. J. Physiol. 263: 513-538.

Yoshikami, S., George, J. S. and Hagins, W. A. 1980. Light-induced calcium fluxes from outer segment layer of vertebrate retinas. Nature 286: 395-398.

Zeki, S. M. 1978. The third visual complex of rhesus monkey prestriate cortex. J. Physiol. 277: 245-272.

Zeki, S. M. 1980. The response properties of cells in the middle temporal area (area MT) of owl monkey visual cortex. Proc. R. Soc. Lond, B. 207: 239-248.

Zeki, S. and Shipp, S. 1988. The functional logic of cortical connections. Nature 335: 311-317.

5. Motor Systems

Neuromuscular Control

The relationship between motor and sensory systems

Behavior is produced by motor systems. They allow the movement of the body and its parts, stabilize posture, and generate the drive for contractile inner organs. Motor systems translate neuronal activity into mechanical energy by controlling muscle activation in a precise way. In a sense this is the opposite process to sensory transduction, where stimulus energy is converted into neuronal signals. Despite this, motor and sensory processes are not really opposites. Neuromuscular control is expressed as a change in muscle contraction, but this requires a continuous flow of sensory information. This information flow is provided by exteroceptors, which monitor the interaction between the animal and its surroundings; and from proprioceptors, which monitor the position and relative movement of body parts.

Motoneurons control the activity of muscle fibers

Special nerve cells, the motoneurons, transmit neuronal signals to muscle fibers (Fig. 5.1). The skeletal motoneurons of vertebrates are among the most intensively studied of all neurons. They have a multipolar cell body which lies in the ventral horn of the spinal cord. Their efferent axon leaves the spinal cord via the ventral root and projects to the muscle fibers in the periphery. These spinal motoneurons receive synaptic input mainly on their dendrites and cell body where they also integrate these inputs, and then generate action potentials at the axon hillock, near the cell body. The skeletal motoneurons in invertebrates have a fundamentally different structure. These neurons are mostly unipolar, have a cell body which is often electrically inexcitable, and lies spatially isolated from synaptic inputs outside the integration zone of the neuropil. A thin neurite connects the cell body with the actual dendritic integrating segment where most of the synapses are formed. The membrane areas in this region of the neuron can be very heterogeneous. They can be excitable, inexcitable, or specialized for dendrodendritic synaptic transmission. The integrating segment is also the site where action potentials originate, and from which the efferent axon departs to innervate the musculature.

Not only the morphology of motoneurons, but also the types of neuromuscular signal transduction are surprisingly diverse. This diversity is obvious, for example, in the way in which a motoneuron makes contact with muscle fibers. Those motoneurons which innervate striated muscle fibers form synapses directly with the muscle cells. By contrast, those motoneurons which innervate smooth muscle do not form direct synapses, but terminate in axonal swellings (varicosities), from which transmitter is released nondirectionally. In many (but not all) vertebrate striated muscle fibers, only one synaptic contact region is form-

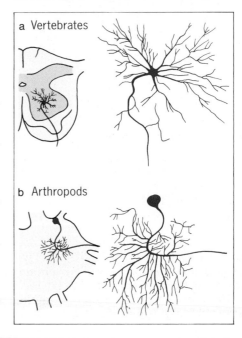

a Vertebrates

b Arthropods

Fig. 5.**1** Structure of motoneurons in vertebrates and arthropods (after Cullheim and Kellerth, and Reichert)

ed per muscle fiber, and is termed the *neuromuscular synapse or motor endplate.* In other striated muscle fibers, like the *multiterminally* innervated muscle fibers of many invertebrates or the tonic muscle fibers of vertebrates, each fiber is contacted by many synapses which can be distributed over the whole fiber. Finally, in invertebrates a muscle fiber can also be *polyneuronally* innervated by several motoneurons (Fig. 5.2).

In general, a single motoneuron innervates several muscle fibers so that the motoneuron and its postsynaptic muscle fibers form a *motor unit.* The number of muscle fibers belonging to a motor unit can vary from one to more than a thousand.

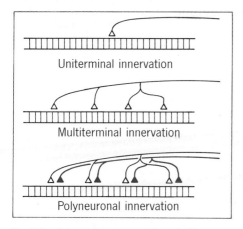

Fig. 5.2   Schematic representation of different patterns of neuromuscular innervation. Uniterminal and multiterminal innervation occur in vertebrates and invertebrates; polyneuronal innervation occurs in invertebrates

The motor endplate is a specialized synapse

In the skeletal muscles of vertebrates each action potential in the presynaptic motoneuron produces an action potential in the postsynaptic muscle fiber. This action potential then propagates regeneratively along the whole muscle fiber. In this case the neuromuscular synapse is structurally and functionally specialized for 1:1 signal transfer (Fig. 5.3). This synaptic signal transmission is an all-or-nothing phenomenon, like the signal conduction in an axon. The requirement for an all-or-nothing transmission explains why the *endplate potential* (a postsynaptic potential) that is evoked in the muscle fiber by a presynaptic action potential has to be so unusually large (p. 77).

At other neuromuscular synapses like the multiterminally innervated tonic vertebrate muscles, a presynaptic action potential produces only a postsynaptic depolarization in the muscle fiber. However, since these are generated at numerous synaptic contact points, they can spread electrotonically over the whole muscle fiber. The greatest diversity in the types of neuromuscular transmission is seen in the invertebrates, where a presynaptic action potential can lead to a graded postsynaptic potential, a regenerative all-or-nothing action potential, or a graded regenerative postsynaptic response, depending on the type of muscle fiber innervated.

Apart from the various electrical properties of the muscle fiber membrane, the contractile and morphological properties of the different muscle fiber types also contribute significantly to the diversity of possible neuromuscular control mechanisms. There are fast-contracting, phasic, muscle fibers. There are also slow-contracting, tonic, muscle fibers. There are muscle fibers which can be induced into a maintained contraction state *(catch),* and in the asynchronous flight muscles of some insects there are even muscles whose contraction must be triggered by prior stretching.

An excitation–contraction process in the muscle fiber converts the neuronal signal into mechanical contraction

The contraction of a muscle fiber is initiated by the depolarization of the muscle cell membrane. But exactly how does this occur? The coupling between membrane depolarization and mechanical contraction has been most intensively studied in the skeletal muscle fibers of vertebrates. The depolarization of the cell membrane is assumed to invade the muscle fiber via the T-tubules, and from there cross over to the sarcoplasmic reticulum. As a result, Ca^{2+} channels in the membrane of the sarcoplasmic reticulum open transiently, and Ca^{2+} flows out of the sarcoplasmic reticulum and into the cytoplasm. This results in a temporary increase in the Ca^{2+} concentration in the cytoplasm, which in turn activates regulatory Ca^{2+}-binding proteins, especially the troponin–tropomyosin complex. Conformational changes in these regulatory proteins allow the cross-bridges between actin and myosin to form, and the active sliding between actin and myosin filaments can occur; the muscle fiber contracts. The contraction is ended when the level of free Ca^{2+} in the cytoplasm is lowered again by the active uptake of Ca^{2+} into the sarcoplasmic reticulum. Just as in signal transmission at chemical synapses, Ca^{2+} channels and changes in the intracellular Ca^{2+} concentration also play critical roles here.

Although the excitation–contraction coupling in phasic skeletal muscle fibers of vertebrates has been analyzed down to the molecular level, two facts must be emphasized:

— A complete reaction chain has not yet been formulated for the electromechanical coupling in these muscle fibers.
— The excitation–contraction process does not proceed in the same way in all muscle fiber types. In the muscles of molluscs, for example, there is no troponin. In the muscle fibers of protochordates the T-tubule system is missing. Many smooth muscle cells

even have no sarcoplasmic reticulum. The diversity of neuromuscular control mechanisms is obvious even at this level.

Neuromuscular control involves complex neural integration

Depolarization of the muscle cell membrane initiates the contraction of a muscle fiber. But how is the size of this depolarization, and therefore the strength of the contraction, controlled? In vertebrate striated muscles, an action potential in the motoneuron evokes a muscle action potential which generally leads to a single contraction of all the muscle fibers of the motor unit. As the frequency of action potentials increases there is a transition from single to maintained contractions. The prolonged activation of the muscle fibers by a rapid repetition of action potentials is called a tetanus. The strength of contraction of the motor unit can thus be controlled by *modula-*

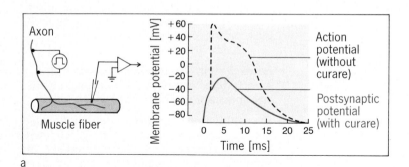

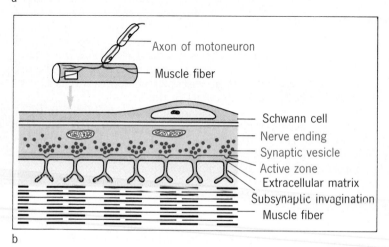

Fig. 5.3 Vertebrate neuromuscular synapse. **a** An action potential in the motoneuron leads to an action potential in the innervated muscle fiber. The large amplitude postsynaptic potential (endplate potential) can be revealed by blocking the action potential with curare. **b** Schematic representation of a cross section through the neuromuscular synapse (after Katz)

tion of the firing rate of the motoneuron. The tension which is produced by a motor unit can only be regulated over a certain range by modulation of action potential frequency in the motoneuron. This is because there is no gradation between inactivity and single contractions. A graded increase in the total tension of the muscle is therefore achieved by other means. A weak muscle contraction is typically controlled by motoneurons which belong to small motor units. Increasingly stronger contractions are achieved by additional activation of more or larger motor units. This method of regulating the muscle tension by progressively increasing the number of activated motor units is called *recruitment* (Fig. 5.**4a**). Since the size of a motoneuron (soma and axon) often increases with the size of the innervated population of muscle fibers, it is mostly the small motoneurons which are activated first during a muscle contraction; larger motoneurons only come into play with increased strengths of contraction.

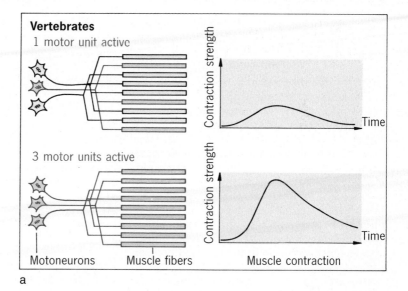

a

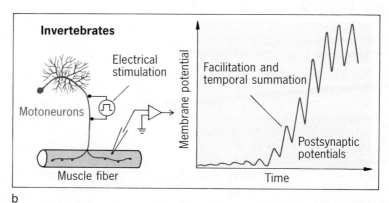

b

Fig. 5.**4**   Neuromuscular integration. **a** In vertebrates muscle tension is often controlled by changes in the number of active motor units. **b** In invertebrates the strength of muscle contractions is controlled over a broad range by modulating the frequency of presynaptic action potentials. This can occur because the neuromuscular synapse shows temporal summation and facilitation

In invertebrates, flexibility in neuromuscular control cannot be achieved through a large number of gateable motor units. In arthropods and some annelids, for instance, a given muscle is innervated by only one or a few motoneurons. In such cases the strength of contraction is regulated largely by modulating the frequency of presynaptic action potentials. This is also true for the tonic muscle fibers in vertebrates. Finely graduated and variable muscle contractions are possible because the neuromuscular synapses involved show a high degree of temporal summation and facilitation (Fig. 5.4b). The depolarization of the muscle fiber increases in a graduated way when the interval between presynaptic action potentials decreases. Additionally, in polyneuronal innervation, every muscle fiber is innervated by different excitatory motoneurons and sometimes also by inhibitory motoneurons. In such cases the neuromuscular synapses of the various motoneurons can have different properties. Excitatory motoneurons can evoke strong depolarizations with little facilitation and summation, or small depolarizations with considerable facilitation and summation. The activation of inhibitory motoneurons can even counteract a simultaneous excitation of the muscle fibers. This inhibitory action can result from direct postsynaptic inhibition of the muscle fibers, or from presynaptic inhibition of the excitatory motoneuron, or from both mechanisms together.

The motoneuron is the final common pathway in motor control circuits

What is special about motor systems is that the end result of all the motor information processing is directed onto a single target element, namely onto the motoneuron. As Sherrington pointed out, the motoneuron is the final common pathway, the final link, in the chain between stimulus and response. All neuronal signals, regardless of where they originate, must go via motoneurons if they are to have an influence on the musculature and therefore on behavior.

The requirement for simultaneous and coordinated activation of many muscles necessitates the orchestration of a whole ensemble of motoneurons, even for the simplest of movements. For every movement, even just turning over this page, agonistic, antagonistic and postural muscles must be controlled in a finely graded way, in the right sequence, and with the correct weighting. A few, out of the many possible options for making movements, must be selected and carried out. Adaptive responses must occur even to conflicting sensory stimuli. It is clear from this that a large number of neuronal control networks must act on the motoneurons to produce coordinated motor actions.

It is therefore no surprise that a single motoneuron can receive up to 10 000 synaptic input connections involving electrical transmission, chemical postsynaptic excitation, chemical postsynaptic inhibition, and chemical presynaptic inhibition. Through these synapses information from the whole body and from higher nervous centers converges onto the motoneuron. Each individual synapse only has a very small effect on the motoneuron, typically in the range of a few 100 µV. The suprathreshold excitation of a motoneuron therefore requires the more or less simultaneous input from many converging fibers. Important sources for this information are the peripherally situated proprioceptors, as well as central nervous motor centers, which in mammals are found in the brain stem, cortex and cerebellum.

Reflexes Are the Elementary Units of Motor Action

Principle and occurrence

Although the motoneuron is the final common pathway for motor action, this action is mostly controlled and coordinated by *premotor networks*. These networks can be quite complex. Early efforts to understand their mode of action were concerned with identifying the basic building blocks from which the motor control systems are constructed. In many respects the *reflex pathway* can be considered as one of these building blocks. In its simplest form a reflex pathway consists of a direct connection between a presynaptic sensory neuron and a postsynaptic motoneuron. Reflex pathways of this type are found in the most primitive of coelenterate nervous systems. Similar simple reflex circuits lie embedded in the complex motor circuits of the most highly evolved vertebrates. The concept of a reflex, first formulated in an overly mechanistic way by Descartes, acquired major significance through the work of

Sherrington on mechanisms of spinal integration. The finding that the reflex is the *fundamental unit of reaction* in neuronal integration also originates from Sherrington.

Motor activity is a graded function of the reflex-releasing stimulus

A reflex action is a simple, largely stereotyped, motor action evoked by a sensory stimulus. In general, it is a graded function of the releasing stimulus, both in its strength, and in its spatial and temporal extent (Fig. 5.5). In a sea anemone, a light touch to one of the tentacles leads to a slow tentacle retraction which generally lasts only a short while. Strong mechanical stimulation of the same tentacle, however, leads to a rapid (for an anemone) and maintained withdrawal of this tentacle and the neighboring tentacles, as well as the stalk. The extension of the reflex action to larger and larger areas of the motor apparatus as the stimulus strength increases is called *radiation*. Reflexes can proceed "automatically," that is, without being initiated by higher nervous centers. Consider the familiar knee-jerk reflex which cannot be consciously initiated or suppressed. However, this does not mean that reflex pathways function in isolation from other parts of the nervous system. The opposite is the case.

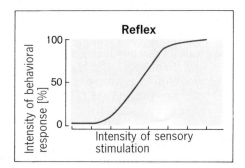

Fig. 5.**5**   The strength and extent of reflex actions are generally a graded function of the initiating stimulus (after Kandel)

The monosynaptic reflex is the simplest form of motor control

Monosynaptic extension reflexes belong to the most elementary form of motor responses. Figure 5.6 shows two examples. The *stretch receptors* in the abdomen of the crayfish are excited

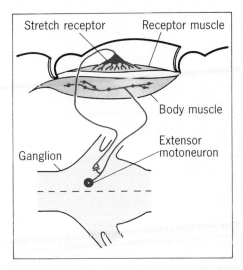

Fig. 5.**6a**   Monosynaptic stretch reflexes. Crustacean stretch receptors respond to bending of the abdomen. The stretch receptors form monosynaptic connections with extensor motoneurons which mediate the extension of the abdomen

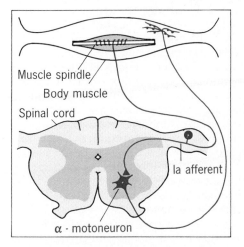

Fig. 5.**6b**   The Ia afferents of the vertebrate muscle spindle respond to muscle stretch. Ia afferents form monosynaptic connections with α-motoneurons which mediate a contraction of the functional working muscle

by bending of the abdomen. These stretch receptors make direct, monosynaptic, connections with extensor motoneurons which cause a stretching of the abdomen. As a result of this simple monosynaptic reflex pathway, a bending of the abdomen caused by external influences can be automatically compensated for. In vertebrates the large, fast-conducting, sensory neurons which innervate the muscle spindles of the skeletal musculature are called *Ia afferents*. They are excited by stretching of the intrafusal receptor muscle fibers of the muscle spindles. The motoneurons which innervate the extrafusal functional musculature are called α *motoneurons*. Ia afferents make direct, monosynaptic, connections with the α motoneurons, which in turn innervate those muscles in which the relevant muscle spindles lie. If a muscle is stretched by external influences, then the Ia afferents are activated. These excite the α motoneurons via the monosynaptic reflex pathway, and the motoneurons then cause a compensatory contraction of the musculature.

There is a feedback system present in both the extension reflex of crustacea and the *myotactic reflex* of vertebrates, which produces a reflex contraction in response to a stretching of the muscle. Such a compensating system could serve to keep a given muscle length constant (length-stabilizing control system), and thereby contribute to the maintenance of a body position. But this is not the only function of this reflex pathway. The synaptic excitation which continually impinges on the α motoneurons from the Ia afferents also contributes, for example, to maintaining the motoneurons at a base level of excitation. This is important for the maintenance of *muscle tone,* that is, the partially contracted state which is present in muscle even without active movement.

Even this simplified account shows that the monosynaptic connection between sensory and motor neurons can fulfill various motor control functions. This becomes clearer on closer examination of the synaptic connections which are formed between Ia afferents and spinal motoneurons.

Stretch reflexes control and coordinate the activity of musculature

The Ia afferents are the starting point for considerable neuronal divergence. In the gastrocnemius muscle of the cat, a given Ia afferent sensory neuron forms monosynaptic connections with all the α motoneurons which innervate the muscle—about 300 motoneurons. In addition, this sensory neuron forms monosynaptic connections with α motoneurons which innervate other, synergistically active, muscles. Finally, via monosynaptic excitatory connections with *Ia inhibitory interneurons,* which themselves inhibit the α motoneurons of antagonistically acting muscles, a disynaptic inhibition of antagonists occurs. The Ia afferents therefore contribute directly to the regulation of tension in their own muscle, and to the activation of synergistic, and inhibition of antagonistic, muscles. They are also involved indirectly and polysynaptically in the excitation and inhibition of many other motoneurons. The activation of the Ia afferents by a deformation of the muscle can therefore have widespread motor effects. However, this is not all just a "one-way street." The Ia afferents can themselves be influenced by motor efferents.

The sensory terminals of the Ia afferents lie embedded in the intrafusal muscle fibers of the muscle spindles. These intrafusal muscle fibers are innervated in many cases by γ *motoneurons* (Fig. 5.**7a**). The γ motoneurons and the intrafusal muscle fibers together are called the *fusimotor system.* An activation of the γ motoneurons effects a contraction of the intrafusal musculature at both ends of the muscle spindle. This leads to a stretching of the dendrites

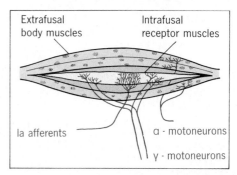

Fig. 5.**7a**   The fusimotor system. Ia afferents of the muscle spindle lie embedded in intrafusal receptor muscle fibers. The receptor muscle fibers are innervated by γ motoneurons

of the Ia afferents which lie in the middle of the muscle spindle, and therefore to their excitation.

During a neuronally driven muscle contraction, both α and γ motoneurons are activated together. This makes sense because during contraction of only the extrafusal musculature, the muscle spindles would slacken and therefore not be in a position to register changes in muscle length. By contrast, the *coactivation of α and γ motoneurons* provides for a contraction of the extrafusal body musculature while simultaneously keeping the muscle spindles at a sensitive setting (Fig. 5.**7b**). Ia afferents are therefore continually in a position to detect small changes in the established length of the muscle and compensate for these via reflex pathways. A similar type of control probably occurs in those muscles in which both the extrafusal and intrafusal muscle fibers are innervated by the same motoneurons ("β innervation").

Apart from those muscle extension reflexes which originate with the Ia afferents, a whole series of reflex pathways are activated by the *Ib afferents*. Ib afferents, also called Golgi tendon organs, have their sensory endings in the tendons of skeletal muscles. Due to their anatomical arrangement they are connected in series with the muscle fibers, and therefore better suited for registering muscle tension. This contrasts with the Ia afferents which are connected in parallel to the muscle fibers, and preferentially detect changes in muscle length. All the Ib afferent reflex pathways are polysynaptic. They act on motoneurons principally via spinal interneurons, and are spatially much more extensive than the Ia afferents. Further muscle reflex pathways originate from

— numerous joint receptors whose messages can be consciously (painfully) perceived
— smaller afferent fibers (II afferents) which innervate the intrafusal muscle fibers in a similar way to the Ia afferents
— receptor cells deep in the musculature
— cutaneous sensory cells

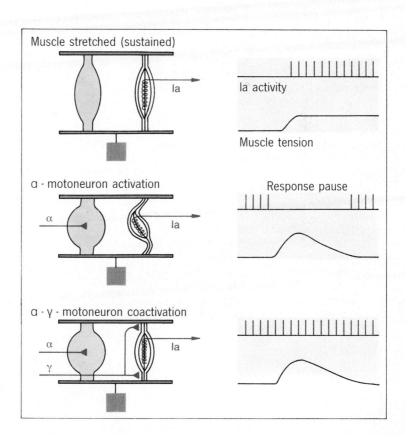

Fig. 5.**7b**   Ia afferents are excited by passive stretching of the muscle (top). Activation of the α motoneurons alone would lead to a relaxation of the muscle spindles and thereby to a decrease in their sensitivity (middle). Coactivation of α and γ motoneurons maintains the sensitivity of the muscle spindles (bottom) (after Camhi, and Hunt and Kuffler)

What purpose do the extension reflexes, the Golgi tendon reflexes, and other reflexes which commence with the muscle-associated proprioceptors, serve? Earlier ideas about an "efferent control via the γ loop" or an "inverse myotactic reflex via Ib afferents" are today being questioned. More recent results indicate rather that the primary function of the muscle receptor reflexes could lie in the regulation of muscle stiffness. But can there really be such a thing as only one function for a given reflex pathway? Considering the many circuits in the spinal cord which can be potentially activated, it is wise to be cautious with any single functional interpretation of reflex pathways.

Spinal reflexes are based on interneuronal connections

There is no doubt that elementary reflex pathways play important roles in motor control. In addition, there are many other interneuronal connections in the spinal cord which relay sensory information back to motoneurons, and so allow complex reflex actions to be generated. Although we are only now beginning to understand the diversity of spinal networks in vertebrates, some of these polysynaptic reflex pathways are already known:

— *Recurrent inhibition* (Fig. 5.**8a**). Reflex activation of an α motoneuron leads via the axon collaterals of this motoneuron to a prolonged excitation of an interneuron called the Renshaw neuron. The Renshaw neuron

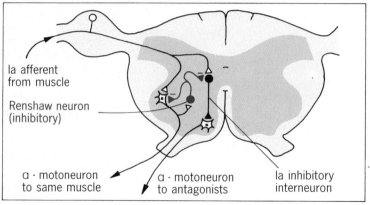

la afferent
from muscle

Renshaw neuron
(inhibitory)

α - motoneuron
to same muscle

α - motoneuron
to antagonists

la inhibitory
interneuron

a

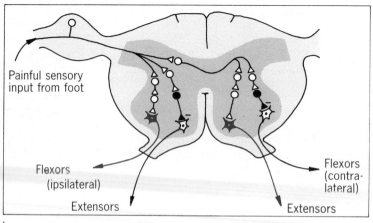

Painful sensory
input from foot

Flexors
(ipsilateral)

Extensors

Flexors
(contra-
lateral)

Extensors

b

Fig. 5.**8** Spinal reflex circuits, simplified. **a** Recurrent inhibition via the Renshaw neuron. **b** Interneuronal connectivity for the crossed extension reflex

then inhibits the motoneuron which excited it (negative feedback). Moreover, it inhibits many other synergistically acting motoneurons and inhibits Ia inhibitory interneurons, which themselves inhibit antagonistic motoneurons. The Renshaw inhibition could have several functional consequences. These include shortening the active phase of excited motoneurons; emphasizing the activity of strongly excited motoneurons as compared to weakly excited motoneurons; and disinhibiting antagonistically acting motoneurons.

— *Positive support reflex.* A light stimulation of the sole of the foot elicits a reflex activation of extensor motoneurons which encompasses the whole leg. This also activates spinal interneurons in several segments of the spinal cord. If the stimulus source is slowly moved, then the stimulated extremity follows the stimulus with an extension response. If contact is made along the way with a resistance, for example with the ground, then Ib afferent pathways are activated which elicit a co-contraction of extensors and flexors. This produces a pillar-like stiffening of the leg and can contribute to the support of the body.

— *Crossed extension reflex* (Fig. 5.**8b**). A painful stimulus to the sole of the foot of one leg can lead to the retraction of this leg, and a simultaneous reflex extension of the contralateral leg. This occurs because in addition to excitation of the flexor motoneurons and inhibition of the extensor motoneurons of the stimulated leg, there is a simultaneous excitation of the extensor motoneurons and inhibition of the flexor motoneurons of the contralateral leg. For this to happen, afferent information is conducted via spinal interneuron networks to the contralateral side of the spinal cord where it is transmitted in "inverted" form to extensor and flexor motoneurons.

The latter two examples show that differential stimulation of the same body part can activate completely different, and even opposed, spinal reflex pathways. This is feasible because of the many possible alternative connections which can occur at the level of the spinal cord. Taken together, the spinal networks can be compared with a huge train yard which consists of many, partially intersecting, tracks. The way in which a reflex-evoking stimulus travels through the spinal reflex networks and leads to a motor response may compare with the way in which an incoming train traverses the set of train tracks. Depending on the positioning of the switches, a different trajectory can result each time. But who sets the switches in the nervous system, and how?

Reflexes are subordinate to segmental coordination and descending control

The neuronal elements of the spinal cord constitute circuits which can generate coordinated motor activity. Coordinated activity at the level of a single spinal segment is mediated by *axon collaterals* which derive from the motoneurons and interneurons, as well as by local interneurons and local circuits. Intersegmental coordination is facilitated by short *propriospinal interneurons* which exchange information between homologous regions of neighboring segments. Long propriospinal interneurons which form extensive descending and ascending projections in the spinal cord are involved in the coordinated control of extensive regions of the body musculature (for example, the whole axial musculature).

In addition, control can also be exerted by descending fibers from the brain. Descending information channels which exit supraspinal centers can influence different components of the spinal circuitry to allow certain reflexes while suppressing others (Fig. 5.**9**). One way this can occur is via the direct action of descending fibers on the presynaptic terminals of the afferent neurons. Such axoaxonal connections can mediate a presynaptic inhibition of particular afferent information channels, and so establish an input selectivity. Descending control can also act directly on motoneurons and thereby strengthen or weaken reflexes. Descending excitation of a motoneuron can increase the effectiveness of a simultaneous sensory input (summation). Descending inhibition of a motoneuron can reduce the effectiveness of a sensory input.

Reflex selection and *gain control* can be achieved above all by descending control of spinal interneurons. The reflex pathway which a sensory input follows can be set in advance by the selective excitation of some interneurons and the selective inhibition of others. This optimizes the information processing during the

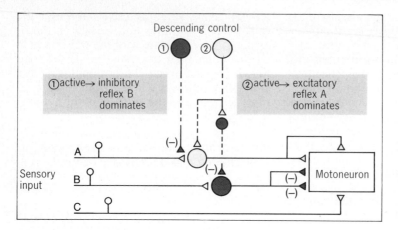

Fig. 5.**9**   Descending control over reflex pathways. A hypothetical, extremely simplified schematic for selection of a coordinated reflex by different descending control fibers. White circles = excitatory neurons, black circles = inhibitory neurons

short interval between stimulus and response. Descending control can activate certain populations of interneurons in changing combinations appropriate to ongoing motor activity. In this way reflexes can be centrally modulated in amplitude and polarity, as well as in their spatial and temporal expression. In this sense, the selection of different reflex pathways by descending connections resembles the selection of various subroutines in a complex computer program, or as said before, the setting of switches.

Neuronal Programs for Episodic Motor Activity

Relationship to behavior

The fact that spatially and temporally structured behavioral patterns can be preprogrammed into the networks of the nervous system is an important finding in neuroethology. An appropriate stimulus can activate these programs and so elicit the behavioral pattern. In the case of a few nonrhythmical, episodic behavioral responses, such motor programs have already been accounted for at the level of individual neurons. What is surprising is that even apparently simple episodic actions are based on a whole series of interacting neuronal mechanisms.

Motor responses of the all-or-nothing type are centrally preprogrammed

The search for the basic elements of behavior has revealed a second mode of action alongside the reflex mechanism. This motor response, termed the *fixed action pattern,* contrasts with the reflex in that it has all-or-nothing properties (Fig. 5.**10**). This means that the intensity of the releasing stimulus must first reach a critical threshold before the response is evoked. Above this stimulus threshold the response is generally elicited at full strength and with a stereotyped course. Dramatic examples of such motor actions are sneezing, vomiting, or orgasm. However, the classification of a behavioral response as being all-or-nothing does not mean that it always occurs in the same way. The response parameters can be influenced within certain limits by internal or external factors.

In a formal sense the release of a fixed action pattern can be considered the same as making a simple decision. Following the decision there is an activation of motor circuits which then evoke a coordinated discharge of neuromuscular excitation. In some cases the motor coordination can occur independently of further sensory input, for example, in rapid, ballistic attack or escape responses. Motor pattern generation in these circumstances is largely the product of central, "hard wired" circuits. In other fixed action patterns sensory feedback and synaptic plasticity play important organizational roles.

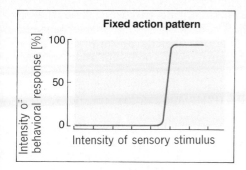

Fixed action pattern

Fig. 5.**10**   All-or-nothing properties of a fixed action pattern. Below the threshold value there is no response; above threshold the response occurs at full strength (after Kandel)

Command neurons can evoke coordinated motor response components

In some cases important neuronal elements of the circuits which activate a fixed action pattern can be localized within the CNS. For example, in the escape responses controlled by giant fiber systems, identifiable neurons initiating the response are, by virtue of their position in the circuit, the "decision-makers." Most of the giant fiber systems which have been studied in annelids, molluscs, insects and a few lower vertebrates function along similar principles (Fig. 5.**11**). Escape-initiating input signals synapse convergently onto the giant fiber, having first passed through a sensory filter network. Activation of the giant fiber, in some cases by a single action potential, is then sufficient to initiate what appears to be a complete behavioral response element.

Often the activation of the "command-ing" giant fiber is not only sufficient, but also necessary for the initiation of a particular component of the escape response. This means that the corresponding behavior can only be evoked by activation of that giant fiber. In other cases the activity of whole aggregates of neurons, rather than of single cells, is necessary to evoke particular responses. Further, there are neurons which do not function as initiators, but which must be tonically active for particular motor responses to occur. Permissive command elements like these are often involved in the control of body posture or limb position.

Strictly speaking, giant fibers are neither sensory nor premotor interneurons, but should rather be seen as interneurons with decision-making and command functions. In the simplest case they are the focus of sensory convergence, and so function as decision-making elements in that they respond to preprocessed sensory information in either a subthreshold or suprathreshold way. If the neurons are excited above threshold then the decision falls in favor of a preprogrammed action. The command function of these neurons becomes effective in this case because of their hierarchically dominant position in the motor pathway.

Although certain components of the response can be initiated by giant fibers or functionally similar neurons in other systems, it should be emphasized that single command neurons never produce a complete behavioral response. No single neuron alone can evoke a behavior. The cells which are called command neurons produce their amazing effects by activating a whole chain of neuronal circuits. In the final instance, it is the state of these circuits as determined by sensory feedback and feedforward, by motor control networks acting in parallel, by neuromodulators and hormones, and by a multitude of descending signals from the brain, which is decisive for the evoked behavior.

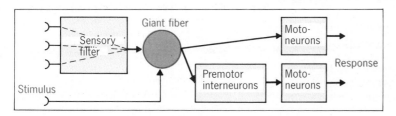

Fig. 5.**11**   Simplified representation of the organization of the giant fiber systems for escape behavior

Spatial coordination can be represented in synaptic connectivity

Preprogrammed episodic motor activity, even when it is initiated by single neurons, can proceed in a highly coordinated way. A good example is the escape response of the crayfish which is initiated by giant fiber systems. There are two pairs of giant fibers in the crayfish which can initiate rapid tailflips. Both giant fibers of each pair are coupled into a single functional unit by reciprocal electrical synapses. The two medial giant fibers receive their input from sensory cells in the anterior region of the animal. They initiate a tailflip that moves the animal rapidly backward. The two lateral giant fibers receive their input from sensory cells in the posterior region of the animal. They initiate a tailflip that propels the animal forward. The different orientation of the two escape responses makes behavioral sense and can be explained by the different connectivity patterns the giant fibers make with postsynaptic neurons in the abdomen (Fig. 5.12). The medial giant fibers form electrical synapses with the giant flexor motoneurons in all abdominal segments. The lateral giant fibers on the other hand only form synapses of this type with the giant flexor motoneurons in the first three abdominal segments. If the medial giant fibers fire, then all flexor motoneurons are excited. This leads to a flexion of all abdominal segments, the abdomen bends, and a tailflip is generated which drives the animal backward. If on the other hand the lateral giant fibers fire, then the posterior segments of the abdomen receive no motor drive, and they remain extended. Most of the force generated by the tailflip is therefore directed downward, and as a result the animal is propelled forward and away.

The *Mauthner neuron system* of many fish is constructed in a similar way. It is responsible for the startle response of these animals to sudden vibratory stimuli. Every animal has two bilaterally symmetrical Mauthner neurons whose cell bodies and dendrites lie in the medulla oblongata. Each Mauthner neuron receives sensory input from the ipsilateral auditory and vestibular systems. Its axon descends in the spinal cord and projects onto the motoneurons of the contralateral tail musculature. If a Mauthner neuron is excited above threshold, there is a contraction of the tail musculature on the opposite side of the body, which results in a rapid tail flip oriented away from the stimulus source.

In these two cases the trajectory of the response is prefigured by the synaptic connectivity of the giant fiber systems. This is advantageous for escape responses because only a short time is spent organizing an appropriate first response. The threatened animal can respond quickly and in this way gains a little time to "think" about what to do next.

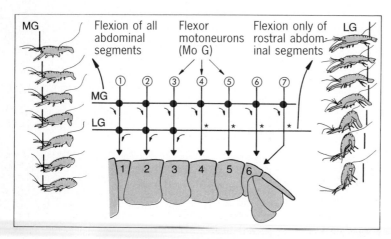

Fig. 5.12 Giant fiber systems in the crayfish. Medial giant fibers (MG) have a rostral receptive field and produce an escape response to the rear. Lateral giant fibers (LG) have a caudal receptive field and produce a forward-directed escape response. The different behavioral responses can be explained by the different connectivity patterns between the two giant fiber systems and postsynaptic motoneurons in the abdomen (after Wine)

Command-dependent inhibition has several functional roles

The job of command neurons does not end with the activation of the appropriate motor systems. As in most other motor systems, inhibition plays just as important a role here as excitation. In the rapid escape response of the crayfish for example, a widely distributed network of inhibitory interneurons is activated (Fig. 5.13). This command-dependent inhibition has at least four different functions:

— *Inhibition of antagonists.* Concomitant with the activation of the abdominal flexors, there is a short duration inhibition of abdominal extensors, and this is initiated both by centrally acting inhibitory interneurons and by peripherally acting inhibitory motoneurons. This inhibition originates from the giant fibers and prevents a disrupting contraction of the antagonistic extensor muscles during the flexion phase. Via as yet undescribed polysynaptic connections, the giant fibers cause an additional longer-term inhibition of all those motor subsystems whose activity could disrupt the escape response. The tonic postural system, for example, undergoes command-dependent inhibition.

— *Temporal scaling of flexion.* Following activation of the abdominal flexor muscles by the giant fibers, and after contraction of the flexor musculature, there is a delayed inhibition of these motoneurons (central inhibition) and muscles (peripheral inhibition). This inhibition also originates from the giant fibers and is distributed by polysynaptic interneuronal networks. This inhibition terminates flexion at the appropriate time and so allows subsequent responses to occur.

— *Termination.* The giant fiber system is designed to initiate an episodic response and is not suited for the generation of cyclically repeated responses. For this purpose other, rhythmically active, motor systems are employed. Recurrent inhibition mediates an auto-suppression of the giant fiber to prevent it from firing repetitively on sensory stimulation, something which would otherwise significantly disrupt the response.

— *Sensory protection.* A rapid tailflip produces an enormous amount of sensory feedback which could swamp the highly sensitive mechanosensory system. The ensuing adaptation would greatly reduce the sensitivity of this system. To prevent such a loss of sensitivity, the giant fibers produce both a presyn-

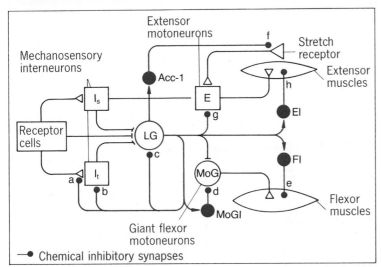

Fig. 5.**13**   Schema showing command-dependent inhibition in the escape system of the crayfish. An extensive inhibitory network emanates from the giant fiber (LG). Sensory afferents are presynaptically inhibited (a). Sensory interneurons (I_t) are postsynaptically inhibited (b). The giant fiber is recurrently inhibited (c). The giant motoneuron MoG is inhibited by the motor inhibitor (MoGI) (d). Flexor muscles are peripherally inhibited by the flexor inhibitor (FI) (e). Stretch receptors are peripherally inhibited by an accessory interneuron (Acc1) (f). Extensor motoneurons (E) are centrally inhibited (g). Extensor muscles are peripherally inhibited by the extensor inhibitor (EI) (f) (after Wine and Hagiwara)

aptic inhibition of sensory afferent terminals, and a postsynaptic inhibition of primary sensory interneurons.

The teleost Mauthner neuron system contains command-dependent inhibitory interactions which have a similar functional significance. In addition, the two Mauthner neurons interact via reciprocal inhibitory connections. This ensures that only one of the two neurons can be active at a given time. This is important since water-borne vibrations could otherwise excite both neurons, which would produce a simultaneous contraction of the whole tail musculature, and therefore result in an effective paralysis of the animal. This reciprocal inhibition is polysynaptic and occurs via both chemical and electrical inhibitory synapses, the latter having an unusual structure (Fig. 5.**14**).

Multiple levels of control ensure the flexibility of motor behavior

Animals are not robots. Fixed action patterns can proceed in a stereotyped way because they are centrally preprogrammed. However, this does not mean that the appearance of an adequate stimulus automatically results in the initiation of the corresponding fixed response. There is a set of conditions which codetermine the expression of episodic behavior. For example, the neuronal system required for a fixed action pattern might only be available for a limited period during the life of the animal. Further, this system might be blocked by the lack of activating neuroactive substances. The release of a fixed action pattern can also be subordinate to a circadian control. The stimulus threshold for the release of the response can be activity-dependent; for instance, it can be raised by habituation. Finally, competing motor programs can exert an internal control.

The most common form of internal control over episodic behavior is that emanating from higher centers in the CNS. Such centers are often the source of a *descending inhibition* of the circuits that initiate the response. This inhibition allows the release of a fixed action pattern to be flexible and adapted to the current behavioral state of the animal. For example, the escape response of the crayfish is suppressed by descending inhibition when the animal finds itself in the clutches of a predator, or out

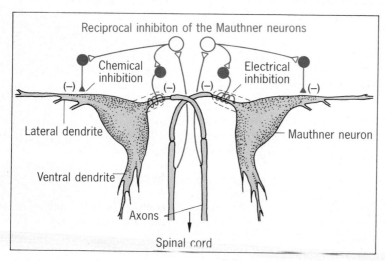

Fig. 5.**14**   Simplified representation of reciprocal inhibition in the Mauthner neuron system. Inhibitory neurons are activated via axon collaterals from each Mauthner neuron, and then chemically and electrically inhibit the contralaterally homologous Mauthner neuron

of the water. Tailflips under these circumstances are meaningless. The inhibition in this case is directed onto the giant fiber itself, which means that the rapid escape response is specifically suppressed, but not the sensory or motor system in general. The animal therefore remains capable of action and response. For obvious good reasons, an inhibition of the tailflip also occurs in gravid females whose eggs are attached to the underside of the tail.

Neuronal Oscillators Produce Rhythmic Motor Activity

Historical perspective

There are a multitude of motor responses which consist of rhythmically repeated units of action. Consider the different forms of locomotion like flying, swimming, and walking; or other rhythmically occurring motor activities like breathing or chewing. How are these behavioral units generated by the nervous system? Two very divergent concepts for the neuronal control of rhythmical motor activity arose around the turn of the century (Fig. 5.**15**). The hypothesis of peripheral control, founded by Sherrington, postulated the dominant role of coupled reflexes. Like a chain reaction, the initiating stimulus in a *chain reflex* should lead to an initial response via reflex action. This response itself forms a second stimulus which would then lead to a second response, and so on. By contrast, in the hypothesis of central control Brown postulated that rhythmical activity is produced by central circuits, by *neuronal oscillators*. These neuronal oscillators, also called *central pattern generators,* should be able to function rhythmically independent of sensory feedback.

Experimental evidence supporting both hypotheses has appeared over the years. However, what has become clear largely through the work of von Holst on swimming in fish and of Wilson on insect flight, is that there are neuronal oscillators which can produce rhythmical motor activity without depending on sensory feedback. We know today how widespread neuronal oscillators are. Every rhythmical motor activity which has been studied in detail can be traced back to the operation of a central neuronal oscillator. However, we also know that sensory information plays important roles in the expression of rhythmical activity. The controversy "peripheral or central control" has, thus, been resolved by a synthesis.

Pacemaker neurons are rhythmically active due to intrinsic cellular properties

Cellular properties can lead to a single neuron being rhythmically active on its own. The endogenous activity of such a *cellular oscillator* or *pacemaker neuron* is generally based on a cyclical interaction between various ion currents and channels. This interaction can be very complex (Fig. 5.**16a**). The result is a polarizing *endogenous rhythm*. There is no generally applicable scheme that can explain the mechanism of all cellular oscillators. Different endogenous cellular oscillators possess different ion channels, and function differently in their fine details. In addition, a range of other intrinsic cellular properties can contribute to the generation of rhythmical activity in individual neurons (Fig. 5.**16b**). These include

– the tonic baseline activity of the cell,
– accommodation of the spiking response evoked by depolarization,
– postinhibitory rebound, where neuronal firing is triggered by termination of inhibition, and
– the capacity to generate bistable membrane potentials. Besides the normal resting potential, some neurons can also assume a stable "plateau potential" above the threshold for action potentials. Extrinsic input can switch these cells backward and forward between the two potentials.

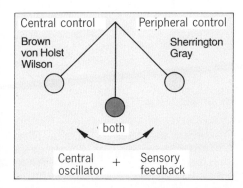

Fig. 5.**15**   Rhythmical behaviors are produced by central neuronal oscillators whose activity is modulated by sensory feedback. Earlier concepts emphasized either the central nervous, or peripheral sensory, component in rhythm production

Some cellular oscillators are not totally capable of firing rhythmically by themselves, and require an initial activation. This form of activation can be either synaptic or hormonal in nature. Such cells are termed *conditional* cellular oscillators. The activity of all pacemaker neurons studied to date can be influenced by synaptic input. This is because synaptic currents can interact directly with the rhythm-generating currents. It is through such interactions that a neuronal control of pacemaker cells is possible.

A rhythmically active pacemaker neuron could control the activity of a complete system. This requires the neuron to have appropriate connections with the system being driven. However, although endogenous oscillators are found embedded in rhythmically active motor networks, these cells do not dictate the whole rhythm. They are more like members in a "cooperative"; they contribute their capacity for endogenous oscillation to the cause of rhythm production.

Network oscillators can be rhythmically active due to specific connectivity

Neurons which produce rhythmical motor activity never do this in isolation. They are always incorporated into neuronal circuits. Such circuits often have properties which can lead to rhythmical activity even when no cellular oscillators are involved. Such emergent oscillatory properties are based on matching combinations of synaptic characteristics and specific connectivity patterns. In these cases we speak of *network oscillators*.

Various patterns of neuronal connectivity can lead to rhythmical activity. The principles on which they work can best be understood by considering some simplified model circuits. We will consider three types of rhythmically active circuits (Fig. 5.17). All three share the fact that, in addition to specific connectivity, various special properties have to be fulfilled for rhythmical activity to occur.

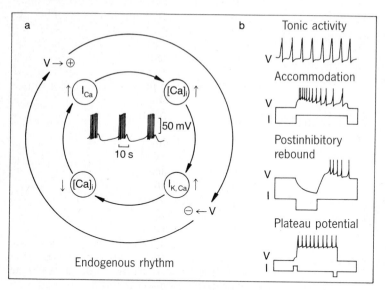

Fig. 5.**16**   Cellular oscillators. **a** The cyclical activity in a hypothetical endogenous oscillator can arise as follows. A slow depolarization leads to activation of a depolarizing Ca^{2+} current. This is regenerative and depolarizes the cell up to the threshold for action potentials. The cell begins to fire. The intracellular Ca^{2+} concentration increases, and Ca^{2+}-dependent K^+ channels become activated. An outwardly directed K^+ current repolarizes the cell to below threshold for the action potentials. The cell stops firing. Voltage-dependent Ca^{2+} channels become inactivated, the intracellular Ca^{2+} concentration drops, and the Ca^{2+}-dependent K^+ channels become inactivated. The cycle begins anew. **b** Further cellular properties which can contribute to the expression of endogenous rhythms in pacemaker neurons (after Gorman et al., and Selverston et al.)

In *self-excitatory networks* two or more neurons are linked to one another by excitatory synaptic connections. If the network has some preexisting tonic activity then positive feedback can lead to fluctuations in the activity of the neuronal assembly. This can then be converted to periodic activity if there is a restorative process which ensures that the network always returns to its initial state on reaching a critical discharge frequency. This restorative termination process can be realized, for example, by an inhibitory neuron which only reaches threshold at higher discharge frequencies of the excitatory neuronal assembly. Specialized ion channels in individual neurons can also function restoratively. Self-excitatory networks can only be monophasically active—all the neurons alternate rhythmically between being active or inactive.

Reciprocally inhibitory networks consist of neurons which are reciprocally connected to one another by inhibitory synapses. In the sim-

plest case such a network can comprise two reciprocally inhibitory neurons. These types of negative feedback networks oscillate when there is a constant maintained excitation of the reciprocally inhibitory neurons on the one hand, and there is a built-in process which allows the activity of single neurons to decrease following prior activity on the other hand. The tonic excitation can be produced by a third neuron which forms excitatory connections with the elements of the inhibitory network. The decline in activity can result from synaptic depression, from adaptation or from postinhibitory reactivation of the inhibiting partner neuron. Reciprocally inhibitory networks produce biphasic rhythms. There is an alternation of rhythmicity, with one part of the network active and the other inactive.

The generation of polyphasic rhythms is one of the features of *recurrent cyclical inhibitory networks*. These networks consist of several elements which are connected to one another in the shape of a ring by inhibitory synapses. In order to oscillate, the network must simply receive a tonic excitatory drive. One can follow the functioning of such a network in the form of a simple ring circuit consisting of three neurons as represented in Figure 5.17. Cyclically inhibitory networks do not require an additional restorative process. They can produce as many activity phases as there are ring elements, provided that there is an uneven number of elements.

In this simplified description we have assumed that network oscillators consist of "uniform" neurons which are connected to one another either excitatorily or inhibitorily in a stereotyped way. However, based on the cellular analysis of real neuronal oscillators, we know that the functioning of network oscillators can only be understood when the synaptic properties of the individual neurons are also considered. There is a whole spectrum of synaptic properties which various neurons employ to generate rhythmical activity in network oscillators. These include

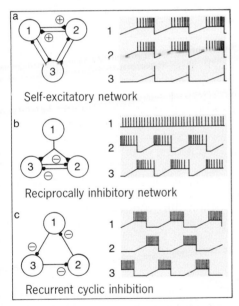

Self-excitatory network

Reciprocally inhibitory network

Recurrent cyclic inhibition

Fig. 5.**17** Types of rhythmically active circuits. **a** Excitatory connections between neurons 1 and 2 cause augmentations in their activity which are periodically terminated by the activity of an inhibitory neuron 3. **b** Inhibitory connections between neurons 3 and 2 produce periodically alternating activity. Neuron1 is responsible for tonic drive. **c** Three neurons which are linked into a ring by inhibitory connections produce triphasic rhythmical activity. Inhibitory synapses = black circles, excitatory synapses = black triangles (after Stent and Kristan)

— variability in the amplitude and time course of synaptic currents,
— synaptic transmission of passive, electrotonic potentials,
— variability in the coupling coefficients and rectifying properties of electrical synapses,
— transmitter-dependent activation of voltage-

gated ion channels in the postsynaptic cell, and

- multicomponent PSPs. These are characterized by the fact that the same transmitter substance has different effects on the postsynaptic cell, or that the same presynaptic cell releases two transmitter substances with different postsynaptic effects.

Central pattern generators are complex and integrate intrinsic, synaptic, and network properties during the production of rhythmical activity

To date, no known rhythmically acting motor system is controlled by a neuronal oscillator which employs just a *single* mechanism for rhythm generation. All the central pattern generators studied to date are *hybrid systems*. This can be exemplified using the neuronal oscillator for the rhythmical swimming movements of the sea snail *Tritonia*. As this is one of the few neuronal oscillators for locomotion to have been sufficiently explained at the cellular level, we shall consider it here in some detail.

Tritonia withdraws from the attacks of predatory starfish using a swim behavior which consists of rapid, alternating, dorsal and ventral flexions of the body (Fig. 5.**18a**). This relatively simple cyclical behavior is produced by an interneuronal central pattern generator which alternately drives the dorsal and ventral flexor motoneurons. Four bilaterally symmetrical groups of interneurons contribute to the neuronal oscillator. These are called C2, DSI, VSI-A, and VSI-B (Fig. 5.**18b**). The DSI activate the dorsal motoneurons, the VSI the ventral motoneurons. These interneurons are connected together in a complex network (Fig. 5.**18c**). Characteristic of this network is the presence of mainly chemical synapses with very different action times. Many of these synapses produce multicomponent PSPs. Thus the synapse from C2 onto DSI causes an excitation followed by an inhibition, while the synapse from C2 onto VSI-A produces an inhibition followed by an excitation. These multicomponent synapses play an important role in the temporal scaling of the oscillation. For example, in the early phase of a cycle they cause neuron C2 to excite its synergist DSI, and inhibit the antagonist VSI-A, while a little later the same C2 inhibits DSI and excites VSI-A. When VSI-A becomes active it in turn excites VSI-B, and both then contribute to the inhibition of the antagonistic DSI. One can also see that both self-excitatory connections (between VSI-A and VSI-B), and reciprocally inhibitory connections (between DSI and VSI-B), are built into this network.

This synaptic connectivity is important for the production of the rhythm; there are, however, several additional important factors. These are

- the type of adaptation of the action potential frequency in the individual neurons,
- the level of the activation threshold for neuron C2, and
- an intrinsic mechanism for delayed excitation in neuron VSI-B. This involves an intrinsic K^+ current ($I_{K,A}$) which is activated by synaptic depolarization and then slowly inactivates. This K^+ current leads to a delay in the formation of synaptically initiated action potentials and so forms a delay element in the network.

A coordinated rhythm is produced by the interplay of all these factors (Fig. 5.**18d**). It is possible to model the operation of this neuronal oscillator mathematically and generate a computer reconstruction of it. However, this is only successful when the experimentally obtained connectivity data, the membrane properties of the individual neurons, and the time course of the respective synaptic potentials are taken into account. Information about the activity pattern of the neurons alone is not sufficient for either a qualitative understanding, or a realistic simulation, of the network.

The neuronal organization of several other central pattern generators in various invertebrates is also quite well understood. These include the control network for the swimming behavior and the rhythmic heartbeat of the leech, the flight behavior of the locust, as well as the rhythmic gastric movements and heartbeat of the lobster. A complex organization is a distinguishing feature of all of these. Given this complexity in invertebrate central pattern generators, it is not surprising that little is as yet known about the cellular organization of neuronal oscillator circuits in vertebrates. What can be said about neuronal oscillators for locomotion in vertebrates is that they seem to be segmentally arranged in the spinal cord, and that they consist of interneuronal networks. The motoneurons seem to be merely ouput elements here and are not involved in rhythm generation.

Sensory feedback has multiple roles in shaping rhythmical activity

Rhythmic motor activity does not proceed in a completely stereotyped way. It must be constantly adapted to the actual behavioral state of the animal and to varying environmental conditions by sensory information. This requires that sensory information about the effector state and about the behavioral consequences of rhythmical activity be fed back into the CNS where it is then appropriately recombined with the activity of the neuronal oscillator. This sensory feedback can modify the *amplitude, phase or frequency* of the rhythmical program produced by the neuronal oscillator so that adaptive behavior results. For instance, sensory information about instabilities during the wingbeat of the locust has several flight-stabilizing consequences. Sensory feedback can lead to the recruitment of flight motoneurons and so influence the power of the wingbeat. It can also cause bilaterally homologous motoneurons to fire at different times in the wingbeat cycle, and so induce phase shifts in the positioning of the wings to influence flight steering. Sensory reflex pathways can even drive the interneurons of the central oscillator directly, and so produce a change in the wingbeat frequency. The end result of sensory feedback is a stabilized, aerodynamic, flight behavior.

The strength of the effects caused by sensory feedback can vary greatly in different rhythmical programs. While the influence of the central neuronal oscillator predominates in rhythmical activity which is largely independent of the environment, like stomach movements, in behaviors which are *strongly environmentally interactive,* like walking, the influence of sensory feedback is clearly dominant. During walking in the cat, sensory feedback changes various parameters involved in coordination in a cycle by cycle way, and so ensures a stable locomotion across uneven terrain. Moreover, sensory feedback is also critical for the transition from one phase to the next, and can even stop the whole rhythm in a particular phase, for example when a further step would endanger the balance of the animal.

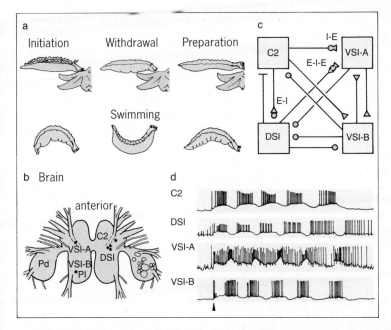

Fig. 5.**18**   The swimming behavior of *Tritonia* is produced by an interneuronal central pattern generator. **a** The escape behavior has several components. **b** Interneurons of the central pattern generator. C2, DSI, and VSI-A lie in the cerebral ganglion, VSI-B lies in the pleural ganglion (Pl). Swim motoneurons are aggregated in the pedal ganglion (Pd). All the neurons occur as bilateral pairs. **c** Circuit for the oscillator interneurons. Apart from simple synapses, multicomponent synapses are also found. (E = excitation, I = inhibition). **d** The rhythmical activity patterns of the oscillator interneurons during swimming behavior (after Getting)

Sensory feedback modulates not only the activity of the central pattern generator; it is itself under rhythmical control. During rhythmical activity, the same "hard-wired" reflex can be adaptive during one phase of the movement, but be non-adaptive during another phase. For this reason the strength of the reflex pathway must be adjusted rhythmically to the ongoing behavior. This adjustment is a product of the central neuronal oscillator. Such rhythmical adjustments can be phase-dependent increments or decrements in the strength of the reflex. It is even possible to have a phase-dependent *reflex reversal*. In a running cat, for example, cutaneous stimulation of the sole of the foot leads to excitation of flexors during one phase of the running cycle, and the same stimulus leads to excitation of extensors during another phase. The rhythmic channeling of sensory information is carried out by circuits in the spinal cord of the animal.

Coordination of oscillators is important for locomotion

The neurobiological analysis of locomotion, particularly in vertebrates, has lead to the concept of *multiple coupled oscillators*. It has been shown in fish and amphibians that all parts of the spinal cord are inherently capable of producing the alternating motor activity of swimming movements. The minimal circuit element required seems to be present in every segment. One therefore assumes that the overall system is built up in a modular way, and consists of unitary oscillators for each segment, or even hemisegment. The intersegmental phase shifts in motor activity characteristic for undulatory swim behavior result from a coordination between segmental unitary oscillators. The coordination can proceed in either a strictly phase-coupled way (absolute coordination) or be more weakly expressed, so that sliding phase shifts can also occur (relative coordination).

This concept also applies to locomotion in tetrapods. Here a separate oscillator is assumed to control each leg. Coordinating circuits ensure that the activity in contralateral and ipsilateral limbs match. The animal's various *gaits* (step, trot, pace, gallop, etc.) could result from changes in the coordination between the unitary oscillators (Fig. 5.**19**). The same is true for the switch from forward to reverse locomotion. Finally, the unitary oscillators for locomotion can be recombined into other behavioral patterns by appropriate coordinating circuits. For example, spinally controlled scratching behavior seems to consist of rhythmically occurring locomotory subroutines, which in this case are restricted to a single limb.

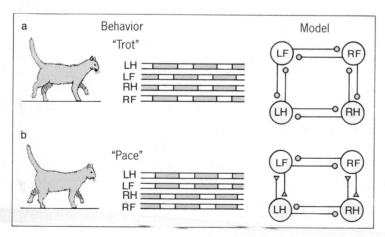

Fig. 5.**19** Coordination of individual oscillators. Very simplified model for the generation of different gaits. **a** Trot **b** Pace. Each leg is controlled by a unitary oscillator. Different gaits are produced by changes in the coordination between individual oscillators. LH = left hindleg, LF = left foreleg, RH = right hindleg, RF = right foreleg (after Pearson and Grillner)

Motor Control Is Hierarchically Organized

Overview of the various levels

In higher invertebrates there are several hierarchically arranged levels of motor control. The lowest level is that of the motoneurons. These are controlled by motor program circuits which are found in the largely segmentally located ganglia. (This group includes the neuronal oscillator circuits described above). These, in turn, are subordinate to the intersegmental command neurons, which are finally under descending control emanating from motor centers in the brain. Clinical studies, electrical brain stimulation of various experimental animals, and studies on the functional neuroanatomy of the vertebrate brain, are all in agreement that motor control systems in vertebrates are constructed in a similar hierarchical way. Higher organizational levels in the brain plan and decide the course of an action. They then influence intermediate levels, which themselves control the lowest levels of premotor interneurons and motoneurons.

Higher command centers activate and control segmentally organized premotor programs

The way in which an hierarchically structured motor system is organized can be clearly shown in higher mammals (Fig. 5.**20**). The neuronal networks in the *spinal cord* can be considered the lowest level of motor control. Simple stereotyped responses are produced here. The serially organized circuits of the spinal cord can generate behavioral components automatically, even when the spinal cord is separated from the brain. The next higher level of the motor hierarchy is the *brain stem*. Here descending motor command signals and ascending sensory information are processed and relayed onward. With the exception of the corticospinal circuits, most of the motor pathways which descend in the spinal cord have their origin in brain stem centers. Above the brain stem is the *motor cortex*. This part of the cerebral cortex lies in the region of the precentral gyrus in humans, and is an important starting point for preprocessed descending motor commands which are transmitted to the spinal

cord, the brain stem, and other subcortical centers. In addition, the behaviorally relevant components of information processing occurring in other cortical regions converge in the motor cortex. The *premotor cortical regions* can be seen as the highest level in the motor hierarchy. This level plays a critical role in deciding on a particular behavioral course of action, in the spatial localization of targets, and in the programming of movements. Intercortical connections, like those connecting the premotor areas to the prefrontal and postparietal regions of the cortex, are also substantially involved in target-oriented motor actions.

Typically, every control level in a motor hierarchy receives input from the body periphery. This allows descending motor commands to be modified by sensory information. The neurons of the motor cortex even have peripheral receptive fields which are similar to those of the somatosensory cortex. This underlines once more the close interdependence between motor and sensory pathways. But in other respects too, the organization of complex motor control systems has properties similar to those found in sensory systems. For example:

— The topographic organization of most motor systems. Neighboring circuit elements influence neighboring body parts. There are multiple copies of these topographic representations in cortical regions.
— The formation of modular neuron aggregations in cortical and subcortical regions.
— The possibility of higher levels in the motor hierarchy regulating the information flow which arrives from lower levels.

Sensory and motor systems are similarly organized in one further respect. In both cases the hierarchically structured organization is supplemented by parallel information processing.

Descending motor control is exerted via serial and parallel circuits

A direct consequence of the hierarchical organization of motor systems can be seen in the sequential way in which control processes occur. The premotor cortex influences the motor cortex, the motor cortex the brain stem, and the brain stem in turn, the spinal cord. However, as well as this type of organization, in which the higher organizational level controls the respective subordinate level, there are also parallel transmission channels through which a superior level can act directly and independently on every subordinate level. In this way higher motor control levels can intervene directly in programs running at the lowest levels: to command, modulate, or refine. For example, *corticospinal projections* allow the motor cortex to act directly on the interneurons, and in primates even on the motoneurons, in the spinal cord (Fig. **5.21**).

Corticospinal projections act on those spinal interneurons which are active during spinal reflexes. In this way the cortex can control entire reflexes. The direct connections between the cortex and spinal motoneurons allow the independent control of individual muscles. This is important for fine, manipulative performances which are carried out by the distal muscles of the body extremities. The extent and importance of the corticospinal connections increase with phylogeny in the mammals, and peak in the highest primates.

The parallel cooperation of numerous control centers allows not only the division of labor and specialization of motor subsystems, but also facilitates the functional recovery of motor control following lesions in the nervous system. For example, a partial coordination can still be carried out after the loss of a control center, by using intact motor systems acting via parallel channels.

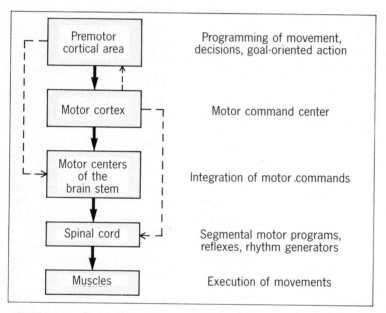

Fig. 5.**20** Simplified representation of hierarchically structured information transfer in the motor control system of higher vertebrates

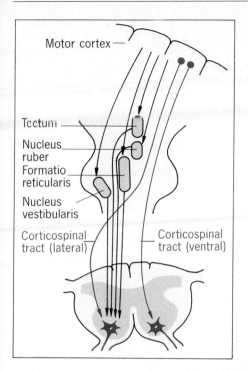

Motor cortex —

Tectum

Nucleus ruber

Formatio reticularis

Nucleus vestibularis

Corticospinal tract (lateral)

Corticospinal tract (ventral)

Fig. 5.21 Schematic showing descending motor control in primates. The motor cortex controls the spinal moto-neurons via parallel connections which project onto moto-neurons either indirectly via different brain nuclei, or directly via corticospinal pathways

Central feedback informs higher control centers about the implementation of programs at lower levels

The hierarchical organization of motor control systems differs from a rigid military hierarchy in at least two ways:

— In motor systems a subordinate level is not only controlled by its direct "superior," but also by all the other superior levels.
— The information flow in a motor hierarchy is not only unidirectional from top to bottom. Feedback circuits are widespread and en-sure that information is also transmitted from below to above (Fig. 5.22).

An important task of the motor cortex is the ini-tiation of movements. The motor cortex is in-formed about the implementation of these movements by multiple feedback circuits. One part of this feedback comes from the body pe-riphery. This sensory feedback originates from the activated muscles, or from proprioceptors in the joints and neighboring integument. However, there is also an *internal feedback* to higher centers from those interneuronal cir-cuits which are active during the implementa-tion of a given motor program. This internal feedback keeps higher centers informed about what is happening in subordinate processing levels. In this case the brain is following the motto "Trust is fine, control is better."

The cerebellum and basal ganglia are motor integration centers

Two processing centers which do not belong directly to the motor control hierarchy are im-portant for the coordination of motor activity in vertebrates: the cerebellum and the basal ganglia. The *cerebellum* has no direct connec-tions with the spinal cord. It contributes to the coordination of processing in the brain stem and motor cortex in that it acts as a comparator, comparing the descending motor command signals with the sensory messages coming from the motor response actually carried out. If a dis-crepancy arises between the "intended" and the "actual" values, the cerebellum can, via on-going error detection and correction, intervene in a regulatory way in the implementation of a movement. Apart from its role in sensorimotor coordination, the cerebellum also fulfills im-portant functions in the maintenance of bal-ance and the setting of muscle tone.

The exact way in which the *basal ganglia* function is not yet known. They receive signals from all cortical regions and act above all on the premotor areas of the cortex. Their basic ar-rangement is modular, and they are somato-topically organized. Diseases of the basal gan-glia lead to characteristic defects in motor per-formance. These are abnormal, uncontrolled, movements like tremor, chorea or ballism, a slowed occurrence of intended movements, and disturbances of muscle tone and postural reflexes. Some of these diseases are character-ized by disturbances in chemical transmitter systems. In Parkinson's disease there is a meta-bolic defect in the dopaminergic system. In Huntington's disease groups of cholinergic and GABAergic neurons in the striatum die.

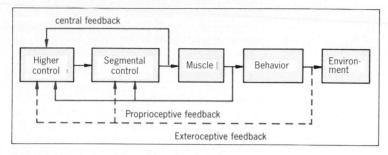

Fig. 5.**22** Simplified representation of information feedback in motor control systems

References

General Reviews

Barnes, W. J. P. and Gladden, M. H. (eds.) 1985. Feedback and Motor Control in Invertebrates and Vertebrates. Croom Helm, London

Bentley, D. and Konishi, M. 1978. Neural control of behavior. Annu. Rev. Neurosci. 1: 35-59

Bliss, D. E., Atwood, H., Sandeman, D. C. (eds.) 1982. The Biology of Crustacea. Academic, New York

Bush, B. M. H. and Clarac, F. (eds.) 1985. Coordination of Motor Behavior. Cambridge University Press, Cambridge

Camhi, J. M. 1984, Neuroethology. Sinauer, Sunderland

Carpenter, D. O. 1982. Cellular Pacemakers. Wiley, New York

Eaton, R. C. (ed.) 1984. Neural Mechanisms of Startle Behavior. Plenum, New York

Freund, H. J. 1983. Motor unit and muscle activity in voluntary motor control. Physiol. Rev. 63: 387-436

Friesen, W. O. and Stent, G. S. 1978. Neural circuits for generating rhythmic movements. Annu. Rev. Biophys. Bioeng. 7: 37-61

Gallistel, C. R. 1980. The Organization of Action: A New Synthesis. Wiley, New York

Getting, P. A. 1989. Emerging principles governing the operation of neural networks. Annu. Rev. Neurosci. 12: 185-204

Gewecke, M. and Wendler, G. (eds.) 1985. Insect Locomotion. Parey, Berlin

Grillner, S. and Wallén, P. 1985. Central pattern generators for locomotion, with special reference to vertebrates. Annu. Rev. Neurosci. 8: 233-262

Hasan, Z. and Stuart, D. G. 1988. Animal solutions to problems of movement control: The role of proprioceptors: Annu. Rev. Neurosci. 11: 119-224

Hoy, R. R. 1989. Startle, categorical response, and attention in acoustic behavior of insects. Annu. Rev. Neurosci. 12: 355-376

Hoyle, G. (ed.) 1977. Identified Neurons and Behavior of Arthropods. Plenum, New York

Hoyle, G. 1983. Muscles and Their Neural Control. Wiley, Somerset

Kandel, E. R., Schwartz, J. H. and Jessel, T. M. (eds.) 1991. Principles of Neural Science, 3rd edition. Elsevier, New York

Lorenz, K. 1970. Studies in Aninal and Human Behavior, Vols, I and II. Harvard University Press, Cambridge.

Lundberg, A. 1979. Multisensory control of spinal reflex pathways. Progr. Brain Res. 50: 11-28.

Mountcastle, V. B. (ed.) 1980. Medical Physiology, 14th edition Mosby, St. Louis

Pearson, K. G. 1976. The control of walking. Sci. Am. 235: 72-86.

Rothwell, J. C. 1987. Control of Human Voluntary Movement. Croom Helm, Beckenham.

Selverston, A. I. (ed.) 1985. Model Neural Networks and Behavior. Plenum, New York,

Selverston, A. I. and Moulins, M. (eds.) 1986. The Crustacean Stomatogastric System. Springer, New York.

Original Publications

Akazawa, K., Aldridge, J. W., Steeves, J. D. and Stein, R. B. 1982. Modulation of stretch reflexes during locomotion in the mesencephalic cat. J. Physiol. 329: 553-567.

Arbuthnott, E. R., Ballard, K. J., Boyd, I. A., Gladden, M. H. and Sutherland, F. I. 1982. The ultrastructure of cat fusimotor endings and their relationship to foci of sarcomere convergence in intrafusal fibres. J. Physiol. 331: 285-309.

Atwood, H. L. and Bittner, G. D. 1971. Matching of excitatory and inhibitory inputs to crustacean muscle fibers. J. Neurophysiol. 34: 157-170.

Atwood, H. L. and Morin, W. A. 1970. Neuromuscular and axoaxonal synapses of the crayfish opener muscle. J. Ultrastruct. Res. 32: 351-369.

Banks, R. W., Barker, D., Bessou, P., Pages, B. and Stacey, M. J. 1978. Histological analysis of muscle spindles following direct observation of effects of stimulating dynamic and static motor axons. J. Physiol. 283: 605-619.

Barker, D., Emonet-Dénand, F., Laporte. Y. and Stacey, M. J. 1980. Identification of the intrafusal endings of skeletofusimotor axons in the cat. Brain Res. 185: 227-237.

Barker, D., Stacey M. J. and Adal, M. N. 1970. Fusimotor innervation in the cat. Phil. Trans. R. Soc. Lond. B 258: 315-346.

Barrett, J. N. and Crill, W. E. 1974. Specific membrane properties of cat motoneurones. J. Physiol. 239: 301-324.

Barrett, J. N. and Crill, W. E. 1974. Influence of dendrite location and membrane properties on the effectiveness of synapses on cat motoneurones. J. Physiol. 239: 325-345.

Berthold, C.-H., Kellerth, J.-O. and Conradi, S. 1979. Electron microscopic studies of serially sectioned cat spinal α-motoneurons. J. Comp. Neurol. 184: 709-740.

Boyd, I. A. 1962. The structure and innervation of the nuclear bag muscle fibre system and the nuclear chain muscle fibre system in mammalian muscle spindles. Phil. Trans. R. Soc. Lond. B 245: 81-136.

Brigant, J. L. and Mallart, A. 1982. Presynaptic currents in mouse motor endings. J. Physiol. 333: 619-636.

Brown, A. G. and Fyffe, R. E. W. 1981. Direct observations on the contacts made between 1a afferent fibres and α-motoneurones in the cat's lumbosacral spinal cord. J. Physiol. 313: 121-140.

Brown, T. G. 1911. The intrinsic factors in the act of progression in the mammal. Proc. R. Soc. Lond. B 84: 308-319.

Buchtal, R. and Schmalbruch, H. 1980. Motor unit of mammalian muscle. Physiol. Rev. 60: 90-142

Buller, A. J., Eccles, J. C. and Eccles, R. M. 1960. Differentiation of fast and slow muscles in the cat hind limb. J. Physiol. 150: 339-416.

Burke, R. E., Walmsley, B. and Hodgson, J. A. 1979. HRP anatomy of group 1a afferent contacts on alpha motoneurones. Brain Res. 160: 347-352.

Burrows, M. 1980. The control of sets of motoneurones by local interneurones in the locust. J. Physiol. 298: 213-233.

Burrows, M. and Siegler, M. V. S. 1982. Spiking local interneurons mediate local reflexes. Science 217: 650-652.

Cheney, P. D. and Fetz, E. E. 1980. Functional classes of primate corticomotoneuronal cells and their relation to active force. J. Neurophysiol. 44: 773-791.

Crago, P. E., Houk, J. C. and Rymer, W. Z. 1982. Sampling of total muscle force by tendon organs. J. Neurophysiol. 47: 1069-1083.

Critchlow, V. and von Euler, C. 1963. Intercostal muscle spindle activity and its γ-motor control. J. Physiol. 168: 820-847.

Crowe, A. and Matthews, P. B. C. 1964. The effects of stimulation of static and dynamic fusimotor fibres on the response to stretching of the primary endings of muscle spindles. J. Physiol. 174: 109-131.

Czarkowska, J., Jankowska, E. and Sybirska, E. 1981. Common interneurones in reflex pathways from group 1a and 1b afferents of knee flexors and extensors in the cat. J. Physiol. 310: 367-380.

Deliagina, T. G., Feldman, A. G., Gelfand, I. M. and Orlowsky, G. N. 1975. On the role of central program and afferent inflow in the control of scratching movements in the cat. Brain Res. 100: 297-313.

Diamond, J. 1968. The activation and distribution of GABA and L-glutamate receptors on goldfish Mauthner neurones: An analysis of dendritic remote inhibition. J. Physiol. 194: 669-723.

Diamond, J. and Miledi, R. 1962. A study of foetal and new-born muscle fibres. J. Physiol. 162: 393-408.

Drew. T. and Rossignol, S. 1984. Phase-dependent responses evoked in limb muscles by stimulation of medullary reticular formation during locomotion in thalamic cats. J. Neurophysiol. 52: 653-675.

Dudel, J., Finger, W. and Stettmeier, H. 1980. ATPase activity in rapidly activated skinned muscle fibres. Pflügers Arch. 387: 167-174.

Dudel, J. and Kuffler, S. W. 1961. Presynaptic inhibition at the crayfish neuromuscular junction. J. Physiol. 155: 543-562.

Eaton, R. C., Bombardieri, R. A. and Meyer, D. L. 1977. The Mauthner-initiated startle response in teleost fish. J. Exp. Biol. 66: 65-81.

Eccles, J. C. and Sherrington, C. S. 1930. Numbers and contraction-values of individual motor-units examined in some muscles of the limb. Proc. R. Soc. Lond. B 106: 326-357.

Eldridge, F. L. 1977. Maintenance of respiration by central neural feedback mechanisms. Fed. Proc. 36: 2400-2404.

Emonet-Dénand, F., Jami, L. and Laporte, Y. 1980. Histophysiological observations on the skeletofusimotor innervation of mammalian spindles Progr. Clin. Neurophysiol. 8: 1-11.

Evarts, E. V. and Tanji, J. 1976. Reflex and intended responses in motor cortex pyramidal tract neurons of monkey. J. Neurophysiol. 39: 1069-1080.

Fatt, P. and Katz, B. 1953.. The effect of inhibitory nerve impulses on a crustacean muscle fibre. J. Physiol. 121: 374-389.

Fields, H. L., Evoy, W. H. and Kennedy, D. 1967. Reflex role played by efferent control of an invertebrate stretch receptor. J. Neurophysiol. 30: 859-874.

Frank, K. and Fuortes, M. G. F. 1957. Presynaptic and postsynaptic inhibition of monosynaptic reflexes. Fed. Proc. 16: 39-40.

Fuchs. P. A. and Getting, P. A. 1980. Ionic basis of presynaptic inhibitory potentials at crayfish claw opener. J. Neurophysiol. 43: 1547-1557.

Fukami, Y. 1982. Further morphological and electrophysiological studies on snake muscle spindles. J. Neurophysiol. 47: 810-826.

Fukami, Y. and Hunt, C. C. 1977. Structures in sensory region of snake spindles and their displacement during stretch. J. Neurophysiol 40: 1121-1131.

Furshpan, E. J. and Furukawa, T. Y. 1962. Intracellular and extracellular responses of the several regions of the Mauthner cell of the goldfish. J. Neurophysiol. 25: 732-771.

Furukawa, T., Fukami, Y. and Asada, Y. 1965. A third type of inhibition in the Mauthner cell of goldfish. J. Neurophysiol. 26: 759-774.

Furukawa, T. Y. and Furshpan, E. J. 1963. Two inhibitory mechanisms in the Mauthner neurons of the goldfish. J. Neurophysiol. 26: 140-176.

Garnett, R. and Stephens, J. A. 1981. Changes in recruitment threshold of motor units produced by cutaneous stimulation in man. J. Physiol. 311: 463-473.

Getting, P. A., Lennard, P. R. and Hume R. I. 1981. Central pattern generator mediating swimming in Tritonia. I. Identification and synaptic interaction. J. Neurophysiol. 44: 151-165.

Georgopoulos, A. P., Kettner, R. E. and Schwarz, A. B. 1988. Primate motor cortex and free arm movements to visual targets in three-dimensional space. II: Coding of the direction of movement by a neuronal population. J. Neurosci. 8: 2928-2937.

Heitler, W. J. 1978. Coupled motoneurones are part of the crayfish swimmeret central pattern oscillator. Nature 275: 231-234.

Henneman, E., Somjen, G. and Carpenter, D. O. 1965. Functional significance of cell size in spinal motoneurons. J. Neurophysiol. 28: 560-580.

Honig, M. C., Collins, W. F. and Mendell, L. M. 1983. α-Motoneuron EPSPs exhibit different frequency sensitivities to single Ia-afferent fiber stimulation. J. Neurophysiol. 49: 886-901.

Horak, F. B. and Nashner, L. M. 1986. Central programming of postural movements: Adaptation to altered support-surface configurations. J. Neurophysiol. 55: 1369-1381.

Houk, J. and Henneman, E. 1967. Responses of Golgi tendon organs to active contractions of the soleus muscle of the cat. J. Neurophysiol. 30: 466-481.

Hunt, C. C. and Kuffler, S. W. 1951. Further study of efferent small nerve fibres to mammalian muscle spindles: Multiple spindle innervation and activity during contraction. J. Physiol. 113: 283-297.

Hunt, C. C. and Kuffler, S. W. 1954. Motor innervation of skeletal muscle: Multiple innervation of individual muscle fibres and motor unit function. J. Physiol. 126: 293-303.

Huxley, H. E. 1969. The mechanism of muscular contraction. Science 164: 1356-1366.

Jack, J. J. B., Redman, S. J. and Wong, K. 1981. The components of synaptic potentials evoked in cat spinal motoneurones by impulses in single group Ia afferents. J. Physiol. 321: 65-96.

Jankowska, E. and McCrea, D. A. 1983. Shared reflex pathways from 1b tendon organ afferents and 1a muscle spindle afferents in the cat. J. Physiol. 338: 99-112.

Jankowska, E., Padel, Y. and Tanaka, R. 1976. Disynaptic inhibition of spinal motoneurones from the motor cortex in the monkey. J. Physiol. 258: 467-487.

Jansen, J. K. S. and Matthews, P. B. C. 1962. The central control of the dynamic response of muscle spindle receptors. J. Physiol. 161; 357-378.

Jones, E. G. and Wise, S. P. 1977. Size, laminar and columnar distribution of the efferent cells in the sensory-motor cortex of monkeys. J. Comp. Neurol. 175: 391-438.

Katz, B. 1949. The efferent regulation of the muscle spindle in the frog. J. Exp. Biol. 26: 201-217.

Katz, B. 1950. Depolarization of sensory terminals and the initiation of impulses in the muscle spindle. J. Physiol. 111: 261-282.

Kirkwood, P. A. and Sears, T. A. 1974. Monosynaptic excitation of motoneurones from secondary endings of muscle spindles. Nature 252: 243-244.

Kirkwood, P. A., Sears, T. A. and Westgaard, R. H. 1981. Recurrent inhibition of intercostal motoneurones in the cat. J. Physiol 319: 111-130.

Kirkwood, P. A. and Sears, T. A. 1982. Excitatory postsynaptic potentials from single muscle spindle afferents in external intercostal motoneurones of the cat. J. Physiol. 322: 287-314.

Korn, H., Triller, A. and Faber, D. S. 1978. Structural correlates of recurrent collateral interneurons producing both electrical and chemical inhibitions of the Mauthner cells. Proc. R. Soc. Lond. B 202: 533-539.

Kuwada, J. Y. and Wine, J. J. 1979. Cryfish escape behavior: Commands for fast movement inhibit postural tone and reflexes and prevent habituation of slow reflexes. J. Exp. Biol. 79: 205-224.

Landgren, S., Philips, C. G. and Porter, R. 1962. Minimal synaptic actions of pyramidal impulses on some alpha motoneurones of the baboon hand and forearm. J. Physiol. 161: 91-111.

Landmesser, L. 1971. Contractile and electrical response of vagus-innervated frog sartorius muscles. J. Physiol. 213: 707-725.

Landmesser, L. 1972. Pharmacological properties, cholinesterase activity and anatomy of nerve-muscle junctions in vagus-innervated frog Sartorius. J. Physiol. 220: 243-256.

Lang, F., Atwood, H. L. and Morin, W. A. 1972. Innervation and vascular supply of the crayfish opener muscle. Z. Zellforsch. 127: 189-200.

Liddell, E. G. T. and Sherrington, C. S. 1925. Recruitment and some other features of reflex inhibition. Proc. R. Soc. Lond. B 97: 488-518.

Lundberg, A., Malmgren, K. and Schomburg, E. E. 1975. Convergence from 1b, cutaneous and joint afferents in reflex pathways to motoneurones. Brain Res. 87: 81-84.

Matthews, B. H. C. 1931. The response of a muscle spindle during active contraction of a muscle. J. Physiol. 72: 153-174.

Matthews, B. H. C. 1933. Nerve endings in mammalian muscle. J. Physiol 78: 1-53.

Matthews. P. B. C. 1981. Evolving views on the internal operation and functional role of the muscle spindle. J. Physiol. 320: 1-30.

Mendell, L. M. and Henneman, E. 1971. Terminals of single Ia fibers: Location, density, and distribution within a pool of 300 homonymous motoneurons. J. Neurophysiol. 34: 171-187.

Mittenthal, J. E. and Wine, J. J. 1973. Connectivity patterns of crayfish giant interneurons: visualization of synaptic regions with cobalt dye. Science 179: 182-184.

Mountcastle, V. B., Lynch, J. C., Georgopoulos, A., Sakata, H. and Acuna, C. 1975. Posterior parietal association cortex of the monkey: Command functions for operations within extrapersonal space. J. Neurophysiol. 38: 871-908.

Muir, R. B. and Lemon, R. N. 1983. Corticospinal neurons with a special role in precision grip. Brain Res. 261: 312-316.

Muller, K. J. and McMahan, U. J. 1976. The shapes of sensory and motor neurones and the distribution of their synapses in ganglia of the leech: A study using intracellular injection of horseradish peroxidase. Proc. R. Soc. Lond. B 194: 481-499.

Nagy, F., Dickinson, P. S. and Moulins, M. 1988. Control by an identified modulatory neuron of the sequential expression of plateau properties of, and synaptic inputs to, a neuron in a central pattern generator. J. Neurosci. 8: 2875-2886.

Nichols, T. R. and Houk, J. C. 1976. Improvement in linearity and regulation of stiffness that results from actions of stretch reflex. J. Neurophysiol. 39: 119-142.

Polit, A. and Bizzi, E. 1978. Processes controlling arm movements in monkeys. Science 201: 1235-1237.

Prochazka, A., Hulliger, M. Zangger and P. Appenteng, K. 1985. "Fusimotor Set": New evidence for α-independent control of γ-motoneurones during movement in the awake cat. Brain Res. 339: 136-140.

Pearson, K. G. 1972. Central programming and reflex control of walking in the cockroach. J. Exp. Biol. 56: 173-193.

Pearson, K. G., Heitler, W. J. and Steeves, J. D. 1980. Triggering of locust jump by multimodal inhibitory interneurons. J. Neurophysiol. 43: 257-278.

Pearson, K. G. and Iles, J. F. 1970. Discharge patterns of coxal levator and depressor motoneurons of the cockroach Periplaneta americana. J. Exp. Biol. 52: 139-165.

Poritsky, R. 1969. Two and three dimensional ultrastructure of boutons and glial cells on the motoneuronal surface in the cat spinal cord. J. Comp. Neurol. 135: 423-452.

Reichert, H. and Wine, J. J. 1982. Neural mechanisms for serial order in a stereotyped behaviour sequence. Nature 196: 86-87.

Reichert, H. and Wine, J. J. 1983. Coordination of lateral giant and non-giant systems in crayfish escape behavior. J. Comp. Physiol. 153: 3-15.

Reichert, H., Wine, J. J. and Hagiwara, G. 1981. Crayfish escape behavior: Neurobehavioral analysis of phasic extension reveals dual systems for motor control. J. Comp. Physiol. 142: 281-294.

Renshaw, B. 1940. Activity in the simplest spinal reflex pathways. J. Neurophysiol. 3: 373-387.

Renshaw, B. 1941. Influence of discharge of motoneurons upon excitation of neighboring motoneurons. J. Neurophysiol. 4: 167-183.

Robertson, J. D. 1963. The occurrence of a subunit pattern in the unit membranes of club endings in Mauthner cell synapses in goldfish brains. J. Cell Biol. 19: 201-221.

Robertson, J. D., Bodenheimer, T. S. and Stage, D. E. 1963. The ultrastructure of Mauthner cell synapses and nodes in goldfish brains. J. Cell Biol. 19: 159-199.

Robertson, R. M. and Moulins, M. 1981. Firing between two spike thresholds: Implications for oscillating lobster interneurons. Science 214: 941-943.

Robertson, R. M., Pearson, K. G. and Reichert, H. 1982. Flight interneurons in the locust and the origin of insect wings. Science 217: 177-179.

Sherrington, C. S. 1898. Decerebrate rigidity, and reflex coordination of movements. J. Physiol. 22: 319-332.

Sears, T. A. 1964. Efferent discharges in alpha and fusimotor fibers of intercostal nerves of the cat. J. Physiol. 174: 295-315.

Sears, T. A. 1964. The slow potentials of thoracic respiratory motoneurones and their relation to breathing. J. Physiol. 175: 404-424.

Shik, M. L., Severin, F. V. and Orlovsky, G. N. 1966. Control of walking and running by means of electrical stimulation of the mid-brain. Biofizika 11: 659-666.

Stent, G. S., Kristan, W. B., Friesen, W. O., Ort, C. A., Poon, M. and Calabrese, R. L. 1978. Neuronal generation of the leech swimming movement. Science 200: 1348-1357.

von Euler, C. 1977. The functional organization of the respiratory phaseswitching mechanisms. Fed. Proc. 36: 2375-2380.

Wallén. P. and Grillner, S. 1987. N-methyl-D-aspartate receptor induced, inherent oscillatory activity in neurons active during fictive locomotion in the lamprey. J. Neurosci. 7: 2745-2755.

Weinrich, M. and Wise, S. 1982. The premotor cortex of the monkey. J. Neurosci. 2: 1329-1345.

Westbury, D. R. 1982. A comparison of the structures of α- and γ-spinal motoneurones of the cat. J. Physiol. 325: 79-91.

Westin, J., Langberg, J. J. and Camhi, J. M. Responses of giant interneurons of the cockroach Periplaneta americana to wind puffs of different directions and velocities. J. Comp. Physiol. 121: 307-324.

Willard, A. 1981. Effects of serotonin on the generation of the motor program for swimming by the medicinal leech. J. Neurosci. 7: 936-944.

Wine, J. J. and Krasne, R. B. 1972. The organization of escape behaviour in the crayfish. J. Exp. Biol. 56: 1-18.

Wine, J. J. 1977. Crayfish escape behavior. III. Monosynaptic and polysynaptic sensory pathways involved in phasic extension. J. Comp. Physiol. 121: 187-202.

Wiersma, C. A. G. 1938. Function of the giant fibers of the central nervous system of the crayfish. Proc. Soc. Exp. Biol. Med. 38: 661-662.

Zucker, R. S. 1972. Crayfish escape behavior and central synapses. I. Neural circuit exciting lateral giant fiber. J. Neurophysiol. 35: 599-620.

6. Systems Integration

Sensorimotor Integration

Principle

Complex sense organs and motor control systems do not exist in isolation. Sensory information must be suitably recombined with motor activity in order to produce adaptive behavior. The task of carrying out such recombinations is the function of sensorimotor integration networks. Functionally, these networks are neither typically sensory nor motor, nor is the integration produced restricted to single, isolated structures. Coordinated sensorimotor integration is the product of a complex interaction between diverse neuronal processes. To give an impression of the enormous diversity of sensorimotor coordination processes, a few well-studied integration mechanisms will be considered.

Sensorimotor integration is essential for the control of directed locomotor activity

With the exception of a few ballistic movements which occur without sensory feedback, almost all target-oriented locomotory activity is modified by sensory information. This control is essential because a flying insect, a swimming fish, or a walking human will all invariably deviate from their course, either due to inherent asymmetries in their effector structures, or to diverting environmental influences. These course deviations must be detected and then corrected. Sensory messages concerning deviations must be processed and then compensated for at the motor level. This requires relatively complex sensorimotor integration networks. Some aspects of the organization of such networks have been studied on a relatively simple animal, the locust.

The flight steering system of the locust is based on neuronal circuits which can convert information about course deviations into stabilized flight behavior. The animal possesses a type of "autopilot" (Fig. 6.1a). Course deviations in flight are detected by a number of sense organs, such as compound eyes, simple eyes (ocelli), and many wind-sensitive hairs. The relevant information from all these sense organs converges onto a set of descending course-deviation detecting neurons in the brain. Each of these deviation detectors is programmed to signal a very specific type of course deviation, based on its own specific sensory input. The activity of these deviation detectors represents an error message which must subsequently be integrated with the activity of the flight motor to produce a correcting steering response. This requires that the deviation signal be phase-coupled with the oscillations of the flight motor, and then be transmitted with the appropriate synaptic sign to the correct motoneurons.

The correct recombination of sensory information with the centrally generated flight rhythm is carried out by a population of sensorimotor integration neurons. These interneurons receive their input signals from the deviation detectors and relay their output signals to flight motoneurons. These segmental interneurons are not just involved in a simple switching process because, apart from sensory input, they also receive rhythmically alternating excitatory and inhibitory drive from the neuronal flight oscillator. As a result of this rhythmical drive a phase-independent sensory deviation signal is matched to the phase-dependent activity of the flight motoneurons. At the same time the postsynaptic connectivity of these segmental interneurons ensures the automatic distribution of the now phase-coupled information to the currently active motoneurons. The consequences are the changes in phase and amplitude of the wingbeats necessary to produce balanced flight steering behavior.

Many segmental integration neurons are involved in this sensorimotor integration network. Some drive wing elevator motoneurons, others wing depressor motoneurons. The overall network has several important properties which are of general relevance (Fig. 6.1b).

– Sensory information reaches motoneurons only when the oscillator is active; in this

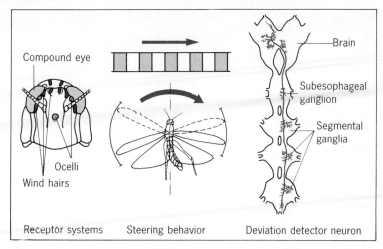

Fig. 6.**1a**   Sensorimotor integration in the locust. The autopilot for flight steering. Several sensory receptor systems detect course deviations (left). Processed information about course deviations is translated into steering behavior (middle). Descending deviation detector neurons relay information about course deviations from the brain to motor control centers in the segmental ganglia (right)

case that means when the animal is flying.
— A copy of the centrally generated motor rhythm is used for controlling the flow of sensory information. By switching rhythmically back and forth, the neuronal oscillator distributes the same sensory information alternatively to different motoneurons.
— The same sensory information can lead to inhibition as well as to excitation of motoneurons since various segmental interneurons can have opposite synaptic effects on different motoneurons.

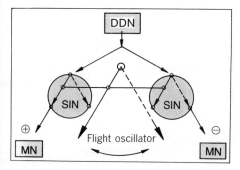

Fig. 6.**1b**   Simplified diagram showing the sensorimotor integration network. Sensory deviation information is channeled to different motoneurons at the flight rhythm. DDN = deviation detector neurons (descending), SIN = sensorimotor integration neuron (segmental), MN = motoneurons (efferent) (after Reichert and Rowell)

— The phase-coupled signal is "automatically" relayed to the correct motoneurons without any prior "decision-making" processes.

The switching of preprocessed sensory information by central oscillators at the level of segmental interneurons, as well as the overall organization of this sensorimotor integration network, are not properties solely of the flight control system of the locust. Descending connections between sensory projection areas in the brain and the premotor level of the spinal cord are also characteristic for the locomotor control systems of vertebrates. In these animals a central neuronal oscillator, together with spinal interneurons, also serve to switch descending sensory signals phase-dependently. Just as in the locust, the end result is the integration of non–phase-coupled sensory messages with rhythmical motor activity.

Oculomotor systems allow target-oriented eye movements

While scanning these lines both your eyes are being moved in a coordinated and precise way in order to image the words being "looked at" on the fovea, which is the region of highest acuity in the retina. These eye movements are among the fastest movements of which the human body is capable. They are carried out by three pairs of muscles which move the eyeball in three different spatial axes.

The coordinated control of the eye muscles is the job of the oculomotor system. This system is responsible for five different functions:

- *Generation of saccades.* These are sudden, ballistic eye movements which can direct both eyes to various spatial targets within fractions of a second, and at velocities of up to 700° per second. Saccades occur during reading, for example.
- *Continuous tracking responses.* Here the image of a target object is maintained on the fovea and visually tracked during object movement.
- *Vestibulo–ocular reflex.* This compensatory reflex serves to stabilize the eyes' line of sight on a fixated target during rapid movements by the head itself.
- *Optokinetics.* If an observer moves his own body in space, then certain objects around him are visually fixated by the optokinetic system and their movement tracked with respect to the body.
- *Convergence movements.* If a visually fixated object approaches or recedes from an observer, then both eyes are moved independently of one another in order to keep the object focused on both foveas.

As expected from such a diversity of functions, the oculomotor system is a complex integration network in which the output signals of the oculomotor nuclei in the brain stem are regulated by signals from various brain regions (Fig. 6.2). Many of the oculomotor system functions feature the integration of visual information with that from the vestibular system. Sensory messages about head movements, which are recorded by the vestibular system, reach the oculomotor nuclei directly from the vestibular nuclei, and indirectly via intercalated neurons in the reticular formation of the pons. The vestibular nuclei play an important role in the performance of all types of eye movements, except saccades. In saccades the superior colliculus coordinates visual information and eye movements. This coordination is again carried out via relay centers in the reticular formation. Intentional, voluntary eye movements are under the control of areas in the frontal cortex.

A characteristic of the oculomotor system is that it is functionally modular. Certain neuron groups are concerned with determining the velocity of eye movements in the three

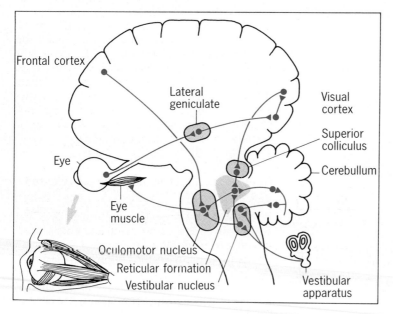

Fig. 6.**2** Oculomotor control system, simplified. Eye movements are controlled by a complex network that extends over several brain nuclei. Visual and vestibular information are processed for the control of eye movements. The three eye muscle pairs are shown schematically (lower left) (after Robinson)

spatial axes, others compute the velocity of head rotation, others again are delegated to compute the error between the actual and the desired eye position, while others are occupied with the spatial coordinates of visually fixated target objects. Despite all this compartmentalization there is still an intensive exchange of information between the various neuronal computing units in the oculomotor system. All these subsystems also have a common site of action, namely the oculomotor motoneurons, onto which all the preprocessed information converges.

The high velocity, accuracy, and reliability of oculomotor responses may create the impression that the underlying neuronal circuits are rigid and to some extent hard-wired. This is not the case! All eye movements, especially the vestibuloo-cular reflexes, exhibit considerable plasticity. If an image displacement occurs on the retina during a head movement despite the oculomotor compensation mechanism, then motor learning can lead incrementally to a recalibration of the vestibulo-ocular reflex. A further important sensorimotor integration structure, namely the cerebellum, is involved in these motor learning processes.

Repetitively organized circuit modules in the cerebellum serve sensorimotor coordination

The cerebellum is an amazing structure. More than half of all the neurons in our brain lie in the cerebellum. These neurons are arranged with almost crystal-like regularity in repetitive microscopic circuit modules, particularly in the cerebellar cortex. The multiple repetition of similar neuronal connectivity patterns indicates that large regions of the cerebellum carry out very similar information processing tasks.

The three main regions of the cerebellum are phylogenetically of different ages, and can be distinguished on the basis of the site of origin of their inputs, and their output target regions (Fig. 6.3a). The *archicerebellum* receives its input signals largely from the vestibular system and is important for the control of eye movements and balance. In the *paleocerebellum*, which contains complete, multiple, motor and somatosensory representation of the body, somatosensory signals from the spinal cord as well as input from the motor cortex are processed. Finally, the *neocerebellum* receives input from many cortical regions, particularly from sensory and motor areas, after these inputs have been preprocessed in the medulla. The neocerebellum is involved in the preparation and performance of coordinated movements of the limbs. In higher vertebrates the output signals of the cerebellum are relayed to

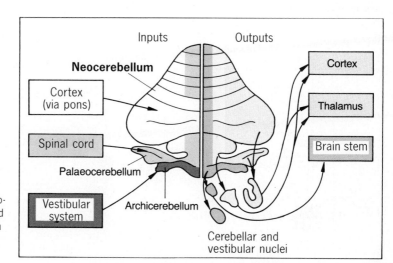

Fig. 6.**3a**   Cerebellum. Input–output relationships shown according to a comparative, phylogenetic viewpoint (left half), and according to efferent projection areas into the cerebellar and vestibular nuclei (right half)

the vestibular nuclei and a series of cerebellar nuclei which have motor and promotor projection sites.

The microanatomy and microphysiology of the cerebellar cortex is based on five neuron types which are arranged in three layers (Fig. 6.**3b,c**). The only efferent neurons of the cerebellar cortex are the *Purkinje cells,* whose cell bodies lie in the middle *Purkinje cell layer,* and whose regularly arranged, fan-shaped dendritic trees arborize two-dimensionally in one plane of the outer *molecular layer.* Purkinje cells have an inhibitory effect on postsynaptic neurons in the cerebellar nuclei.

The input signals to the cerebellar cortex arrive mainly via two types of afferents, the *climbing fibers* and the *mossy fibers.* Climbing fibers have their cell bodies in the inferior olive of the medulla. The dendritic tree of each Purkinje cell receives synaptic input from one single climbing fiber, although each climbing fiber forms synapses with numerous different Purkinje cells. The synaptic connection between climbing fibers and Purkinje cells belongs to the strongest excitatory connections yet found in the brain. An action potential in a single climbing fiber produces a series of action potentials in the postsynaptic Purkinje cell. Mossy fibers have their cell bodies in several different nuclei in the brain stem. They form

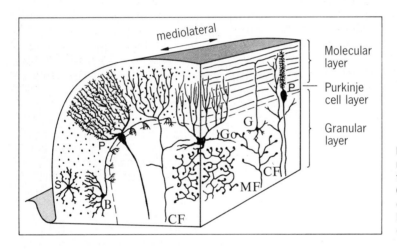

Fig. 6.**3b** Three-dimensional representation of the cytoarchitecture of the cerebellum. Go = Golgi cell, B =basket cell, CF = climbing fiber, G = granule cell, MF = mossy fiber, P = Purkinje cell, S = stellate cell

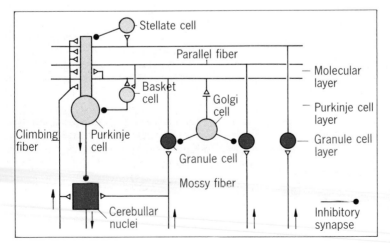

Fig. 6.**3c** Circuit diagram of the excitatory and inhibitory connections in the cerebellum (after Brodal, Shepherd and Fox)

excitatory synaptic connections with *granule cells,* which lie in the lowermost *granular layer* of the cerebellar cortex. (In the human cerebellum there are about 10^{11} granule cells!) The axons of the granule cells ascend to the topmost molecular layer where they make a T-shaped bifurcation and form the *parallel fibers,* which run orthogonally to the fan-shaped dendritic tree of the Purkinje cells. Many mossy fibers converge onto each granule cell. Up to 200 000 granule cells converge in turn onto each Purkinje cell, and each single parallel fiber synapses with about 100 different Purkinje cells. The single synapse which a parallel fiber forms with a Purkinje cell is excitatory, but has a much weaker effect than that of the climbing fiber.

Apart from the excitatory pathways from the climbing and mossy fibers to the Purkinje cells, the cerebellar cortex also contains inhibitory pathways. *Basket cells* and *stellate cells* lie in the molecular layer, are activated by parallel fibres, and lead to a feedforward inhibition of the Purkinje cells. *Golgi cells* lie in the granular layer, are also activated by parallel fibers, and lead to a feedback inhibition of the parallel fibers by inhibiting the granule cells. These inhibitory circuits carry out a sort of lateral inhibition in the cerebellum.

Climbing and mossy fibers not only form synapses in the cerebellar cortex, but also have collaterals which run to the cerebellar nuclei. These resulting "direct" information channels to the cerebellar nuclei can, thus, be modulated by the "indirect" information channels which run from the climbing and mossy fibers via neuronal circuits in the cerebellar cortex. This subdivision into different information channels is important. A cooperation between these two parallel pathways could allow the cerebellum to function as a comparator, as mentioned above, and compare intended with effected motor actions. It is also likely that many of the circuits in the cerebellum can be modified by experience and that this plasticity is critical for motor learning.

Voluntary motor control: insight into intentional actions

Intuitively, it is clear to everyone what an "intentional" or "conscious" motor act is. Reaching for the morning cup of coffee is a voluntary act. But how are such purpose-oriented actions generated and initiated in the central nervous system? We can assume that such acts are centrally preprogrammed; but we are only just beginning to understand how such "program routines" are organized. The first hints come from experiments on single neurons in the motor cortex of monkeys. The experimental animal is first trained to move a lever in one direction or the other, but only after it has received two successive signals. The first signal tells the animal in which direction to move the lever. This is a preparatory signal for action. The subsequent second signal means "carry out the act." What can be seen is that certain neurons in the motor cortex of these animals become active after the first signal, but well before the second signal and the undertaken act. This activity takes place completely within the system and precedes any overt action. We therefore assume that these cells are controlled by central programs for preparatory action, and that the activity of these cells signals an internal readiness to carry out a certain motor act. Extracellular field potentials which point to this sort of motor intentionality (readiness potentials) can be recorded in an electroencephalogram using surface electrodes.

An insight into neuronal preprogramming of voluntary actions can also be obtained from the human brain using a noninvasive experimental method. This method is based on the fact that those brain regions which are currently especially active have a raised blood supply. Following the injection of radioactively labeled xenon into the circulatory system of a test subject, the local blood supply of the brain can be monitored using detectors placed on the head surface. If the test subject now carries out a simple motor act, for example bending a finger, then an increase in neuronal activity in the motor and somatosensory cortex is recorded. If, on the other hand, the test subject carries out a complex sequence of finger movements, then regions in the supplementary motor area also become active, in addition to those in the motor and somatosensory cortex. When the test subject is now instructed to rehearse the complex sequence of finger movements "mentally," then no activity increase is recorded in the motor and somatosensory cortex. There is, however, an increase in activity in the supplementary motor area, and this even though absolutely no motor activity is undertaken (Fig. 6.4). This shows that one can analyze the central nervous activity correlated with a coordinated act and that of its preparation.

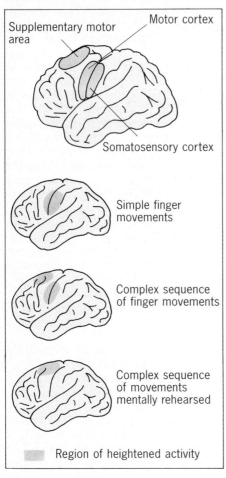

Region of heightened activity

Fig. 6.**4**   Regions of heightened activity in the human cortex during the performance of various tasks (after Roland et al.)

Autonomic Integration

Principle and significance

The brain is not just concerned with the outside world. As a control center it is critically involved in regulating the course of internal functions within its own body. Just how important the exact neuronal control of internal homeostatic systems is only becomes clear to us when something goes wrong with this control mechanism. The performance of the autonomic integration networks which monitor and coordinate the activity in most of the internal organs is only rarely consciously noticed. Only, for example, when the neuronal adjustment of the heartbeat rhythm is disturbed during body exertion or when the coordinated movements of the gastrointestinal tract breakdown, or when the activity of the endocrine glands can no longer be regulated, does the exceptional importance of autonomic integration become clear. The regulation of the "internal milieu" requires extensive sensory input, integrative information processing in the peripheral and central nervous systems, and coordinated efferent pathways.

Autonomic integration can be investigated at the cellular level in invertebrates

A reasonably precise description of visceral control mechanisms has been obtained in several invertebrates because in these animals neuronal integration can be studied at the level of identified neurons. An example is the way in which rhythmical heartbeats are generated in some invertebrates. Coordination in the control of heartbeat can come about either exclusively neuronally or via an interaction between neuronal circuits and heart musculature. The heartbeat of the lobster is generated neurogenically by the neurons of the cardiac ganglion. These neurons are themselves controlled by the CNS via an inhibitory and two excitatory neurons. In the leech, the rhythmical heartbeat is regulated both neurogenically by a segmentally distributed neuronal oscillator, and myogenically by the intrinsic contractile properties of the muscles in the major blood vessels.

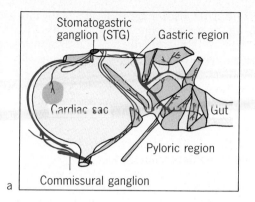

a   Stomatogastric ganglion (STG) · Gastric region · Cardiac sac · Gut · Pyloric region · Commissural ganglion

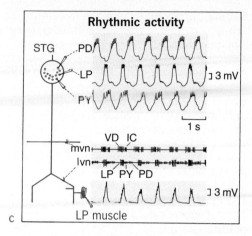

c   **Rhythmic activity**

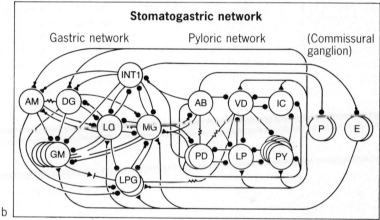

b   **Stomatogastric network**

Gastric network   Pyloric network   (Commissural ganglion)

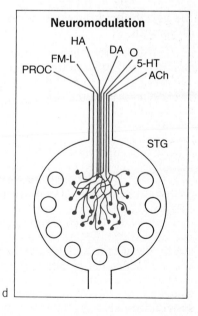

d   **Neuromodulation**

Fig. 6.**5**   Stomatogastric system of the lobster. **a** Diagrammatic overview of the stomatogastric system with nerves and innervated target tissues. **b** Neuronal circuit diagram of the gastric and pyloric networks. Black circles = inhibitory synapses, black triangles = excitatory synapses, resistors = electrical synapses. Individual neurons are identified by letters. **c** Rhythmic motor activity in the pyloric network. Intracellular and extracellular recordings from different neurons as well as from an innervated muscle. LP muscle = muscle innervated from the lateral pyloric neuron, mvn = median ventricular nerve, lvn = lateral ventricular nerve. **d** Neuromodulatory input. Input fibers with different neurotransmitters have diffusely branched terminals in the neuropil of the stomatogastric ganglion (after Selverston, and Marder et al.)

Even relatively simple visceral control requires quite complex integration systems, as can be seen by analyzing the *stomatogastric* system of the lobster. The neuronal network of the stomatogastric system consists of two subsystems, the gastric and the pyloric networks (Fig. 6.**5**). The pyloric subsystem can be viewed as a network of coupled cellular oscillators. The gastric subsystem generates its rhythmical activity largely on the basis of network properties. Both subsystems contribute to the generation of motor control rhythms which drive the muscles in the gastric and pyloric regions of the lobster's stomach.

The stomatogastric nervous system can assume several activity states. The ongoing motor activity rhythm is not determined solely by the intrinsic properties of one or the other subsystem. Hierarchically superior neuronal oscillators in other ganglia, signals from proprioceptors in the stomach wall, hormonal input from other ganglia and endocrine glands, as well as locally acting neuromodulators, are all involved in the generation of the active rhythm. The coordinated regulation of the stomach musculature requires all these integration mechanisms to be flexible, so that, depending on the circumstances, it can be switched from one stable activity mode to another according to what is necessary for the processing of different foodstuffs.

The vertebrate autonomic nervous system is bipartite

In most vertebrates the autonomic system can be subdivided into a *parasympathetic* and a *sympathetic* part (Fig. 6.**6**). Both subsystems can have excitatory or inhibitory effects on the target organs they innervate. The ganglia of the parasympathetic nervous system generally lie near the innervated visceral structure. They receive their innervation from preganglionic neurons which lie in certain brain stem nuclei or in the sacral spinal cord. The postganglionic neurons in these ganglia form spatially restricted synaptic connections with the target tissue they innervate. In higher vertebrates the ganglia of the sympathetic nervous system are largely arranged in a chain near the spinal cord, and are innervated by preganglionic neurons from the thoracolumbar spinal cord. The postganglionic neurons of the sympathetic nervous system form spatially extensive synaptic connections with visceral target tissue. Many internal organs are innervated by both the parasympathetic and the sympathetic nervous systems. The action of the two subsystems is generally antagonistic, whereby sympathetic activation often has a more extensive effect. A few innervated regions, however, are predominantly or even exclusively controlled by only one subsystem.

Simplifying considerably, the sympathetic subsystem may be said to have a generally excitatory function, a system geared to preparing for stress. Its activation, for example, causes an increase in heart rate and blood pressure, as well as a mobilization of the body's energy stores. Correspondingly, one can view the parasympathetic nervous system, again greatly simplified, as a generally calming subsystem, preparing for rest. Parasympathetic activation lowers heart rate and blood pressure, and leads to a reestablishment of the resting homeostasis of the body. An overall, coordinated regulation of the whole autonomic nervous system, as well as the integration of autonomic and somatic activation, is performed by centers in the hypothalamus.

The different neuronal components of the autonomic nervous system have, to some extent, characteristic transmitter systems. The presynaptic, preganglionic neurons of both subsystems release acetylcholine as a transmitter. The postganglionic neurons of the parasympathetic nervous system also use acetylcholine, whereas those of the sympathetic system use norepinephrine (noradrenaline). However, in many cases different neuropeptides are also released in addition to these classic transmitters. The co-release of a neuropeptide with acetylcholine or norepinephrine can lead to complex postsynaptic interactions. The different cellular mechanisms which are initiated as a result can evoke postsynaptic potentials with very different kinetics, duration, and strength in the target cells (smooth muscle cells, heart muscle cells, glandular cells) of the autonomic nervous system.

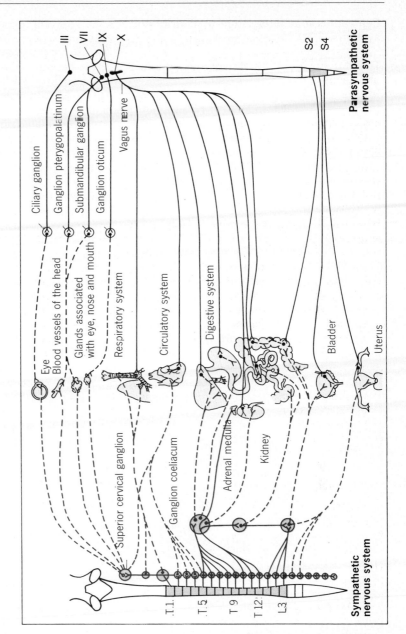

Fig. 6.**6** Human autonomic nervous system, simplified. Sympathetic part (left), parasympathetic part (right), and target organs (middle). Postganglionic neurons are represented by dashed lines (after Eckert)

Central nervous integration by distributed systems

The vertebrate autonomic nervous system is often considered a motor system because its efferents act directly on effectors. However, there are also other integrative systems which are critical for the coordinated control of the whole organism and which lie completely within the confines of the brain. These systems can be partially mapped using transmitter-specific histochemistry and immunocytochemical staining methods. Such aggregations of neurons in the brain can be shown to form extensive distributed projections (Fig. 6.7). The coordination of autonomic functions, the setting of central nervous excitatory states, as well as the modulation of pain messages, are among the many possible roles of these networks.

Several populations of noradrenergic neurons whose somata lie in mesencephalic nuclei have projections of this type. One of these neuron aggregations is in the locus coeruleus whose few hundred projection neurons form highly branched axons which ramify into almost all regions of the brain. The extensive innervation area of these neurons is an indication that the noradrenergic system is involved in the control of integrative activity in many different central nervous circuits. As a result the noradrenergic system is often seen as a central nervous "autonomic system." Groups of serotonergic neurons whose cell bodies lie in the mesencephalon and rhombencephalon have similarly widespread innervation areas.

Transmitter-specific projection systems forming more limited innervation areas are known for almost every transmitter type. These

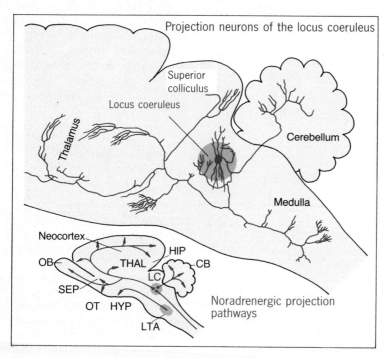

Fig. 6.**7**   Neurons with extensive projections. A neuron in the locus coeruleus of the mouse with collaterals in various brain regions (top). Site of origin and projection areas of noradrenergic neurons with widespread projection areas in the rat brain (bottom). LC = locus coeruleus, LTA = lateral tegmental area, CB = cerebellum, HIP = hippocampus, HYP = hypothalamus, OB = olfactory bulb, OT = olfactory tubercle, SEP = septum, THAL = thalamus (after Scheibel and Scheibel)

include projection systems which utilize dopamine, acetylcholine, glutamate, aspartate, GABA or glycine. In addition there are numerous peptidergic projection systems such as the hypothalamic neuron groups which have endorphins as neurotransmitters, as well as those neuron groups distributed throughout the brain with enkephalins as neurotransmitters. Endorphins and enkephalins have evoked particular interest because they bind as agonists to opioid receptors.

Central nervous integration by widely distributed systems also occurs in invertebrates, as shown by the amine-containing neuron systems which contribute to the control of posture in the lobster. In this animal, a serotonergic as well as an octopaminergic population of neurons act in a coordinated way at several sites in the motor control system. The activation of the serotoninergic system results in the animal assuming an aggressive body posture. The activation of the octopaminergic system leads to a body posture which signals a submissive behavior.

Circadian rhythms are centrally driven

The body does not perform at the same activity level at all hours of the day, and that includes the nervous system. It is subject to endogenously generated biorhythms. The most important of these biorhythms is the approximately 24-hour *circadian diurnal rhythm*. The nervous system is not only influenced by this diurnal rhythm, it is also involved in its regulation. In many cases central nervous structures can be identified which are responsible for the autonomous expression of the circadian rhythm. These neuronal pacemakers form an internal clock which can produce a regular circadian succession of activity and rest phases even in "free-running" mode, without pacemaker information from the environment. Sensory information can couple the endogenously generated activity rhythm to the natural day-night succession, which sets up a precise 24-hour rhythmicity.

In invertebrates the neuronal pacemakers are often closely associated with the visual system. In molluscs like *Aplysia* or *Bulla* the internal clock is actually located in the eye itself. A population of neurons in the eyestalk generates the baseline circadian oscillations. The rhythmical activity of this neuron cluster is then matched to the exact sequence of the natural light-dark cycle by visual input from the retina. Interestingly, the neuronal pacemaker in these molluscs can be modulated by efferent fibers from an extensively distributed serotoninergic neuron system in the brain that influences the overall excitatory state of the animal.

Circadian activity-rest cycles are also known in arthropods. A series of behavioral and electrophysiological experiments show that bees undergo a sleep-like resting phase during the night. Classic experiments on the orientation of bees via a "sun compass" even demonstrate the existence of a very precise internal clock in these insects. In *Drosophila* there are mutants which have a defective diurnal rhythm. Certain mutants have a shortened diurnal rhythm (19 hours), others have a lengthened one (29 hours), and others again have absolutely no diurnal rhythm. In all these mutants, not only the circadian rhythm but also other, faster-running activity rhythms, are affected. The mutations responsible are all in the *per* gene.

Virtually all vertebrates have a circadian activity rhythm which can be coupled to the natural day-night cycle by the influence of light. The neuronal centers which are responsible for the generation of the endogenous diurnal rhythm form a distributed system whose main oscillator lies in the paired *suprachiasmatic nucleus* at the anterior border of the hypothalamus. The suprachiasmatic nucleus receives visual input from the optic nerve via the retinohypothalamic tract. Along with other pacemaker neuronal oscillators having somewhat different endogenous rhythms, the suprachiasmatic nucleus forms a system of multiple oscillators which together control the cyclical changes in body and brain functions during the sleep and waking states.

In humans, the analysis of the neuronal phenomena accompanying sleep and waking states is based mainly on measurements from the electroencephalogram (EEG). The EEG basically represents the summated synaptic field potentials from the apical dendrites of cortical neurons, but also provides information about the activity of thalamic centers, since thalamocortical connections relay the synchronized rhythmical activity present in certain nuclei in the thalamus to cortical neurons. EEG analyses have contributed to an accurate characterization of various sleep states. During sleep, several characteristic frequencies and amplitudes appear in the EEG and can be correlated with well-defined sleep phases. The α and β waves which occur in the EEG during wakefulness for instance, are replaced during sleep by δ and θ waves. From a neuronal viewpoint, sleep represents an extraordinarily complex cyclic sequence of activity states. In general, falling asleep is followed by a phase of particularly deep sleep which is then replaced by a regular sequence of light and deep sleep phases (Fig. 6.8). Since fast eye movements occur during light sleep, this phase is called REM *(rapid eye movement)* sleep. Increased dreaming usually occurs in the REM-sleep phase. The brain remains receptive to sensory information from the environment during the entire sleep period. Motor commands also continue to be relayed to motoneurons in the spinal cord. However, in most cases there is no activation of the skeletal musculature because the motoneurons are actively inhibited (particularly during the REM sleep). The complex nature of nightly sleep, which is generally not consciously perceived, indicates that multiple neuronal subsystems are involved in this active behavioral state.

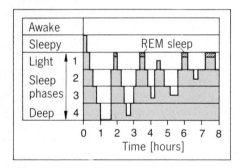

Fig. 6.**8**   Sleep pattern of a young adult human. REM sleep phases are shown cross-hatched (after Ottoson)

Neuroendocrine Integration

Similarity between transmitter release and neurosecretion

Since glands, like muscles, are effector structures they are generally subject to nervous regulation. Many exocrine glands, for example, are controlled by the autonomic nervous system. The endocrine system is very closely linked to the nervous system. The many endocrine glands which produce hormones and then release these into the blood circulation are partly innervated by nerve cells, and they themselves consist partly of nerve cells which are specialized for hormone release. Such *neuroendocrine* cells, often also called *neurosecretory* cells, have typical neuronal properties. They receive synaptic input, produce action potentials and release messenger substances from their terminals in a Ca^{2+}-dependent manner. The often massive release from specialized neurosecretory terminals of hormones synthesized in the cell body is not directed at neighboring postsynaptic cells, but occurs mostly into the vessels of the blood circulatory system. In this way the hormones released can act in a coordinated way on multiple, widely separated, target cells. Generally, neurosecretion occurs much more slowly than transmitter release, but it then has a typically much longer reaction time. This should not, however, lead to the impression that the mechanisms of neurosecretion and transmitter release are contradictory in nature. They are much more like two extreme organizational forms of a continuum. Neuroendocrine cells which occur at the phylogenetic level of coelenterates probably arose early in evolution. They could even have been the precursors of real nerve cells (Fig. 6.**9**).

Neurosecretion plays a key role in the invertebrates

In all higher animals neurosecretory cells are the essential link between the nervous system and the endocrine system. This is especially true for many invertebrates where neuroendocrine systems are directly responsible for the control of growth and reproduction. In insects, for example, the great majority of hormones are produced by neurosecretory cells. Important exceptions are juvenile hormone and ecdysone, whose synthesis and release however, are again regulated by the neuroendocrine system. In insects, neurosecretory cells are found in every ganglion of the central nervous system as well as in the peripheral nervous system (Fig. 6.**10**). Many neurosecretory axons terminate in structures specialized for storage and release called *neurohemal organs*. The classic insect neurohemal organs are the corpora cardiaca and the corpora allata which store hormones synthesized in the neurosecretory cells of the brain. These neurohemal organs receive their neurohormones via special brain nerves. However, they also produce their own hormones via intrinsic neurosecretory cells. The neurohormonal signals which emanate from the brain, corpora cardiaca and corpora allata, respectively, are critical for the coordination of growth, molting, and metamorphosis.

A detailed insight into the way in which neurohormones are synthesized has been obtained for the egg-laying hormone (ELH) of the sea snail *Aplysia*. This peptide hormone is synthesized in the bag cells. The bag cells are paired neuroendocrine cell aggregates which lie attached to the connectives of the abdominal ganglion. ELH and other related neurohormones initiate the egglaying process, as well as the coordinated behavioral sequence the an-

imal undergoes during egg-laying (Fig. 6.**11a**). On the one hand ELH itself acts as a neurohormone which is released into the blood circulation and evokes a contraction of the musculature in the genital pore. On the other hand, ELH acts as a neurotransmitter which influences certain identified neurons in the abdominal ganglion.

The amino acid sequence for ELH is determined by a gene which codes for a large polyprotein. Following translation this polyprotein is cleaved into numerous small peptides. One of these peptides is ELH; however, two further neuroactive peptides, α- and β-factor, are also produced by cleavage of the polyprotein (Fig. 6.**11b**). The coding of all three neuroactive peptides by the same gene could lead to the coordinated activation of the multiple neuronal systems which are involved in the same behavior. Interestingly, other neuroactive peptides which are also involved in the regulation of egg-laying behavior are coded on two further genes which themselves show a high degree of sequence homology with the ELH gene. One therefore assumes that all three genes belong to a small multigene family with a common evolutionary origin.

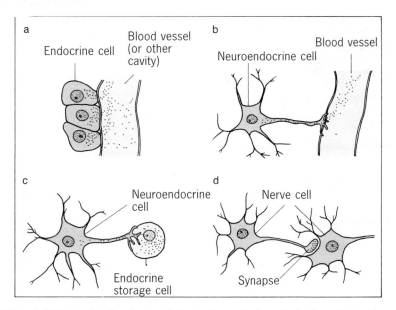

Fig. 6.**9**   Diagrammatic representation of various mechanisms for chemical signal transmission. **a** Endocrine cells secrete hormones into a neighboring blood vessel. **b** Neuroendocrine cells release hormones from specialized terminals into the blood system. **c** Neuroendocrine cells transfer hormones to storage cells. **d** Neurons secrete neurotransmitter directly onto neuronal target cells

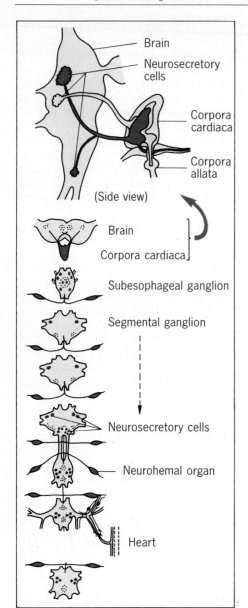

Brain

Neurosecretory
cells

Corpora
cardiaca

Corpora
allata

(Side view)

Brain

Corpora cardiaca

Subesophageal ganglion

Segmental ganglion

Neurosecretory cells

Neurohemal organ

Heart

Fig. 6.**10**   Neurosecretion in insects. Neurosecretory cells in the brain synthesize hormones and transport hormones to the corpora cardiaca and corpora allata which serve as neurohemal organs for the storage and release of the hormones (top). Neurosecretory cells and neurohemal organs occur in the brain, subesophageal ganglion, and in the segmental ganglia (bottom) (after Orchard)

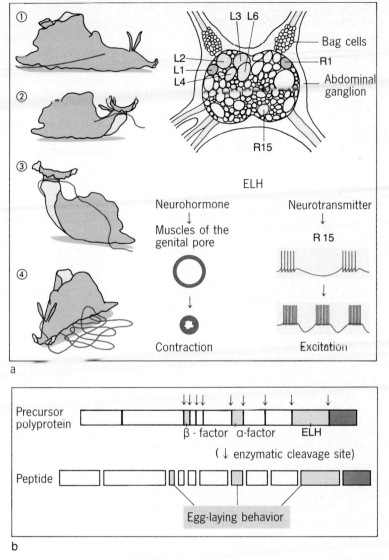

Fig. 6.**11**   Action and synthesis of the egg-laying hormone ELH in *Aplysia*. **a** The coordinated sequence of actions the animal uses to lay a ribbon-shaped egg mass (left). The major sites of synthesis of ELH are the bag cells of the abdominal ganglion (right top). ELH acts like a neurohormone on muscle contractions in the genital pore, and as a neurotransmitter on neuron R15 (bottom right). L1–L4, L6, R1 and R15 are neurons. **b** The precursor molecule for ELH is a polyprotein that is enzymatically cleaved into numerous smaller peptides. At least three of these peptides (α-factor, β-factor, ELH) are neuroactive and are released by the bag cells (after Scheller)

The hypothalamus and pituitary are the neuroendocrine control centers of vertebrates

In humans the hypothalamus comprises less than 1% of the volume of the brain. Despite this, the greater part of the endocrine system is regulated from here. This control, which is carried out via the pituitary, occurs in two ways (Fig. 6.**12**).

- Neurosecretory cells project from the supraoptic and paraventricular nucleus of the hypothalamus to the posterior pituitary lobes and release the two peptide hormones oxytocin and vasopressin from their terminals into the body's circulatory system. Oxytocin produces a contraction of the smooth musculature of the uterus and the mammary glands. Vasopressin raises the blood pressure by acting on the musculature of the blood vessels. It also has an antidiuretic action by stimulating water resorption in the kidney.
- Neurosecretory cells in several other nuclei of the hypothalamus (ventromedial, dorsomedial, infundibular, arcuate, and preoptic nuclei) form a range of hormone-releasing and hormone-inhibiting factors. These peptide factors are initially released into a type of portal vein system and rapidly enter the network of vessels in the anterior pituitary lobe where they influence the release of several hormones which are produced in the secretory cells of the anterior pituitary lobe. These hormones are synthesized under the influence of the releasing and inhibitory factors and secreted into the circulatory system.

The neuroendocrine cells of the hypothalamus which regulate hormone release are themselves influenced by hormones. There is a negative feedback onto the cells of the hypothalamus from some of the somatic hormones as well as from the releasing and inhibitory factors. The neurosecretory cells of the hypothalamus receive neuronal input from many regions of the CNS, including the cerebral cortex and the limbic system. The hypothalamus is therefore at the center of a complex functional network which includes the the pituitary and the endocrine system, the limbic system, the cerebral cortex, the autonomic nervous system, as well as various sensory and motor systems. Due to its central role in this network, the hypothalamus is not only involved in the control of many internal, homeostatic regulatory processes, but also in the production of complex behaviors. Many of the behavioral states regulated by the hypothalamus have a clear emotional content. These include fear, rage, aggression, pleasure and sexual activity. The central, integrative role of the hypothalamus can also be seen in its interactions with an important nonneural system, the immune system.

Interactions between the nervous and immune systems

The mechanisms of the immune system, which extend from recognition of an antigen to secretion of antibodies, differ considerably from those involved in electrochemical signal processing in the nervous system. Nevertheless, the cells of the immune system form a distributed network whose function it is to receive (molecular) information, process this via cell-cell interactions, and produce a (molecular) response. Thus, the basic elements of molecularly expressed "sensory," "integrative," and "motor" processes are contained in the immune system. One can even speak of "memory" in the immune system.

The similarity between the immune system and the nervous system is even more evident at the subcellular level. Voltage-dependent ion channels responsible for depolarizing Na^+ and Ca^{2+} inward currents, and hyperpolarizing K^+ outward currents, are found in the cell membrane of lymphocytes. Certain cells in the immune system even have receptors for peptide neurotransmitters. The presence of these receptors raises the possibility that the cells of the immune system can be influenced by neurohormones in the circulatory system, or even directly by neurons. This does in fact occur.

It has long been known that the proliferation of lymphocytes can be inhibited by psychological stress. However, this immune suppression is only one product of an extensive neuronal regulation of the immune system. The nervous system exerts its control over the immune system partly as a result of sympathetic and parasympathetic innervation of certain immune organs. The major influence of the brain on the immune system, however, is exerted via the hypothalamus and the endocrine system associated with the pituitary. Since the hypothalamus itself is influenced by many structures in the brain, one ends up with a complex network of central nervous immune-regulatory mechanisms. As in most hypothalamic control systems, feedback mechanisms are also involved here. Using specific messenger substances like lymphokines and thymokines, the immune system can exert feedback control over the cells of the hypothalamus and pituitary.

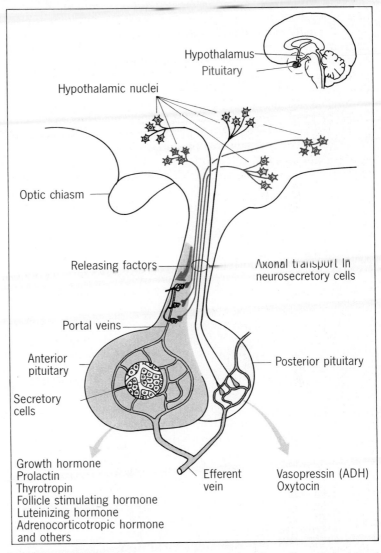

Hypothalamus
Pituitary

Hypothalamic nuclei

Optic chiasm

Releasing factors

Axonal transport in neurosecretory cells

Portal veins

Anterior pituitary

Posterior pituitary

Secretory cells

Growth hormone
Prolactin
Thyrotropin
Follicle stimulating hormone
Luteinizing hormone
Adrenocorticotropic hormone
and others

Efferent vein

Vasopressin (ADH)
Oxytocin

Fig. 6.12   The human pituitary. The anterior lobe of the pituitary consists of nonneural gland tissue; the posterior lobe of the pituitary is an evagination of the brain. Neurosecretory cells in several nuclei of the hypothalamus produce *releasing* factors which reach the anterior lobe via a portal system and control the secretion of a range of hormones there. Other neurosecretory cells in the hypothalamus project into the posterior lobe of the pituitary where they release oxytocin and vasopressin

Sex hormones produce dimorphisms in the nervous system

Sex hormones are responsible for the maturation of the gonads and the secondary sex characteristics. They also have a further important function. They are involved in the generation of sex-specific behaviors like mating or brood care. Sexually dimorphic behaviors have a neuronal correlate in the sex-specific biochemical, anatomical, and physiological differences in the nervous system of male and female conspecifics. These differences are the product of sex-specific differentiation of the brain and result from interactions between sex hormones, and neuronal as well as neuroendocrine regulatory mechanisms. In some cases, sex-specific neuronal differentiation extends to the regulation of behaviors which are not di-

rectly related to reproductive behavior.

In the early stages of embryonic development the brain has in most cases not yet been sexually determined. The mechanisms leading to sexual differentiation of the nervous system are initiated by hormones acting within a restricted critical phase in development. These differentiating mechanisms are the result of a complex interaction between the sex-dependent concentration of sexual hormones, and sex-specific differences in the sensitivity of the neuronal target tissue for these hormones. Disturbances in this interaction can lead to the development of nonadaptive sexual behavior. Thus, in most mammals the females show male behavioral traits when they are treated with certain steroid sexual hormones during the critical phase.

Sexual differentiation of the nervous sys-

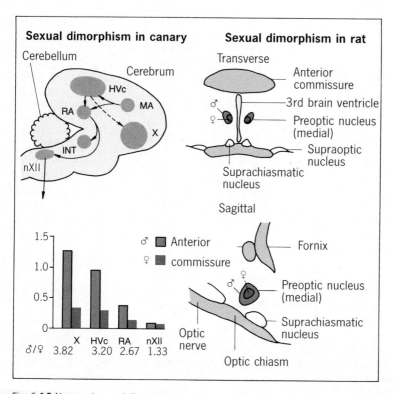

Fig. 6.13 Neuronal sexual dimorphism. **a** Neuronal control centers for the song behavior of songbirds. HVc = nucleus hyperstriatus ventralis, INT = nucleus intercollicularis, MA = nucleus magnocellularis anterior, X — Area X, RA = nucleus robustus archistriatalis, n XII = neural area of the twelfth brain nerve. **b** Volumes of various brain structures involved in song control in canaries. Gray = male, brown = female. **c** Different sizes of a preoptic nucleus in male and female rats. Transverse and sagittal sections through the rat brain. Gray = male, brown = female (after Nottebohm, and Gorski et al.)

tem might be assumed to involve only subtle changes in neuronal connections. However, in many cases the different sex-specific behaviors are associated with dramatic structural differences in the brains of male and female conspecifics. Some of these neuronal *sexual dimorphisms* can even be demonstrated macroscopically with the appropriate staining methods (Fig. 6.13). In certain songbirds where only the male produces a complex song repertoire, some of the brain nuclei which are important for song behavior are up to 4 times as large in males as in females. Neuronal sexual dimorphisms of comparable significance are found in mammals. The medial preoptic nucleus in the thalamus of rodents is 8 times as large in males as it is in females. The neurons in this nucleus are differently organized, cellularly and molecularly, in the two sexes. There are also distinct sexual dimorphisms in the human brain. In women the corpus callosum has a much larger cross-sectional area relative to total brain mass than in men. The cerebral hemispheres of women also seem to be functionally less asymmetric than in men.

Neural Specializations for Complex System Performance

Principle and examples of such specialized neurons

Individual neurons can have astounding properties. In the hippocampus of the rat there are "place cells" which respond to the spatial location of the animal. These nerve cells always seem to be selectively excited when the animal assumes a particular position with respect to its spatial surround. In the temporal cortex of the monkey there are neurons which respond in a specific way to complex visual stimulus configurations. This includes cells which apparently only become active on seeing a monkey's hand. Others respond specifically to individual monkey faces. In the medial and temporal brain lobes of humans there are groups of neurons which respond to individual words in an amazingly selective way during language tasks. An analysis of these nerve cells suggests that words are represented neuronally in the human brain by a type of population coding.

Although the neuronal integration that leads to the highly specific response properties of such nerve cells is still largely unresolved,

one thing is clear. These neuronal capacities are based on complex system properties. They result from the cooperation of many neuronal circuits which together have achieved the capacity for abstraction. Some aspects of the complex information processing occurring in such specialized systems are considered below.

Neuronal systems for interindividual communication

Every nervous system processes information via neuronal communication, and also exchanges information with its surroundings. However, in certain highly developed animals there are systems which allow an efficient communication with other conspecifics. Specialized transmitter and receiver structures, as well as the corresponding machinery for neuronal processing, allow these animals to exchange signals with complex information content. Interindividual communication reaches a pinnacle in certain insects, birds, and mammals.

The neuronal networks which are involved in even simple intraspecific forms of communication in insects can reach a considerable level of complexity. In pheromonal communication, for example, special scent receptor cells are used whose messages are processed in the specialized macromolecular complex of the antennal lobe. Information is then relayed from these complexes to a whole range of other centers in the brain (Fig. 6.14).

Communication by sound is particularly prevalent in the Orthoptera (Fig. 6.15). The songs of crickets are produced by rhythmical movements of the elevated forewings (stridulation). The chirps of the male serve to bring the sexes together and prepare them for mating, as well as to defend his territory, and have a different acoustic structure according to the information they contain. The various song types differ in the duration and repetition rate of their individual sound stimuli. The motor commands for song production are generated by central pattern generators in the segmental ganglia. These segmental circuits are under the hierarchical control of higher brain centers which themselves receive sensory and hormonal input, as well as central feedback information. The brain centers, together with various sensory organs, determine the type and duration of the song. The sound-receiving apparatus consists of a tympanal membrane and

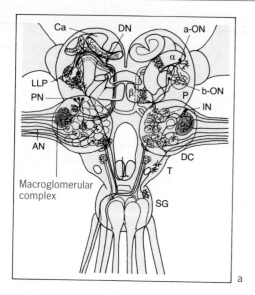

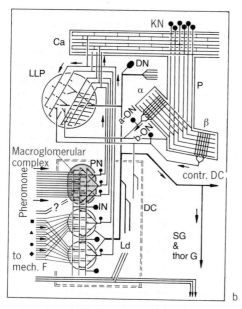

Fig. 6.**14** Olfactory system of the cockroach. **a** Diagrammatic representation of the male brain with several identified neuron types. **b** Diagram of the neuronal networks which process pheromonal and other olfactory signals. In the male, afferent information about pheromones is processed in a special macroglomerular complex. AN = antennal nerve, Ca = calyx, DC = deuterocerebrum, DN = descending neuron, KN = Kenyon cells, IN = local interneuron, Ld = dorsal lobe, I I P = lobus lateralis protocerebralis, mech F = mechanosensory fibers, P = protocerebrum, PN = projection neuron, a-ON = α-lobe output neuron, b-ON = β-lobe output neuron, T = tritocerebrum, thor G = thoracic ganglion, SG = subesophageal ganglion, α = α-lobe, β = β-lobe (after Boeckh)

the auditory receptor cells in the forelegs of the animal. The auditory signals are first transmitted from the receptors to the prothoracic ganglion where they are processed and then relayed to auditory centers in the brain. In these centers there are neurons which are involved in song recognition, and may also be responsible for initiating the subsequent responses of the females. Interestingly, the structures which subserve song production are evolutionary derivatives of the locomotory apparatus, while the structures which subserve sound reception are of proprioceptive origin.

Specialized communication systems are also found in lower vertebrates. The weakly electric fish, for example, not only use their self-produced electric fields for object detection and orientation, but also for social communication. However, complex acoustic communication between conspecifics first appears in songbirds. In many cases only the males produce a specially structured song which can signal territory defense and readiness for mating. In certain bird species the male learns a part of his song repertoire while growing up. This auditory learning process can precede actual singing by several weeks—singing is only perfected by repeated "song practice." In canaries the capacity for learning extends into adulthood. These animals can learn a new song repertoire every year.

The central nervous control of bird song involves several interconnected brain nuclei (Fig. 6.**13a**). The largest of these nuclei is the HVc nucleus in the forebrain. This is connected to another forebrain nucleus, the RA nucleus. Many of the neurons in the RA nucleus project to the medulla where they contact motoneurons which innervate the sound-producing syrinx. In male canaries the HVc and RA nuclei change in size according to a yearly cycle. This size change is at least partly based on the regeneration and degeneration of neurons. At the end of the breeding season more than a third of the neurons in the HVc nucleus degenerate. At the beginning of the next breeding season the same number of neurons become newly incorporated. This neurogenesis is assumed to be important for the recognition or learning of new songs. According to this hypothesis the new song repertoire learned each year has its structural correlate in a song system in the brain which is partly renewed in a yearly rhythm. The amazing anatomical

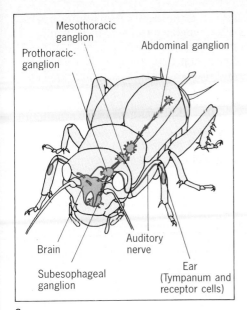

a

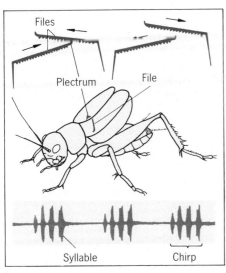

b

Fig. 6.15   Sound communication in the cricket. **a** CNS and peripheral auditory system. **b** Stridulation. Sound production results from rapid, rhythmical, wing closure. With each wing movement a short 5 kHz tone, termed a syllable, results as the plectrum and file rub against one another. The whole song typically consists of numerous chirps, which themselves consist of individual syllables (after Huber and Thorson)

changes in these brain nuclei are at least partially initiated by androgenic sexual hormones, whose titer also undergoes a strong yearly fluctuation.

The centers for the comprehension and generation of language are separated in the human brain

Many mammals have evolved vocalization systems and use them for communication. Consider, for example, the highly complex songs of whales. In primates like chimpanzees and gorillas there is a primitive understanding of language, as their ability to represent simple objects conceptually with symbols shows. However, no other animal possesses a communication system which is nearly as highly developed, and so powerful, as human language. Our language forms not only an important basis for conceptual thinking, it is also the basis for the explosive cultural evolution of our species.

Surprisingly, we know very little about the motor side of speech production in humans. Vocalization requires a coordinated activation of many muscles in the facial region, the larynx, and the chest. The motoneurons of all these muscles are assumed to be coordinated by commands from the motor cortex. This control runs in part directly, via corticospinal connections, and partly indirectly, via the basal ganglia and the cerebellum.

Knowledge about the integrative mechanisms which are responsible for our capacity for speech comes mainly from studies on patients with spatially restricted brain lesions. These studies show that the human cerebral cortex has two important language areas (Fig. 6.16). *Wernicke's area* lies in the temporal lobe. The perception of a read or heard word is assumed to be synthesized and stored in a still unknown form in this area. The functional loss of Wernicke's area results in a serious disturbance in speech comprehension. Patients who have this type of *sensory aphasia* can speak fluently, but their speech makes no sense. These patients are incapable of understanding the speech of others, and because speech comprehension is lacking, they also have serious writing and reading difficulties.

Information from Wernicke's area is relayed via a projection tract to a second language center, *Broca's area,* which lies near the

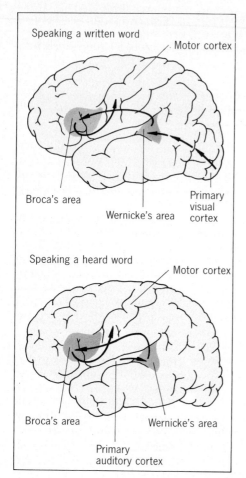

Speaking a written word

Motor cortex

Broca's area

Wernicke's area

Primary visual cortex

Speaking a heard word

Motor cortex

Broca's area

Wernicke's area

Primary auditory cortex

Fig. 6.**16**   Primary language areas in the human cortex. During vocalization of a read or heard word, sensory information first reaches Wernicke's area and from there Broca's area. Wernicke's area is important for language comprehension. Broca's area is important for motor generation of speech. A fiber tract (fasciculus longitudinalis superior [arcuatus]) connects Wernicke's and Broca's areas (after Geschwind)

motor cortex and is important for speech production. There are indications that the grammatical relationships in language, as well as the motor programs for speaking, are stored in this center. During speech these programs are assumed to be relayed to the motor cortex so that the appropriate articulation is carried out. The functional loss of Broca's area leads to an incapacity for speech, termed *motor aphasia,* despite an intact speech motor system. The ability to write is also seriously affected by this

loss. However, the comprehension of spoken and written language remains mostly intact in patients with motor aphasia.

From a structural point of view, Wernicke's and Broca's areas have a remarkable feature. Both are found only in the left cortical hemisphere. This is one example of the extensive asymmetric lateralization of brain functions.

The functional organization of the two brain hemispheres is asymmetric

The two cerebral hemispheres are linked to one another by the fiber bundles of the corpus callosum. What happens when this connection is disrupted? Animal experiments show that each hemisphere can function separately. Information can be processed in one half of the cortex, but is no longer transferred to the other half. For example, when a visual input is restricted to one half of the brain, then visual perception and visually induced learning can occur in this half without the other half knowing anything about it. A type of "split consciousness" occurs. This also applies to the human cortex as studies with patients whose corpus callosum has been transsected for clinical reasons have shown.

These studies, initially carried out by Sperry on such "split-brain" patients, have led to a further surprising discovery. It appears that many higher brain functions are carried out predominantly in one or the other brain half (Fig. 6.17). In most people the left hemisphere predominates in the control of linguistic functions, mathematical ability, and complex movements. By contrast, the right hemisphere is often specialized for spatial perception, complex pattern recognition and intuitive performance. The lateral dominance of either side is never absolute. Both brain halves have the basics necessary to carry out sensory information processing, learning or memory.

A functional lateralization of the brain hemispheres is not only present in humans, but also in monkeys, cats and rats, among others. There is even a clear asymmetry in the nervous system of birds. The central nervous control of the sound-producing syrinx originates mainly in the left half of the brain.

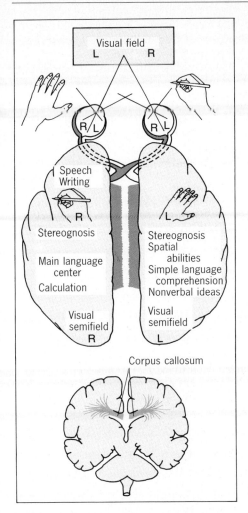

Visual field
L   R

Speech
Writing

R

Stereognosis

Main language
center

Calculation

Visual
semifield
R

Stereognosis
Spatial
abilities
Simple language
comprehension
Nonverbal ideas

Visual
semifield
L

Corpus callosum

Fig. 6.17   Asymmetric organization of the two brain hemispheres in humans. The functional specialization of the two hemispheres can be demonstrated in patients whose corpus callosum has been surgically transected (after Sperry)

Mental illnesses are disturbances of the nervous system

The human brain is unique. It is without doubt the most complex organ that evolution has ever produced. It is our brain that really makes us human beings. However, unfortunately even this organ can become ill. Given the immense significance of the brain, the effects of pathological disturbances of the nervous system can be catastrophic. The changes in consciousness and personality that accompany certain pathological brain disturbances were once considered the work of the devil, and "treated" accordingly. Today we know that mental illnesses are in fact systemic disturbances in the highly complex neuron system of the human brain. It is an important task of modern neuroscience to explain these systemic disturbances and work out methods for their cure.

The human suffering caused by mental illness is immense. It is estimated that in the USA about 20% of all hospital beds are occupied by patients suffering from *schizophrenia* or related disturbances. *Depression* occurs in about 4% of the world's population. Disturbances which can be traced back to *senile dementia* occur in as many as every fourth person who reaches the age of 80. What do we know about these pathological disturbances?

Schizophrenic illness leads to grave aberrations in consciousness, perception, emotional stability and the capacity for social interaction. In many cases schizophrenia can be successfully treated with psychopharmacological agents. Since many of the pharmacologically active substances act as inhibitors in dopaminergic synaptic transmission, it is assumed that schizophrenia is the result of overactivity in the dopaminergic system of the brain. This agrees with experimental results which show that drugs which increase the action of dopamine can induce a schizophrenic-like state. However, a precise explanation for the causes of schizophrenia is still lacking.

Depressions are also at least partly the result of disturbances in certain transmitter-specific systems. The serotoninergic and noradrenergic systems of the brain, especially those of the hypothalamus, are implicated in depressive disease. Depressive states can be successfully treated pharmacologically by antidepressant drugs (monoamine oxidase inhibitors and tricyclides) as well as by lithium. Genetic components play an important role in the tendency to suffer from depression and schizophrenia.

Senile dementia causes an advancing decline in general mental capacity and memory in older people. The most important and most common dementia is *Alzheimer's disease*. In patients suffering from this disease several neuronal anomalies occur more frequently than is usual for this age group.

- Extracellular plaques containing amyloid deposits, neurofibrillary tangles, lipofuscin granules, and granular vacuoles occur more frequently in the nerve cells of the demented than in the normal population.
- Dendrites and neuronal cell bodies swell. In many cases there is a considerable loss of dendrites. Often an abnormal general atrophy of the brain is observed.
- A selective degeneration of cholinergic neurons occurs, mainly in the nucleus of Meynert.

We do not yet know if these phenomena are the cause of the disease or only represent symptoms. At the moment there is no specific treatment for Alzheimer's dementia. Since the life expectancy of the population is constantly rising, more and more people will suffer from this disease. A better understanding of this and other age-related diseases of the brain is therefore urgently required.

References

General Reviews

Andersen, R. A. 1989. Visual and eye movement functions of the posterior parietal cortex. Annu. Rev. Neurosci. 12: 377-404.

Arnold, A. P. and Gorski, R. A. 1984. Gonadal steroid induction of structural sex differences in the central nervous system. Annu. Rev. Neurosci. 7: 413-442.

Bentley, D. and Hoy, R. R. 1974. The neurobiology of cricket song. Sci. Am. 231: 34-44.

Breakefield, X. O. and Cambi, F. 1987. Molecular genetic insights into neurologic diseases. Annu. Rev. Neurosci. 10: 535-594.

Caramazza, A. 1988. Some aspects of language processing revealed through the analysis of acquired aphasia: The lexical system. Annu. Rev. Neurosci. 11: 395-422.

Creutzfeld, O. D. 1983. Cortex Cerebri. Springer, Berlin.

Damasio, A. R. and Geschwind, N. 1984. The neural basis of language. Annu. Rev. Neurosci. 7: 127-147.

Davis, J. M. and Mass, J. W. (eds.) 1983. The Affective Disorders. American Psychiatric Press, Washington.

Edelman, G. M., Gall, W. E. and Cowan, W. M. (eds.) 1990. Signal and Sense: Local and Global Order in Perceptual Maps. Wiley-Liss, New York.

Edelman, R. R. 1990. Magnetic resonance imaging of the nervous system. Discuss. Neurosci. 7: 11-63.

Elfvin, L. G. (ed.) 1983. Autonomic Ganglia. Wiley, New York.

Fuchs, A. F., Kaneko, C. R. S. and Scudder, C. A. 1985. Brainstem control of saccadic eye movements. Annu. Rev. Neurosci. 8: 307-338.

Geschwind, N. 1979. Specializations of the human brain. Sci. Am. 241: 180-199.

Glick, S. D. (ed.) 1985. Cerebral Lateralization in Non-Human Species. Academic, Orlando.

Goodwin, F. K. and Jamison, K. R. 1990. Manic-Depressive Illness. Oxford University Press, New York.

Guillemin, K., Cohn, M. and Melnechuk, T. (eds.) 1985. Neural Modulation of Immunity. Raven, New York.

Harris-Warrick, R. M. and Marder, E. 1991. Modulation of neural networks for behavior. Annu. Rev. Neurosci. 14: 39-57.

Heiligenberg, W. 1977. Principles of Electrolocation and Jamming Avoidance in Electric Fish. Springer, Berlin.

Hobson, J. A. 1988. The Dreaming Brain. Basic Books, New York.

Hopkins, C. D. 1988. Neuroethology of electric communication. Annu. Rev. Neurosci. 11: 497-536.

Huber, F. and Markl, H. 1983. Neuroethology and Behavioral Physiology. Springer, Berlin.

Huber, F. and Thorson, J. 1985. Cricket auditory communication. Sci. Am. 253: 60-68.

Ito, M. 1985. The Cerebellum and Neural Control. Raven, New York.

Jeannerod, M. 1988. The Neural and Behavioural Organization of Goal-Directed Movements. Oxford University Press, New York.

Jones, G. and Peters, A. A. (eds) 1985. The Cerebral Cortex. Plenum, New York.

Kalmring, K. and Elsner, N. 1985. Acustic and Vibratory Communication in Insects. Parey, Berlin.

Kelly, D. B. 1988. Sexually dimorphic behaviors. Annu. Rev. Neurosci. 11: 225-252.

Konishi, M. 1985. Birdsong: from behavior to neuron. Anno. Rev. Neurosci. 8: 125-170.

Lisberger, S. G., Morris, E. J. and Tychsen, L. 1987. Visual motion processing and sensory-motor integration for smooth pursuit eye movements. Annu. Rev. Neurosci. 10: 97-130.

Marr, D. 1969. A theory of cerebellar cortex. J. Physiol. 202: 437-470.

Menzel, R. and Erber, J. 1978. Learning and memory in bees. Sci. Am. 239: 80-87.

Muller, K. J., Nicholls, J. G. and Stent, G. S. (eds.) 1981. Neurobiology of the Leech. Cold Spring Harbor, New York

Ottoson, D. 1983. Physiology of the Nervous System. Macmillan, London.

Prichard, J. W. and Shulman, R. G. 1986. NMR spectroscopy of brain metabolism in vivo. Annu. Rev. Neurosci. 9: 61-86.

Price, D. L. 1986. New perspectives on Alzheimer's disease. Annu. Rev. Neurosci. 9: 489-512.

Raichle, M. E. 1983. Positron emission tomography. Annu. Rev. Neurosci. 6: 249-267.

Robinson, D. A. 1989. Integrating with neurons. Annu Rev. Neurosci. 12: 33-46.

Scharrer, B. 1987. Neurosecretion: Beginnings and new directions in neuropeptide research. Annu. Rev. Neurosci. 10: 1-18.

Selkoe, D. J. 1989. Biochemistry of altered brain proteins in Alzheimer's disease. Annu. Rev. Neurosci. 12: 463-490.

Selkoe, D. J. 1991. The molecular pathology of Alzheimer's disease. Neuron 6: 487-498.

Selverston, A. I. (ed.) 1985. Model Neural Networks and Behavior. Plenum, New York.

Selverston, A. I. and Moulins, M. (eds.) 1986 The Crustacean Stomatogastric System. Springer, New York.

Silverman, A. J. and Zimmerman, E. A. 1983. Magnocellular neurosecretory system Annu. Rev. Neurosci. 6: 357-380.

Snyder, S. H. 1986. Drugs and the Brain. Scientific American Books, New York.

Stellar, J. R. and Stellar, E. 1985. The Neurobiology of Motivation and Reward. Springer, Berlin.

Steriade, M. and McCarley, R. W. 1990. Control of Wakefulness and Sleep. Plenum, New York.

Swanson, L. W. and Sawchenkeo, P. E. 1983. Hypothalamic integration: Organization of the paraventricular and supraoptic nuclei. Annu. Rev. Neurosci. 6: 269-324

Original Publications

Abraham, C. R., Selkoe, D. J. and Potter, H. 1988. Immunochemical identification of the serine protease inhibitor α_1-antichymotrypsin in the brain amyloid deposits of Alzheimer's disease. Cell 52: 487-501.

Adrian, E. D. 1943. Afferent areas in the cerebellum connected with the limbs. Brain 66: 289-315.

Arnold, A. P. 1980. Quantitative analysis of sex differences in hormone accumulation in the Zebra finch brain: methodological and theoretical issues. J. Comp. Physiol. 189: 421-436.

Arnold, A. P., Nottebohm, F., and Pfaff, D. W. 1976. Hormone concentrating cells in vocal control and other areas of the brain of the Zebra finch. J. Comp. Neurol. 165: 487-512.

Aserinsky, E. and Kleitman, N. 1953. Two types of ocular motility occurring during sleep. J. Appl. Physiol. 8: 1-10.

Ayoub, D. M., Greenough, W. T. and Juraska, J. M. 1983. Sex differences in dendritic structure in the preoptic area of the juvenile macaque monkey brain. Science 219: 197-198.

Blackman, J. G. and Purves, R. D. 1969. Intracellular recordings from ganglia of the thoracic sympathetic chain of the guinea-pig. J. Physiol. 203: 173-198.

Boeckh, J. and Boeckh, B. 1979. Threshold and odor specificity of pheromone-sensitive neurons in the deutocerebrum of Antheraea pernyi and A. polyphemus (Saturnidae). J. Comp. Physiol. 132: 234-242.

Breedlove, S. M. and Arnold, A. P. 1980. Hormone accumulation in a sexually dimorphic motor nucleus of the rat spinal cord. Science 210: 564-566.

Brody, H. 1955. Organization of the cerebral cortex. IV. A study of aging in the human cerebral cortex. J. Comp. Neurol. 102: 511-556.

Bruce, C. J., Goldberg, M. E. 1985. Primate frontal eye fields: I. Single neurons discharging before saccades. J. Neurophysiol. 53: 603-635.

Calabrese, R. L. 1979. The roles of endogenous membrane properties and synaptic interaction in generating the heartbeat rhythm of the leech, Hirudo medicinalis. J. Exp. Biol. 82: 163-176.

Dearry, A., Gingrich, J. A., Falardeau, P., Fremeau, R. T., Jr., Bates, M. D. and Caron, M. G. 1990. Molecular cloning and expression of the gene for a human D_1 dopamine receptor. Nature 347: 72-76.

Deecke, L., Scheid, P. and Kornhuber, H. H. 1969. Distribution of readiness potential, pre-motion positivity, and motor potential of the human cerebral cortex preceding voluntary finger movements. Exp. Brain Res. 7: 158-168.

Dement, W. and Kleitman, N. 1957. Cyclic variations in EEG during sleep and their relations to eye movements, body motility, and dreaming. Electroencephalogr. Clin. Neurophysiol. 9: 673 690.

Dickinson, P. S., Mecsas, C. and Marder, E. 1990. Neuropeptide fusion of two motor-pattern generator circuits. Nature 344: 155-158.

Dodge, R. 1903. Five types of eye movement in the horizontal meridian plane of the field of regard. Am. J. Physiol. 8: 307-329.

Ehrlich, B. E. and Diamond, J. M. 1980. Lithium, membranes, and manic-depressive illness. J. Memb. Biol. 52: 187-200.

Evarts, E. V. and Tanji, J. 1976. Reflex and intended responses in motor cortex pyramidal tract neurons of monkeys. J. Neurophysiol. 39: 1069-1080.

Fuchs, A. F. 1967. Saccadic and smooth pursuit eye movements in the monkey. J. Physiol. 191: 609-631.

Furness, J. B. and Costa, M. 1980. Types of nerves in the enteric nervous system. Neuroscience 5 : 1-20.

Geschwind, N. and Levitsky, W. 1968. Human brain: Left–right asymmetries in temporal speech region. Science 161: 186-187.

Gibson, A. R., Robinson, R. R., Alam, J. and Houk, J. C. 1987. Somatotopic alignment between climbing fiber input and nuclear output of the cat intermediate cerebellum. J. Comp. Neurol. 260: 362-377.

Gilbert, P. F. C. and Thach, W. T. 1977. Purkinje cell activity during motor learning. Brain Res. 128: 309-328.

Goldman, J. E. and Yen, S.-H. 1986. Cytoskeletal protein abnormalities in neurodegenerative diseases. Ann. Neurol. 19: 209-223.

Gonshor, A. and Melville Jones, G. 1976. Short-term adaptive changes in the human vestibulo-ocular reflex arc. J. Physiol. 256: 361-379.

Gordon, B. 1973. Receptive fields in deep layers of cat superior colliculus. J. Neurophysiol. 36: 157-178.

Gorski, R. A., Gordon, J. H., Shryne, J. E. and Southam, A. M. 1978. Evidence for a morphological sex difference within the medial preoptic area of the rat brain. Brain Res. 148: 333-346.

Gravel, C. and Hawkes, R. 1990. Parasagittal organization of the rat cerebellar cortex. Direct comparison of Purkinje cell compartments and the organization of the spinocerebellar projection. J. Comp. Neurol. 291: 79-102.

Grinvald, A., Cohen, L. B., Lesher, S. and Boyle, M. B. 1981. Simultaneous optical monitoring of activity of many neurons in invertebrate ganglia using a 124-element photodiode array. J. Neurophysiol. 45: 829.840.

Grinvald, A., Hildesheim, R., Farber, I. C. and Anglister, L. 1982. Improved fluorescent probes for the measurement of rapid changes in membrane potential. Biophys. J. 39: 301-308.

Grinvald, A., Manker, A. and Segal, M. 1982. Visualization of the spread of electrical activity in rat hippocampal slices by voltage-sensitive optical probes. J. Physiol. 333: 269-291.

Gurney, M. E. and Konishi, M. 1980. Hormone-induced sexual differentiation of brain and behavior in zebra finches. Science 208: 1380-1383.

Hall, J. C. and Rosbash, M. 1988. Mutations and molecules influencing biological rhythms. Annu. Rev. Neurosci. 11: 373-394.

Hamos, J. E., DeGennaro, L. J. and Drachman, D. A. 1989. Synaptic loss in Alzheimer's disease and other dementias. Neurology 39: 355-361.

Henn, V., Lang, W., Hepp, K. and Reisine, H. 1984. Experimental gaze palsies in monkeys and their relation to human pathology. Brain 107: 619-636.

Heston, L. L. 1970. The genetics of schizophrenic and schizoid disease. Science 167: 249-256.

Hikosaka, O. and Wurz, R. H. 1983. Visual and oculomotor functions of monkey substantia nigra pars reticulata. I. Relation of visual and auditory responses to saccades. J. Neurophysiol. 49: 1230-1253.

Hobson, J. A., McCarley, R. W. and Wyzinski, P. W. 1975. Sleep cycle oscillation: Reciprocal discharge by two brainstem neuronal groups. Science 189: 55-58.

Hooper, S. L. and Moulins, M. 1989. Switching of a neuron from one network to another by sensory-induced changes in membrane properties. Science 244: 1587-1589.

Hore, J. and Flament, D. 1986. Evidence that a disordered servo-like mechanism contributes to tremor in movements during cerebellar dysfunction. J. Neurophysiol. 56: 123-136.

Hyman, B. T., Van Hoesen, G. W., Damasio, A. R. and Barnes, C. L. 1984. Alzheimer's disease: Cell specific pathology isolates the hippocampal formation. Science 225: 1168-1170.

Inglis, J. and Lawson, J. S. 1981. Sex differences in the effects of unilateral brain damage on intelligence. Science 212: 693-695.

Ito, M., Sakurai, M. and Tongroach, P. 1982. Climbing fibre induced depression of both mossy fibre responsiveness and glutamate sensitivity of cerebellar Purkinje cells. J. Physiol. 324: 113-134.

Jacklet, J. W. 1981. Circadian timing by endogenous oscillators in the nervous system: towards a cellular mechanism. Biol. Bull. 160: 199-227.

Jacobson, C. D. and Gorski, R. A. 1981. Neurogenesis of the sexually dimorphic nucleus of the preoptic area in the rat. J. Comp. Neurol. 196: 519-529.

Judge, S. J. and Cumming, B. G. 1986. Neurons in the monkey midbrain with activity related to vergence eye movement and accommodation. J. Neurophysiol. 55: 915-930.

Kaplan, E. and Barlow, R. B. 1980. Circadian clock in Limulus brain increases response and decreases noise of retinal photoreceptors. Nature 286: 393-395.

Kellogg, W. N. 1968. Communication and language in home-raised chimpanzee. Science 162: 423-427.

Kelso, S. R., Ganong, A. H. and Brown, T. H. 1986. Hebbian synapses in hippocampus. Proc. Natl. Acad. Sci. USA 83: 5326-5330.

Klarsfeld, A. and Changeux, J. P. 1985. Activity regulates the levels of acetycholine receptor α-subunit mRNA in cultured chicken myotubes. Proc. Natl. Acad. Sci. USA 82: 4558-4562.

Klein, M. and Kandel, E. R. 1980. Mechanism of calcium current modulation underlying presynaptic facilitation and behavioral senitization in Aplysia. Proc. Natl. Acad. Sci. USA 77: 6912-6916.

Kleinschmidt, A., Bear, M. F. and Singer, W. 1987. Blockade of 'NMDA' receptors disrupts experience-dependent plasticity of kitten striate cortex. Science 238: 355-357.

Lee, T., Seeman, P., Rajput, A., Farley, I. J. and Hornykiewicz, O. 1978. Receptor basis for dopaminergic supersensitivity in Parkinson's disease. Nature 273: 59-61

Levy, J., Trevarthen, C. and Sperry, R. W. 1972. Perception of bilateral chimeric figures following hemispheric deconnection. Brain 95: 61-78.

Lincoln, D. W. and Wakerley, J. B. 1974. Electrophysiological evidence for the activation of supraoptic neurones during the release of oxytocin. J. Physiol. 242: 533-554.

Livingstone, M. S., Harris-Warwick, R. M. and Kravitz, E. A. 1980. Serotonin and octopamine produce opposite postures in lobsters. Science 208: 76-79.

Llinás, R. and Sugimori, M. 1980. Electrophysiological properties of in vitro Purkinje cell somata in mammalian cerebellar slices. J. Physiol. 305: 171-195.

Llinás, R. and Sugimori, M. 1980. Electrophysiological properties of in vitro Purkinje cell dendrites in mammalian cerebellar slices. J. Physiol. 305: 197-213.

Lundberg, A. and Weight F. 1971. Functional organization of connexions to the ventral spinocerebellar tract. Exp. Brain Res. 12: 295-316.

Lynch, J. C. and MacLaren, J. W. 1989. Deficits of visual attention and saccadic eye movements after lesions of parietooccipital cortex in monkeys. J. Neurophysiol. 61: 74-90.

Lynch, J. C., Mountcastle, V. B., Talbot, W. H. and Yin, T. C. T. 1977. Parietal lobe mechanisms for directed visual attention. J. Neurophysiol. 40: 362-389.

MacLusky, N. J. and Naftolin, F. 1981. Sexual differentiation of the central nervous system. Science 211: 1294-1303.

McCarthy, R. A. and Warrington, E. K. 1988. Evidence for modality-specific meaning systems in the brain. Nature 334: 428-430.

McCormick, D. A. and Thompson, R. F. 1984. Cerebellum: essential involvement in the classically conditioned eyelid response. Science 223: 296-299.

McCormick, D. A., Steinmetz, J. E. and Thompson, R. F. 1985. Lesions of the inferior olivary complex cause extinction of the classically conditioned eyeblink response. Brain Res. 359: 120-130.

Meyer-Lohmann, J., Hore, J. and Brooks, V. B. 1977. Cerebellar participation in generation of prompt arm movements. J. Neurophysiol. 40: 1038-1050.

Miller, J. P. and Selverston, A. I. 1982. Mechanisms underlying pattern generation in lobster stomatogastric ganglion as determined by selective inactivation of identified neurons. IV. Network properties of pyloric system. J. Neurophysiol. 48: 1416-1432.

Moulins, M. and Nagy, F. 1983. Control of integration by extrinsic inputs in crustacean pyloric circuits. J. Physiol. 78: 739-748.

Mulloney, B. 1977. Organization of the stomatogastric ganglion of the spiny lobster. V. Coordination of the gastric and pyloric systems. J. Comp. Physiol. 122: 227-240.

Mulloney, B. and Selverston, A. I. 1974. Organization of the stomatogastric ganglion in the spiny lobster. I. Neurons driving the lateral teeth. J. Comp. Physiol. 91: 1-32.

Mulloney, B. and Selverston, A. I. 1974. Organization of the stomatogastric ganglion in the spiny lobster III. Coordination of the two subsets of the gastric system. J. Comp. Physiol. 91: 53-78.

Nottebohm, F. 1981. A brain for all seasons: cyclical anatomical changes in song control nuclei in the canary brain. Science 214: 1368-1370.

Nusbaum, M. P. and Marder, E. 1988. A neuronal role for a crustacean red pigment concentrating hormone-like peptide: Neuromodulation of the pyloric rhythm in the crab, Cancer borealis. J. Exp. Biol. 135: 165-181.

Nusbaum, M. P. and Marder, E. 1989. A modulatory proctolin-containing neuron (MPN). I. Identification and characterization. J. Neurosci. 9: 1591-1599.

Nusbaum, M. P. and Marder, E. 1989. A modulatory proctolin-containing neuron (MPN). II. State-dependent modulation of rhythmic motor activity. J. Neurosci. 9: 1600-1607.

Optican, L. M. and Robinson, D. A. 1980. Cerebellar dependent adaptive control of primate saccadic system. J. Neurophysiol. 44: 1058-1076.

Pavlov, I. P. 1906. The scientific investigation of the physical faculties or processes in the higher animals. Science 24: 613-619.

Pearson, R. C. A., Esiri, M. M., Hiorns, R. W., Wilcock, G. K and Powell, T. P. S. 1985. Anatomical correlates of the distribution of the pathological changes in the neocortex in Alzheimer disease. Proc. Natl. Acad. Sci. USA 82: 4531-4534.

Petersen, S. E., Fox, P. T., Posner, M. I., Minton, M. and Raichle, M. E. 1988. Positron emission tomographic studies of the cortical anatomy of single word processing. Nature 331: 585-589.

Posner, M. I., Petersen, S. E., Fox, P. T. and Raichle, M. E. 1988. Localization of cognitive operations in the human brain. Science 240: 1627-1631.

Pycock, D. J., Kerwin, R. W. and Carter, C. J. 1980. Effect of lesion of cortical dopamine terminals on subcortical dopamine receptors in rats. Nature 286: 74-77.

Phelps, M. E., Mazziotta, J. C. and Hueng, S.-C. 1982. Study of cerebral function with positron computed tomography. J. Cerebr. Blood Flow Metab. 2: 113-162.

Rainbow, T. C., Parsons, B. and McEwen, B. S. 1982. Sex differences in rat brain oestrogen and progestin receptors. Nature. 300. 648-649.

Raisman, G. and Field, P. M. 1971. Sexual dimorphism in the preoptic area of the rat. Science 173: 731-733.

Rauschecker, J. P. and Singer, W. 1981. The effects of early visual experience on the cat's visual cortex and their possible explanations by Hebb synapses. J. Physiol. 310: 215-239.

Reichert, H. and Rowell, C. H, F. 1985. Integration of non-phaselocked, exteroceptive information in the control of rhythmic flight in the locust. J. Neurophysiol. 53: 1202-1218.

Reichert, H., Rowell, C. H. F. and Griss, C. 1985. Course correction circuitry translates feature detection into behavioural action in locusts. Nature 315: 142-144.

Robertson, R. M. and Moulins, M. 1981. Oscillatory command input to the motor pattern generators of the crustacean stomatogastric ganglion. I. The pyloric rhythm. J. Comp. Physiol. 143: 453-463.

Robertson, R. M. and Moulins, M. 1981. Oscillatory command input to the motor pattern generators of the crustacean stomatogastric ganglion. II. The gastric rhythm. J. Comp. Physiol. 143: 473-491.

Robinson, D. A. 1970. Oculomotor unit behavior in the monkey. J. Neurophysiol. 33: 393-404.

Roffwarg, H. P., Muzio, J. N. and Dement, W. C. 1966. Ontogenetic development of the human sleep-dream cycle. Science 152: 604-619.

Roland, P. E. and Friberg, L. 1985. Localization of cortical areas activated by thinking. J. Neurophysiol. 53: 1219-1243.

Roland, P. E., Larsen, B., Lassen N. A. and Skinhof, E. 1980. Supplementary motor area and other cortical areas in organization of voluntary movements in man. J. Neurophysiol. 43. 118-136.

Rusak, B., Robertson, H. A., Wisden, W. and Hunt, S. P. 1990. Light pulses that shift rhythms induce gene expression in the suprachiasmatic nucleus. Science 248: 1237-1240.

Schlag, J. and Schlag-Rey, M. 1987. Evidence for a supplementary eye field. J. Neurophysiol. 57: 179-200.

Schwarz, W. J. and Gainer, H. 1977. Suprachiasmatic nucleus: use of ^{14}C-labelled deoxyglucose uptake as a functional marker. Science 197: 1089-1091.

Seeman, P. and Lee, T. 1975. Antipsychotic drugs: Direct correlation between clinical potency and presynaptic action on dopamine neurons. Science 188: 1217-1219.

Selverston, A. I. and Mulloney, B, 1974. Organization of the stomatogastric ganglion of spiny lobster. II. Neurons driving the medial tooth. J. Comp. Physiol. 91: 33-51.

Snider, R. S. and Stowell, A. 1944. Receiving areas of the tactile, auditory, and visual systems in the cerebellum. J. Neurophysiol. 7: 331-357.

Soechting, J. F., Ranish, N. A., Palminteri, R., Terzuolo, C. A. 1976. Changes in a motor pattern following cerebellar and olivary lesions in the squirrel monkey. Brain Res. 105: 21-44.

Sperry, R. W. 1970. Perception in the absence of neocortical commissures. Proc. Res. Assoc. Nerv. Ment. Dis. 48: 123-138.

Starzl, T. E., Taylor, C. W. and Mjagoun, H. 1951. Collateral afferent excitation of the reticular formation of the brain stem. J. Neurophysiol. 14: 479-496.

Swaab, D. F. and Fliers, E. 1985. A sexually dimorphic nucleus in the human brain. Science 228: 1112-1115.

Tanji, J. and Evarts, E. V. 1976. Anticipatory activity of motor cortex neurons in relation to the direction of an intended movement. J. Neurophysiol. 39: 1062-1068.

Tanzi, R. E., Gusella, J. F., Watkins, P. C., Bruns, G. A. P., St George-Hyslop, P., Van Keuren, M. L., Patterson, D., Pagan, S., Kurnit, D. M. and Neve, R. L. 1987. Amyloid β protein gene: cDNA, mRNA distribution, and genetic linkage near the Alzheimer locus. Science 235: 880-884.

Tazaki, K. and Cooke, I. M. 1979. Spontaneous electrical activity and integration of large and small cells in cardiac ganglion of the crab, Portunus sanguinolentus. J. Neurophysiol. 42: 975-999.

Thach, W. T. 1978. Correlation of neural discharge with pattern and force of muscular activity, joint position, and direction of intended next movement in motor cortex and cerebellum. J. Neurophysiol. 41:654-676.

Torebjörk, H. E. and Ochoa, J. 1980. Specific sensations evoked by activity in single identified sensory units in man. Acta Physiol. Scand. 110: 445-447.

Vale, W., Spiess, J., Rivier, C. and Rivier, J. 1981. Characterization of a 41-residue bovine hypothalamic peptide that stimulates secretion of corticotropin and β-endorphin. Science 213. 1394-1397.

Verney, E. B. 1974. The antidiuretic hormone and the factors which determine its release. Proc. R. Soc. Lond. B 135: 25-106.

Weidemann, A., König, G., Bunke, D., Fischer, P., Salbaum, J. M., Masters, C. L. and Beyreuther, K. 1989. Identification, biogenesis, and localization of precursors of Alzheimer's disease A4 amyloid protein. Cell 57: 115-126.

Witelson, S. F. 1976. Sex and the single hemisphere: Specialization of the right hemisphere for spatial processing. Science 193: 425-427.

Yankner, B. A., Dawes, L. R., Fisher, S., Villa-Komaroff, L., Oster-Granite, M. L. and Neve, R. L. 1989. Neurotoxicity of a fragment of the amyloid precursor associated with Alzheimer's disease. Science 245: 417-420.

Yarowsky, P. J. and Ingvar, D. H. Neuronal activity and energy metabolism. Fed. Proc. 40: 2353-2362.

7. Development

Neurogenesis: Neurons Are Born and Acquire an Identity

Early stages in embryology and the developmental program of neurogenesis

The development of the nervous system does not happen all at once. The nervous system is the product of a developmental program which involves neuronal proliferation, migration, differentiation, navigation, recognition, synapse formation and cell death. The way this program operates is precisely controlled by spatially and temporally defined molecular signals. These signals act in a regulatory way on the genes, and also influence other parts of the cellular machinery. They are partly epigenetic and partly genetic in origin. They lead to neuronal cells expressing certain neuronal properties, to growing neuronal processes being directed to the right target areas, and to the formation of the correct synaptic connections. However, the first requirement is neuronal determination. Neurons have to be generated and receive their identity.

The embryological events which precede neuronal determination are similar in many animals. A period of intensive cell division begins immediately after fertilization of the egg. This results, more by cell division than by growth, in the formation of an aggregate of about 1000 cells called a blastula or blastoderm. This is followed by gastrulation which begins as an invagination at one of the poles, and in most species leads to the formation of a three-layered embryo. The outermost of these layers is the ectoderm. The nervous system arises during subsequent development from a defined part of this ectoderm, called the *neuroectoderm*. The way that the complexity and specificity of the adult nervous system develop from a single layered epithelium is one of the most fascinating chapters in modern biology (Fig. 7.1).

Neuronal precursor cells derive from the neuroectoderm

In vertebrates the first sign of the development of the nervous system is a dorsally situated groove which forms on the ectodermal surface of the gastrula (Fig. 7.2). This process is termed neurulation. The groove thickens into a plate-like structure in which the cells of the neuroectoderm become established. Finally the edges of this neural plate arch upward and fuse into a *neural tube*. A swelling forms at the anterior end of this neural tube, and this is the first sign of the future brain. The majority of cells in the brain and spinal cord originate from neuronal precursor cells in the neural tube. By contrast, the peripheral nervous system originates largely from the *neural crest*. The neural crest also originates from the ectoderm and is found as bands of cells along the dorsolateral border of the neural tube. The sensory ganglia of the spinal cord and the ganglia of the autonomic nervous system among others arise from the neural crest. Epidermal plaques from the future head region also contribute cells to several sensory ganglia.

The nervous system originates from the ectoderm in invertebrates as well. This is not only true for the peripheral sensory cells which originate from repeated divisions of precursor cells in the epidermal layer, but also for the neurons of the central nervous system. In insects, for example, the neurons of the segmentally arranged central nervous ganglia develop from the plate-like neuroectoderm which lies ventrally, and extends from the head to the terminal segment (Fig. 7.3a). Certain cells move out of the neuroectoderm into a somewhat deeper layer in the embryo where they form an ordered group of neuronal precursor cells in each segment.

Not all the cells of the neuroectoderm generate neurons. In vertebrates only a part of the cells in the neural tube and neural crests develop into *neuroblasts,* that is into neuronal precursor cells. In invertebrates as well, only one class of cells from the neurogenic region of the ectoderm is converted into neuroblasts; the other cells produce epidermal cell types.

The determination of the neuroectoderm is initiated by inductive interactions

The commitment of a given cell population to a future developmental fate is called *determination.* In vertebrates determination of the neuroectoderm begins with interactions between the embryonic dorsal ectoderm and the em-

bryonic mesoderm, which comes to lie under the ectoderm during the process of gastrulation. This interactive process of neural *induction* is assumed to be initiated by molecular factors released from the mesoderm. The establishment of regional specificity along the anterior-posterior axis of the future nervous system is also the result of interactions between mesoderm and ectoderm. This process establishes the main regions which later produce the cerebral ganglia as well as the spinal cord.

An important consequence of neuronal determination is the decision as to whether a cell in the neuroectoderm will transform itself into a neuronal precursor cell or not. In insects the segregation of neuroectodermal cells into neuronal or epidermal lineages occurs largely

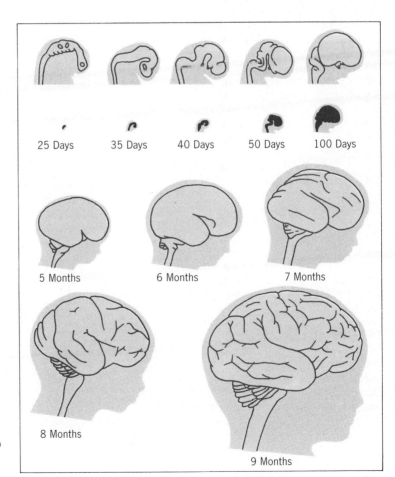

25 Days   35 Days   40 Days   50 Days   100 Days

5 Months   6 Months   7 Months

8 Months

9 Months

Fig. 7.1   Schematic illustration of the embryonic development of the human brain. Developmental sequence of the embryonic and fetal stages. The first 5 stages are shown to scale (bottom) and enlarged to the same size (top) (after Cowan)

via inductive interactions between the initially equivalent cells of the neuroectoderm (Fig. 7.**3b**). When an ectodermal cell first begins to enlarge and differentiate into a neuroblast it produces signals which prevent neighboring cells from also developing into neuroblasts. A group of "neurogenic" genes whose products mediate these cell–cell interactions has been identified in *Drosophila*. The cellular identity of each developing neuroblast is determined by its position in the neuroectoderm. The requisite positional information is at least partly provided by the expression of segmentation genes in the early embryo.

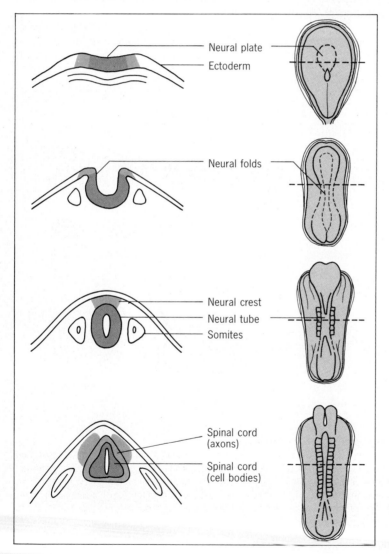

Neural plate

Ectoderm

Neural folds

Neural crest

Neural tube

Somites

Spinal cord
(axons)

Spinal cord
(cell bodies)

Fig. 7.**2**   Genesis of the human nervous system from the ectoderm. A cross-section through the middle of the developing spinal cord (left) and a view from above (right) are shown for various stages (after Cowan)

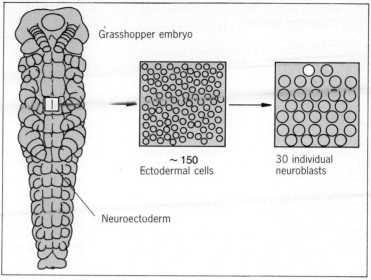

a

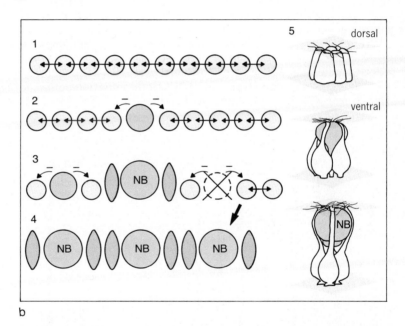

b

Fig. 7.**3**   Neuroblast formation in the grasshopper. **a** Neuroblasts (neuronal precursor cells) originate from a layer of ecto-dermal cells (neuroectoderm) in every segment. **b** The decision as to whether a cell in the neuroectoderm is transformed into a neuroblast or into an epidermal cell largely depends on inductive interactions (1). When one cell begins to develop into a neuroblast it inhibits its neighbors, and prevents them from also differentiating into neuroblasts (2). When a differen-tiated neuroblast is removed, the inhibition falls away (3), and one of the neighboring cells replaces the eliminated neuro-blast (4). During normal development a neuroblast's neighboring cells differentiate into supporting cells (5) (after Kuwada and Goodman, and Doe and Goodman)

Cell proliferation follows a characteristic spatiotemporal pattern

The extent of neuronal proliferation depends on the number of neuronal precursor cells, on the kinetics of the cell division cycle in these precursor cells, and on the overall duration of the proliferative period. Every nerve cell resulting from the proliferation process has a "birthday." This is the time at which a given post-mitotic neuron is produced during the relevant division of the precursor cell. In some cases neighboring neurons (for example neurons in a given cortical layer) have "birthdays" which are close together in time. They arise from cell divisions occurring in a defined, narrow time window. In general, however, the different neuron types in a complex neuronal structure are not all born at the same time, but rather every single cell type is formed during a characteristic phase in development.

In most bilaterally symmetrical animals neuron generation begins at the anterior pole of the developing nervous system and then proceeds caudally. In vertebrates there is a ventro-dorsal gradient as well as a rostrocaudal gradient in neuron proliferation and maturation. This is why the motor systems in the spinal cord are differentiated and functional before the sensory systems. Neuron production not only occurs in an exactly defined spatial and temporal sequence, but is also restricted to certain germinal regions in the brain. In the vertebrate CNS the neuroblasts are largely restricted to the columnar epithelium on the inside (ventricular side) of the neural tube. The increase in cell number during proliferation in this germinal zone results in the neural tube rapidly increasing in thickness from only a single layer of epithelial cells originally.

The progression of the cell division cycle of a neuronal stem cell in the neural tube is interesting (Fig. 7.4). In the G1 phase of the cell cycle the stem cell is connected to the outer and inner surfaces of the neural tube epithelium by cytoplasmic processes, with its cell body lying near the lumen (ventricular zone). The cell body then migrates into the outer layer of the epithelium (marginal zone), where DNA replication subsequently occurs during the S phase. In the G_2 phase that follows, the cell body migrates back into the ventricular zone, and in the M phase the cell then loses contact with the epithelial surfaces and divides. After division both sister cells renew contact with the epithelial surfaces and a new mitotic cycle can

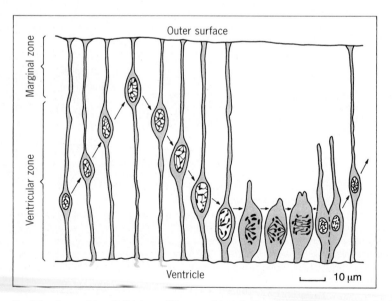

Fig. 7.4   Symmetric cell divisions of the neuroblasts in the neural tube of a vertebrate. Nuclei only divide in the ventricular zone. Some time later the cells switch to asymmetric cell divisions. The postmitotic neurons resulting from asymmetric cell divisions leave the epithelium and migrate to the outer layers of the developing central nervous system (after Sauer)

begin. After a few cell divisions these stem cells stop dividing symmetrically and begin to divide asymmetrically. These asymmetric cell divisions of the neuroblasts then generate the various neuronal cell types. These finally leave the germinal zone as postmitotic neurons (or as glia cells).

Neurons originate from neuronal precursor cells by division and differentiation

The process by which cells acquire more and more different characteristics is termed differentiation. Differentiation processes are the result of many complex interacting mechanisms, and in the final analysis are based on a modulation of gene expression during development. The mechanisms by which a neuron acquires its individual cellular and molecular identity can be divided into two general classes.

— *Lineage mechanisms.* The history of previous cell divisions, and therefore the "position in the family tree," are essential in determining the neuronal properties of cells.
— *Positional mechanisms.* Here the spatial arrangement of cells in the tissue and the resulting interactions with neighboring cells are critical.

In each individual case either one or the other mechanism predominates. The differentiation of neurons in the nematode *Caenorhabditis elegans* is largely lineage-dependent, for example (Fig. 7.**5**). In this animal the nervous system consists of exactly 302 neurons, which fall into at least 118 different differentiated types. All these neurons originate from precursor cells in a stereotyped way. The properties of these neurons are largely (but not completely) determined by their lineage from neuronal precursor cells.

   In general, however, both lineage mechanisms and cell–cell interactions are influential in neurogenesis. The determination of neuronal identity can be followed very clearly in the nerve cells of the segmental ganglia of insects, since many neurons in these ganglia are individually identifiable. The neuroblasts in the segmental ganglia of the grasshopper divide repeatedly and so produce a chain of ganglion mother cells (Fig. 7.**6a**). Each ganglion mother cell divides once more and so produces two ganglion cells which subsequently differ-

entiate into neurons. A single neuroblast can produce between 6 and 100 nerve cells. In this way every neuroblast contributes a whole family of neurons to a ganglion, and then dies. The neurons produced by a neuroblast are not all of the same type, but have structural and functional differences. The relative significance of lineage and of interactions with neighboring cells during this neurogenesis is complex. When a neuroblast begins to divide, lineage initially plays a greater role in determining the identity of its immediate progeny, the ganglion mother cells.

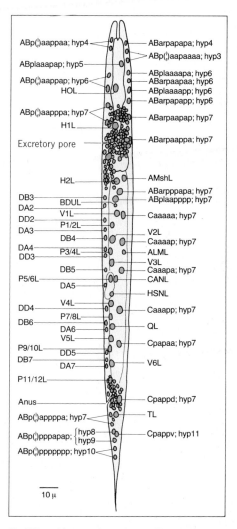

Fig. 7.**5a** Lineage-dependent differentiation in the nervous system of a nematode. Identified neuronal and hypodermal cells of a larva of *Caenorhabditis*

The two neurons which result from the division of the ganglion mother cells are initially equal. Their exact developmental fate is only decided by interactions with each other. However, the properties of the neurons are largely predetermined after this last determination phase.

What is known about the genetic regulation of neuronal differentiation? Insects are favorable model systems for answering this question, too. As in every other nervous system, the development of the insect nervous system depends on the exact spatial and temporal control of the expression of numerous genes

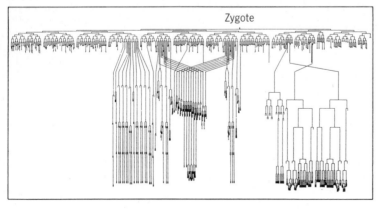

Fig. 7.**5b**   Lineage of all the cells in the animal (after Sulston et al., and Chalfie)

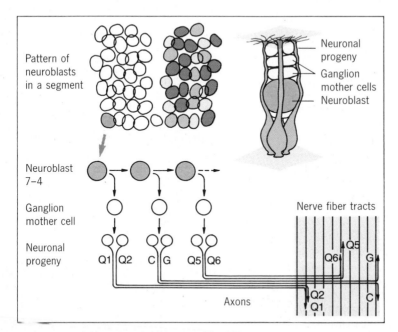

Fig. 7.**6a,b**   Neurogenesis in the grasshopper. **a** The neuroblasts of a body segment are arranged in a stereotyped pattern and divide repeatedly to produce ganglion mother cells, which themselves divide once so that each produces two post-mitotic neurons (top). Neuroblast 7–4 produces about 100 neuronal progeny. These form axons which grow out along nerve bundles in the ganglionic chain (bottom). Q1, Q2, C, G, Q5, and Q6 are neurons

which specify cell fate. Many of these genes are first expressed in a relatively simple spatial pattern during the blastoderm stage, and then reappear in an increasingly complex expression pattern during the course of further embryogenesis. It is interesting that the same segmentation genes which contribute to determining the identity of neuroblasts early in embryonic development are also expressed in later stages in small subgroups of differentiating neurons. If the expression of such genes is disturbed during neurogenesis, for example with molecular genetic manipulation in *Drosophila*, then the identity of some of these neurons is transformed. This can be seen by the fact that the affected neurons develop, among other things, different structures. One can assume that a limited number of these genes are involved in determining neuronal identity by combinatory and regulatory interactions of their gene products.

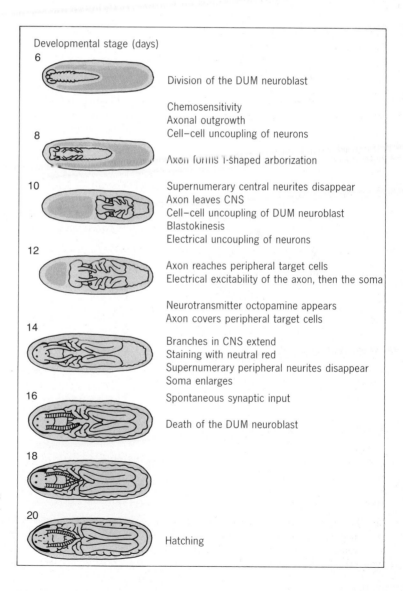

Developmental stage (days)

6 — Division of the DUM neuroblast

Chemosensitivity
Axonal outgrowth
Cell–cell uncoupling of neurons

8 — Axon forms T-shaped arborization

10 — Supernumerary central neurites disappear
Axon leaves CNS
Cell–cell uncoupling of DUM neuroblast
Blastokinesis
Electrical uncoupling of neurons

12 — Axon reaches peripheral target cells
Electrical excitability of the axon, then the soma

Neurotransmitter octopamine appears
Axon covers peripheral target cells

14 — Branches in CNS extend
Staining with neutral red
Supernumerary peripheral neurites disappear
Soma enlarges

16 — Spontaneous synaptic input

Death of the DUM neuroblast

18

20 — Hatching

Fig. 7.**6b** Temporal sequence of appearance of various neuronal characteristics in identified neurons of the grasshopper. The time at which the neuronal phenotype first appears is shown opposite the various embryonic stages. DUM = dorsal unpaired median (after Goodman et al., Goodman and Spitzer)

Individual neurons display a temporal sequence in the differentiation of cellular-neuronal properties

Neuronal differentiation occurs in a series of precisely synchronized orderly steps. An example of such a process can be seen in the development of electrical excitability in neurons. In one of the earliest developmental phases certain neurons form action potentials whose inward current is carried by Ca^{2+} ions. In a subsequent developmental phase they switch to action potentials which are formed by a combination of Ca^{2+} and Na^+ ions. In an even later phase they produce action potentials whose inward current is carried exclusively by Na^+ ions. At the molecular level this means that early in development these neurons mainly employ Ca^{2+} ion channels to generate action potentials, and then later switch to implanting Na^+ channels into their cell membrane.

In invertebrates, the time-dependent appearance of certain cellular properties during development can be followed in detail in identified neurons. These properties include axonal outgrowth, formation of dendrites, electrical coupling, chemosensititvity, and neurotransmitter synthesis. A given neuronal cell type always displays a stereotyped progression in the expression of these various neuronal characteristics (Fig. 7.**6b**).

An orderly temporal progression of neuronal differentiation does not mean that all neurons are strictly preprogrammed from the beginning to have a particular fate. For those neurons deriving from the neural crest, the decision on a neurotransmitter type remains flexible for a long period of time. The neurons of the autonomic ganglia, for example, can develop into cholinergic cells, noradrenergic cells, or cells with two transmitter substances (cholinergic and noradrenergic) depending on the cellular, hormonal, and biochemical nature of their environment.

Cellular migration plays a role in the organogenesis of the nervous system

Relatively early in development neurons must occupy certain positions in the tissue. This is important to allow later processes such as the directed outgrowth of neurites, or the proper formation of synapses, to occur. To achieve this, neurons, or neuronal precursor cells, must often migrate relatively far through the embryonic tissue. These cell migrations can occur at a rate of about 100 µm per day.

The cells of the neural crest are the migratory champions (Fig. 7.7). They migrate from their site of origin to completely different parts of the embryo. In the process they divide and produce neurons, glia and other cell types.

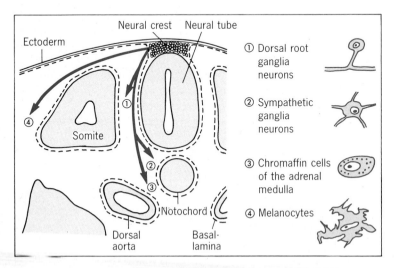

Fig. 7.**7** Migration of the neural crest cells, simplified. Cross-section through the trunk region of a chick embryo at the time of cell migration. Cells taking a deeply ventral migratory path form, among others, the dorsal root ganglia (1), the sympathetic ganglia (2) and the medullary cells of the adrenal gland (3). Cells taking a superficial migratory path form melanocytes (4) (after Sanes)

The process of migration has an important imprinting effect on these cells. This is because their final differentiated state is influenced by interactions with their surroundings during and after migration.

The cells from which the brain and spinal cord derive remain mostly in their ventricular zone of origin until they come into the postmitotic phase. Only then do cell migrations occur. The skeletal motoneurons of vertebrates, for example, derive from cell divisions in the ventricular zone of the neural tube. From there they migrate into the ventral horn of the developing spinal cord. The different layers in the vertebrate cortex also arise from cell migrations. Cortical neurons derive from cell divisions of precursor cells on the innermost ventricular zone and then migrate to finally position themselves in layers at specific regions between the ventricular and marginal zones. Following their migration the "first born" nerve cells settle in a layer near the external surface of the cortex. Nerve cells born subsequently migrate through this first layer and settle only when farther outside. In this way the layers of the cerebral cortex are built up from the inside out. Although most neurons no longer divide following their migration out of the ventricular zone, there are a few exceptions. The neurons in the basal ganglia and in related structures of the cerebrum, as well as some interneurons in the cerebral cortex and the cerebellum, arise from neuronal cells in the subventricular zone via a second wave of proliferation.

Just how important the exact progression of cell migrations is for the organogenesis of the CNS can be seen from the development of the granule cells of the cerebellum. The granule cell precursors first arise in the ventricular zone after the large Purkinje and Golgi cells. They then migrate past the Purkinje and Golgi cells and form the outermost layer in the developing cerebellum. A second wave of proliferation occurs in this external granule layer and generates the basket and stellate cells, in addition to the granule cells. In the primate brain the proliferation of granule cells can extend into the second year of life. Following their

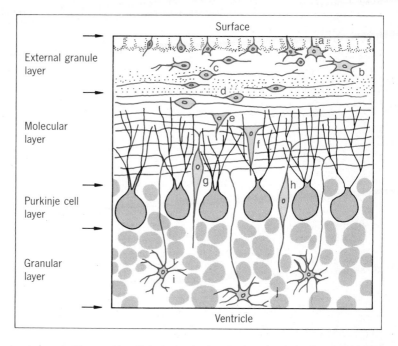

Fig. 7.**8** Cell migration during the development of the granule cells in the cerebellum. Precursor cells migrate from the ventricular zone into the external granule layer where they produce postmitotic granule cells (a). The granule cells develop bipolar processes in the external granule layer (b,c,d), and send a third nerve process into the molecular layer (e,f). The cell bodies of the granule cells then migrate along this outgrowing process (g,h) through the molecular layer and Purkinje layer and finally reach their destination in the granular layer (i,j) (after Jacobson)

formation the granule cells develop two bipolar neurites running parallel to the surface. They then send a third neurite past the Purkinje cells deep into the cerebellum. Finally their cell body migrates along this growing neurite through the molecular and Purkinje cell layers, in order to form the mature granular layer near the ventricular surface (Fig. 7.**8**).

Cell migrations do not always run according to plan. Some of the migrating neurons reach the wrong sites in the nervous system. Most of these "lost" neurons are later eliminated by cell death.

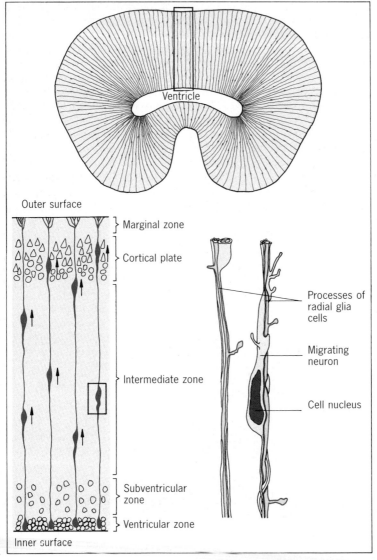

Fig. 7.**9** The role of the radial glia cells in cell migration.
a Processes of the regularly arranged radial glia cells traverse the whole width of the developing cerebral cortex (bottom left). Postmitotic neurons from the ventricular zone migrate along the processes

Cellular scaffolds aid neuronal navigation

How do embryonic neurons determine where they should migrate to, and when they should terminate their migratory phase? In the cerebral cortex migratory neurons appear to move along special nonneural guidance pathways. These are formed by the radial glia cells which extend from the ventricular surface to the external surface of the cortex (Fig. 7.**9a**). These radial glia cells are present while the cortex is developing, but in most cases disappear shortly thereafter. Neurons are closely associated with these radial glia cells during their migration. In mutants in which the glia cells are lacking or improperly organized the development of cortical structures can be extensively disturbed. Radial glia cells are also found in the embryonic spinal cord where they also function as guides for migrating neurons.

An attractive hypothesis for the origin of cortical columns postulates that groups of proliferating cells which arise from symmetrical cell divisions in the ventricular zone are separated from one another by glia, and that each such group is associated with a radial glia cell

(Fig. 7.**9b**). Each proliferating unit then produces various neuron types via asymmetric cell divisions, and an embryonic cortical column results from neuronal migration along the radial glia cell. The number of columns in a given cortical region—and with it the surface of the cortex—is in this model simply determined by the number of proliferating cell aggregates which are formed in early development.

Transiently occurring cellular scaffolds are also found in invertebrates. They also aid in neuronal navigation, although they are more important for the outgrowth of neurites than for cell migration. In the segmental ganglia of *Drosophila*, glia cells are laid down in an orderly pattern. The position of these cells anticipates the course of the connectives between the future ganglia, as well as the course of the major commissures in each segmental ganglion and the location of some of the peripheral nerves. These glial pathways are assumed to serve mainly the outgrowing neurons as guiding structures.

The migration of cells of the neural crest is not only directed by guiding structures. These cells must migrate over relatively long

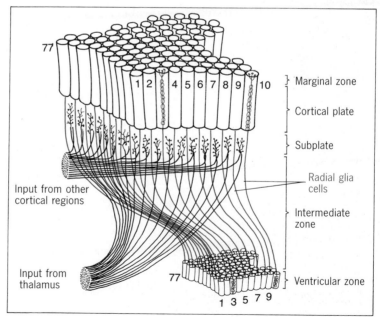

of the radial glia cells (right). **b** Hypothesis for the origin of cortical columns. Proliferative groups of neuroblasts are associated with every glia cell. The neurons generated by a given proliferative group migrate centrifugally along the same radial glia cell and form a column-shaped stack of cells in the cortical plate (after Rakic)

Input from other cortical regions

Marginal zone

Cortical plate

Subplate

Radial glia cells

Intermediate zone

Input from thalamus

Ventricular zone

b

distances through embryonic mesoderm before they reach their targets. The migratory pathways for these cells are assumed to be determined to a great extent by the cell types encountered en route, as well as by the properties of the extracellular matrix. In addition to these locally situated landmarks, positional information is probably also distributed over the entire embryo. However, exactly how the migrating neural crest cells read this information is still unclear.

Axogenesis: How Axons Reach Their Targets

Factors which regulate directed axonal navigation

Nerve cells have to direct their processes with great precision across relatively large distances for neuronal circuits to be established. The axons and dendrites of developing neurons do this by directed navigation rather than by non-directed outgrowth. In doing so they often follow directional cues from the very beginning and make surprisingly few mistakes. Currently we know that directed axonal outgrowth is regulated by many factors, such as the mechanical properties of embryonic tissue, the molecular composition of the substrate, and the cellular organization of the environment, as well

as factors diffusing through the intracellular medium. It is also clear that the relative importance of these factors varies in different developmental stages.

Neurites form growth cones during their development

The structure of a neuron can be viewed as the morphological evidence of the navigational decisions it has made during development. This is because the path followed by each individual neurite, axon and dendrite, is based on a continuous sequence of decisions made by special subcellular structures. These structures, which function as the actual pathfinders during neurite outgrowth, are the growth cones discovered by Cajal at the end of the 19th century (Fig. 7.**10**).

Growth cones are formed at the tips of all outgrowing embryonic neurites. In general the axonal growth cone of a neuron grows out of the cell body first; dendritic processes follow shortly thereafter with their own growth cones. Cell body and growth cone are relatively independent of one another. In many cases the outgrowing growth cones do not cause the cell body to move. Experimentally isolated growth cones, by contrast, can move about independently of the cell body for a period of time.

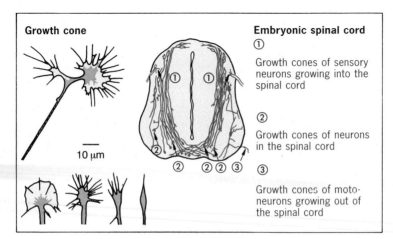

Growth cone

Embryonic spinal cord

① Growth cones of sensory neurons growing into the spinal cord

② Growth cones of neurons in the spinal cord

③ Growth cones of motoneurons growing out of the spinal cord

10 μm

Fig. 7.**10**   Growth cones assume different shapes according to the substrate on which they are growing (left). In the embryonic spinal cord of the chick, growth cones are found on all the outgrowing neurites (right) (after Bray and Cajal)

During their ameboid-like movement within the complex environment of the developing nervous system, the growth cones extend numerous processes which are termed *filopodia* or *lamellipodia* depending on their structure. The tufted filopodia sample the environment directly around the growth cone. In this process they are constantly in motion—they extend and contract cyclically every few minutes. They establish contact with the surfaces of other cells and with the extracellular matrix by means of many fine microspikes. During movement of the growth cone there is an incorporation of cell membrane components near the tip of the growth cone and simultaneously a stabilization of the neurite forming behind it by elements of the cytoskeleton.

Growth cones can be guided by the substrate; they show selective adhesion

The physical properties of the substrate on which the neurite and its growth cones grow can contribute to guidance and pathfinding. An important factor here is the adhesiveness of the substrate. Like fibroblasts, growth cones show a preference for substrates to which they adhere strongly. Since substrates differ in their adhesiveness, directed navigation can result from selective adhesion between outgrowing neurites and the extracellular substrate. This can be demonstrated in a cell culture in which outgrowing neurons are offered a choice of several substrate types. The growth cones grow preferentially on those substrates to which their cell membrane adheres more strongly. In many cases the neurites which form during growth also adhere to the substrate. If the attractive substrate is laid out in a particular geometrical pattern, for example in the culture dish, then the growth cones follow this pattern (Fig. 7.11). The navigational performance of the growth cones on the adhesive substrate is then retained in the morphology of the neurite that is formed during outgrowth.

How can spatial differences in adhesion between growth cone and substrate lead to directed growth? During their repeated extension and retraction the filopodia of a growth cone sample a relatively large area of the substrate. If they preferentially adhere to a given region of substrate, this could produce a tension which might pull the tip of the growth cone in the direction of the site of adhesion. A range of components in the extracellular matrix is adapted for selective adhesion with outgrowing neurites and their growth cones. The two large glycoproteins laminin and fibronectin are the best characterized of these substrate-bound adhesion molecules. A whole

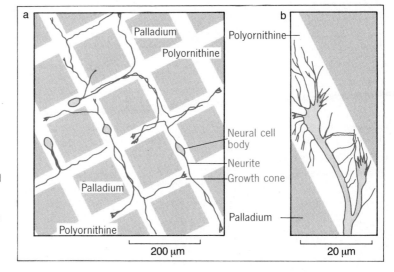

Fig. 7.11 Selective adhesion of growth cones. **a** In cell culture, growth cones show a preference for polyornithine-covered surfaces and avoid palladium-covered areas. **b** An enlargement of the growth cone shows how the filopodia remain in the polyornithine region (after Letourneau)

range of cell-bound receptor molecules, called integrins, which can recognize fibronectin and laminin are currently known.

The motility of growth cones is not only influenced by selective adhesion, but also by a range of other factors like selective contact inhibition, electrical activity, neurotransmitters, and growth substances. Many of these factors are assumed to exert their effect on growth cone behavior via changes in the intracellular Ca²⁺ concentration. The receptors and *second-*

messenger systems involved in translating extracellular chemical signals into a changed intracellular Ca^{2+} concentration are known in a few cases. The intracellular Ca^{2+} concentration could regulate the contractile apparatus within the growth cone, analogous to the situation in muscle cells. In this respect growth cones can be broadly seen as a sort of transducing apparatus which recognizes molecular information in the developing nervous system and transforms it into directed movement (Fig. 7.12).

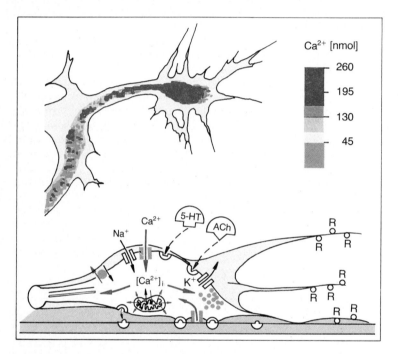

Fig. 7.**12**   The role of Ca^{2+} in the outgrowth of growth cones. The Ca^{2+} concentration in the growth cone is higher than that in other regions of the neuron. Evidence from Ca^{2+}-selective dyes (top). Model of Ca^{2+}-dependent regulation in the growth cone (bottom). Ca^{2+} acts on cytoskeletal elements and on the incorporation of membrane components. Changes in the intracellular Ca^{2+} concentration can result from ion flux across the membrane or via release from intracellular stores. These changes can be regulated by transmitter substances or by the binding of cell surface receptors to substrate regions. 5-HT = 5-hydroxytryptamine, ACh = acetylcholine, R = cell surface receptors (after Kater)

Diffusible molecules evoke chemotactic behavior in growth cones and act as trophic factors

Neuronal navigation mechanisms are most probably not restricted to local interactions. There must also be signals which are active across greater distances. Such signals could consist of a diffusible chemical gradient emanating from a spatially localized source. Although chemical messenger substances of this sort are currently being studied, their biochemical characterization is still incomplete. The way that such chemical signal systems might work can, however, be demonstrated with a model based on the protein *NGF (nerve growth factor)* discovered by Levi-Montalcini, and subsequently well characterized.

NGF is synthesized as part of a larger protein precursor. This precursor consists of two α-, one β-, and two γ- subunits (Fig. 7.13). It is the β-subunit which is neuroactive. This subunit is a dimer with a molecular weight of 26 kDa. The actual NGF, a monomer, consists of 118 amino acids and has sequence homologies with insulin, which also has growth promoting properties.

NGF stimulates the growth and differentiation of certain neurons, especially those in sympathetic and sensory ganglia. Focal injection of NGF into different regions of the CNS during embryonic development can lead to neurons in sympathetic ganglia orienting their outgrowing neurites toward the injection site (Fig. 7.14a). This is probably because the outgrowing axons follow the NGF gradients chemotactically. Cell culture experiments show that growth cones do respond to NGF gradients with directed outgrowth. However, it is still not clear whether NGF acts as a chemotactic substance during the normal development of the nervous system.

NGF seems to be essential for the survival of certain neurons during embryonic development. It has a *trophic function*. This can be seen from the fact that most neurons in the sympathetic and sensory ganglia die when antibodies against NGF are injected into embryos. Moreover, embryonic neurons from these ganglia can only be maintained in culture over

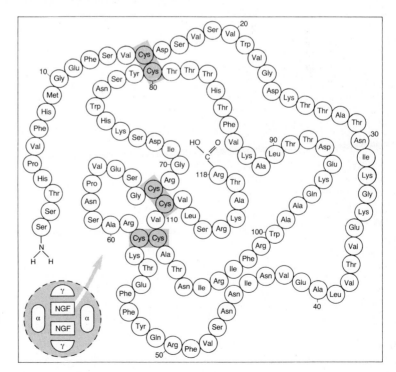

Fig. 7.**13** Structure of NGF. Amino acid sequence of the β-subunit monomer which is the active component of a larger protein precursor (after Angeletti and Bradshaw)

longer periods when NGF is added to the medium (Fig. 7.**14b**). NGF is normally produced and released by the target cells of these neurons. It is then taken up pinocytotically by the neuron terminals and transported via retrograde axonal transport to the cell body where it acts on differential gene expression. A raised NGF concentration increases the amounts of protein and neurotransmitter produced by individual neurons and may also fulfill other important trophic functions in neurons of the CNS.

Many other growth factors which act on specific neurons are known. These include BDNF *(brain-derived neurotrophic factor),* other homologous growth factors known as *neurotrophins,* as well as an undescribed molecular factor which is important for the growth and survival of motoneurons. NGF is probably representative of a variety of retrograde- or anterograde-acting neurogenic substances, all of which have comparable trophic properties.

Pioneer neurons pave the way

Growth cones tend to contact and grow along other nerve cells, and this property can be utilized for neuronal navigation. Small groups of guiding pioneer neurons have been described during the development of the central and peripheral nervous systems in a few invertebrates, and in the spinal cord of lower vertebrates (Fig. 7.**15**). They are the first cells to find their way to their targets, and they then serve as a guiding path for following axons. There are cohesive forces between growth cones and neurites, as well as between different neurites, so that later developing neurites interweave with the axons formed by the pioneer neurons. The end result of this process is that an animal's nervous pathways are mostly made up of parallel axon bundles called *fascicles.*

The process of fasciculation can be followed in detail during the embryonic development of the grasshopper. In this animal pairs of neurons form the first projections from the leg and antennal rudiments into the CNS. Other axons join them, and the individual peripheral nerve pathways form by fasciculation. Pioneer neurons not only grow centrally from the periphery, they also grow from the ganglia of the CNS into the periphery. In many cases inwardly and outwardly growing pioneers meet, and so form the basis of nerve pathways. Finally, the various fiber tracts in the commissures and connectives of the animal are also laid down by pioneer neurons and built up by selective fasciculation of subsequently outgrowing neurites with these axon pathways.

The establishment of nerve pathways by pioneer neurons can only be fully understood when the navigational mechanisms that the pioneers use are also clarified. Navigation in

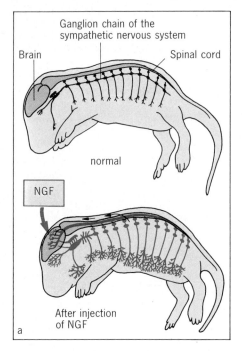

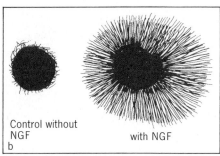

Fig. 7.**14**   Effect of NGF. **a** Neurotrophic actions of NGF following its injection into the brain of a neonatal rat. NGF diffuses from the injection site into the spinal cord and reaches the chain of sympathetic ganglia. This induces an abnormal outgrowth of sympathetic nerve fibers which even reach the brain. **b** NGF induces the outgrowth of neurons in cell culture. An isolated sensory ganglion of an embryonic chick after 24 hours growth with, and without, NGF in the medium (after Levi-Montalcini and Callissano)

early developmental stages is certainly made easier by the fact that the distances which have to be overcome are relatively short. The pioneer neurons can therefore sample their surroundings for likely targets more easily than would be the case after extensive embryonic growth. Cells which are transiently contacted by outgrowing neurites also play an important role. These "guidepost" cells can present the outgrowing axons with molecular signals for correct navigation. Molecular directional information may also be present in the extracellular matrix, on other neurons and neurites, on glia cells, as well as in secreted form in the embryo.

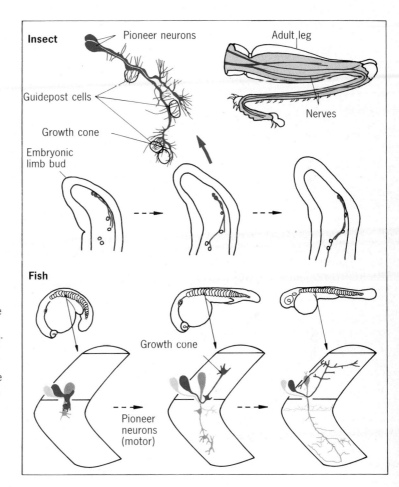

Fig. 7.**15** Pioneer neurons. The earliest neurons in the embryonic limb bud of a grasshopper (top) and in the myotomes of a fish (bottom). In both cases pioneer neurons form the first peripheral nerve pathways. The pioneer neurons of the grasshopper navigate with the help of "guidepost" cells which they contact with their growth cones (after Taghert et al., and Westerfield and Eisen)

Cell-bound adhesion molecules are important for the outgrowth and cohesiveness of nerve fibers

What mediates the adhesion and contact guidance of growth cones to other neurons? Are there interactions apart from adhesion to different extracellular substrates which can also be attributed to cell-bound adhesion molecules? Studies on embryonic neurons in dissociated cell culture have shown that neurons from a given region in the CNS aggregate preferentially with those from certain other regions in the CNS. When cells from various parts of the embryonic nervous system are dissociated and mixed, reaggregation and separation of the cells occurs after a certain time. Neurons from different regions of the retinotectal system of the chicken show this sort of preferential aggregation. Neurons from the temporal region of the retina even show a preferential outgrowth onto particular cell membrane fractions when these are obtained from the appropriate anterior part of the tectum.

Studies characterizing the cell-attached molecules which have adhesive properties have uncovered two families of general membrane-bound adhesion molecules: the Ca^{2+}-independent *N-CAMs (cell adhesion molecules)* and the Ca^{2+}-dependent cadherins. The best studied N-CAM is an integral membrane glycoprotein with a molecular weight of about 200 kDa (Fig. 7.16). N-CAMs have a homophilic adhesion mechanism; the N-CAMs of one cell bind to the N-CAMs of another cell. N-CAMs have N-acetyl neuramino acid and proteoglycan residues which can vary in their stoichiometric composition depending on the tissue and its developmental stage.

The cadherins are functionally similar to the N-CAMs. At present three main groups of cadherins are known: E-cadherin, P-cadherin and N-cadherin. The molecular diversity of the cadherins is not based on changes in the composition of bound carbohydrate residues, but is found at the DNA level in the form of functionally related gene families.

The different cell-bound adhesion molecules are assumed to appear in the various regions of the developing nervous system in a temporally and spatially changing pattern, and act as a "neuronal glue" for the cohesiveness of outgrowing axons. This is supported by the observation that antibodies against N-CAMs inhibit the tendency of growing neurites to stay together. Local changes in the amount, the distribution, or the molecular composition of these molecules can cause changes in adhesiveness, and so contribute to morphogenetic processes in the nervous system. Such dynamic changes in the molecular properties of adhesion molecules could lead to different adhesive patterns being laid down in embryonic tissue without there having to be a large number of adhesion molecules.

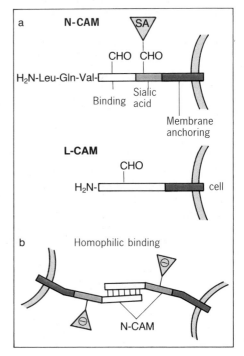

Fig. 7.**16a,b** Cell adhesion molecules. **a** Structure of N-CAM and L-CAM (E-Cadherin), very diagrammatic. The N-CAM glycoprotein is subdivided into an N-terminal part which is responsible for binding, a central portion to which sialic acid residues (N-acetylneuroaminic acid residues) are attached, and a C-terminal part which anchors the molecule in the membrane. **b** Diagram of the homophilic binding between two N-CAM molecules which are located on different cells

Are there target recognition molecules?

A developing nervous system is an absolute maze of neuronal cell bodies, dendrites, neuron fascicles, glia cells and other nonneural elements. It is obvious that outgrowing neurites cannot blindly follow the nearest nerve fiber bundle or glial pathway. Additional mechanisms must operate so that individual neurons can develop their specific structural and connectivity properties. While N-CAMs and cadherins are found throughout the embryo in vertebrates (and in similar form in invertebrates) and participate in morphogenesis at many sites, other molecules have been identified with specific functions in neuronal navigation. There is evidence that these molecules are expressed on the surface of certain groups of embryonic nerve cells, and that the growth cones of particular neurites can specifically recognize these molecules. The distribution of these "recognition molecules" could represent a sort of map for the growth cones.

Specific membrane-associated glycoproteins which label certain axon pathways have been found in the embryonic nervous system of insects. These glycoproteins, termed *fasciclins*, are expressed in a dynamically interactive way on different subgroups of axon bundles during embryogenesis. The axon bundles on whose surfaces these molecules are expressed serve as *labeled pathways* for guiding particular outgrowing neurites. The temporal sequence with which these molecules appear on already developed fibers seems to help the growth cones in making a decision as to which fiber

bundle to follow at a give time. One assumes that individual growth cones can switch from one axon fascicle to another as a result of the sequential change in surface affinities, a phenomenon that can be compared with guiding a travelling train by changing the signal switches. In any case, the cell- and substrate-bound recognition and adhesion molecules, together with the dynamic properties of the growth cones, allow individual neurons to find their way to their respective target areas (Fig. 7.**17**).

The variety of potential recognition and adhesion molecules, as well as the control over their expression on the surfaces of specific cells, is without doubt complex and the subject of intensive research. A series of cell surface molecules which are involved in specific interactions between outgrowing neurites in other systems have already been identified. These include the vertebrate L1, F11, neurofascin, and TAG1 molecule groups. Some of these glycoproteins, which are mainly involved in interactions between growth cones and axons, and in the fasciculation of axons, seem to be interrelated at the molecular level. Surprisingly, one of the insect fasciclins characterized to date displays extensive sequence homology with molecules of the immunoglobulin family. It is interesting that N-CAM and several other adhesion molecules also have molecular similarities with the immunoglobulins. This suggests that the original role of ancestral immunoglobulin-like molecules might have been in adhesion and cell–cell recognition during development.

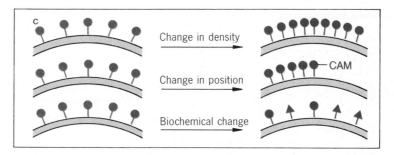

Fig. 7.**16c** Hypothetical model for the change in cell–cell adhesion by local modulation of the cell surface. This modulation can involve a change in the density, distribution, or chemical composition of CAMs (after Edelman)

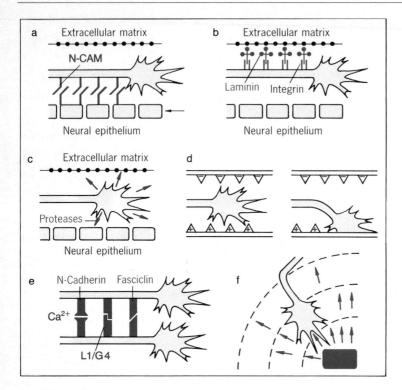

Fig. 7.17 Mechanisms of neuronal navigation. Outgrowing neurites are guided by interactions with their surroundings.
a Adhesion between neurons and neural epithelium by homophilic interactions between cell adhesion molecules. **b** Interactions between glycoproteins of the extracellular matrix and receptor molecules on the axon surface. **c** Progression of a growth cone by release of proteases. **d** Selective attraction or repulsion between growth cones and cell- or substrate-bound molecules. **e** Fasciculation of nerve fibers induced by glycoproteins on different growth cones or neurites. **f** Chemotropic response of a growth cone to diffusible substances (after Dodd and Jessel)

Synaptogenesis: Neuronal Connectivity Is Determined

The principle of how nerve cells search for their targets

Nervous systems are characterized by highly ordered and specific synaptic connectivity patterns. The establishment of such a connectivity pattern necessitates developmental mechanisms which limit the number of possible target cells for each neuron from the very beginning. Part of the specificity with which a neuron recognizes another during development is determined during the prior axonal navigation process. This is because the navigation process restricts the target areas into which an outgrowing neurite is led. A neuron from the retina would normally never send a process into the spinal cord. A ganglion cell in the retina therefore never has to be prevented by restricting programs from forming synapses with α-motoneurons. However, the outgrowing retinal ganglion cell must recognize the correct target cell in the tectum and then be able to initiate synaptogenesis. How does this happen? How can nerve cells which have reached the vicinity of their target cells now, in addition, choose the "right" cell from amongst their many potential partners?

Neurons are to some extent preprogrammed to make connections with their correct partner neurons, but generally not in a very precise way. Connectivity is initially very coarsely developed with an excess of synapses and neurons forming. Selection processes which lay down the correct synaptic connections only come later, and just as in human relationships, communication processes are important here too. Synapse formation is the result of a bidirectional exchange of biochemical information between the presynaptic and postsynaptic cells.

The specificity of neuronal connections is determined by intrinsic neuronal properties and the position of the neuron in the tissue

Specific neurons in one part of the nervous system form synapses preferentially with specific neurons in other parts of the nervous system. For example, axons of retinal ganglion cells from one particular part of the retina form synapses with postsynaptic neurons in well-defined tectal areas, and in so doing ignore neighboring neurons in other regions of the tectum (Fig. 7.18). This phenomenon contributes significantly to the formation of topographic projection systems. A partial explanation for such a neuronal specificity could lie in the fact that pre- and postsynaptic cells are chemically preprogrammed for one another. This corresponds more or less to the *chemoaffinity hypothesis* formulated by Sperry.

As originally formulated, the chemoaffinity hypothesis postulated that neurons undergo a strict molecular labeling during an early developmental stage which produces a biochemical affinity between outgrowing nerve fibers and their complementarily labeled partner cells. A modern version of this hypothesis postulates that the molecular composition of the cell surface facilitates mutual recognition between presynaptic and postsynaptic neurons. Comparable molecular recognition mechanisms could be active both in the specific navigation of growth cones and in partner recognition during synaptogenesis.

How could such a chemical imprinting of partner cells come about? It seems likely that in most animals the genetic information is not sufficient to specify all neuronal connections directly ("one gene—one synapse"). The establishment of neuronal connectivity must therefore include *epigenetic* processes which regulate the sequential activation and modulation of certain parts of the genetic program within the individual neuron. In accordance with the chemoaffinity hypothesis is the notion that neurons acquire their chemical identity according to their position in the embryonic tissue. In the retinotectal system, for example, the chem-

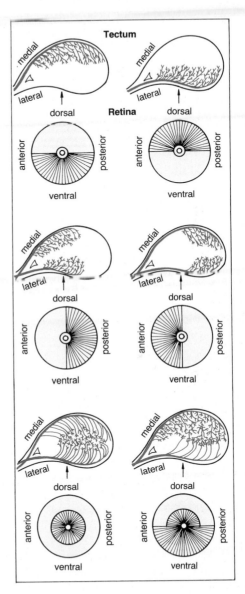

Fig. 7.18 Anatomical evidence for synaptic specificity during regeneration in the retinotectal system of the fish. The pattern of regenerating retinal fibers in the tectum following transsection of the optic nerve and removal of various regions of the retina is shown. Regenerating axons project to the correct tectal areas and form synapses there (after Attardi and Sperry)

ical labeling of future partner cells in the retina and tectum could be established by two orthogonal gradients of morphogenetic substances. Following this chemical predetermination, neurons could locate their partner cells and form appropriate synapses by using a series of chemical and mechanical guidance and recognition mechanisms. Although molecular gradients have been found in the retina, there is as yet no clear indication of their role in coding positional information.

Once neurons have acquired their neuronal specification through biochemical processes, their position in the tissue can then change within certain limits without their losing this specificity. Following the biochemical imprinting phase, intrinsic molecular and cellular factors within the neurons help determine the precision of partner choice, that is, the neu-

ronal specificity. Transplantation experiments show that such intrinsic properties can lead to correct synapse formation even when the outgrowing neurons no longer lie in their original position in the tissue. If a short section of the spinal cord is removed from a chick embryo following the neuronal specification phase and implanted again in the opposite anterior–posterior orientation, then the motoneurons still grow out to their correct target cells (Fig. 7.**19**). The motoneurons are therefore already "predetermined" to make connections with appropriate specific target cells. However, the chemical imprinting of neurons has its limits. If neurons are transplanted too far away from their original position, then they no longer form proper synapses with their correct partner cells. They can then follow incorrect pathways and make synapses with foreign target cells.

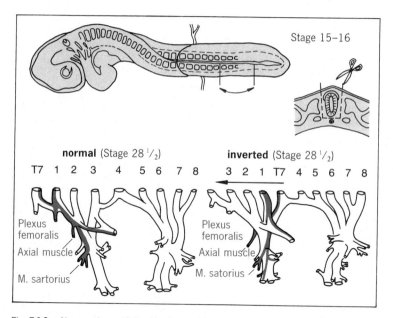

Fig. 7.**19**   Neuronal specificity despite positional change in the tissue. If small regions of the embryonic spinal cord of the chick are removed and reimplanted again in reverse anterior–posterior order, the now ectopic motoneurons compensate for their change in position. They find the correct efferent nerve pathways and innervate the correct muscles (after Lance-Jones and Landmesser)

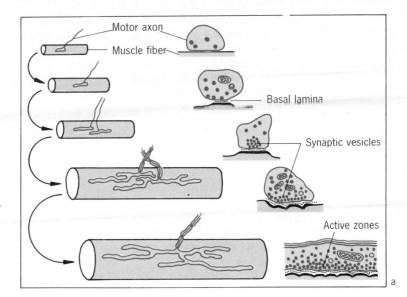

Fig. 7.**20**   Synaptogenesis at the vertebrate neuromuscular synapse. **a** Diagram showing the morphological changes during synapse formation. **b** Change in the distribution of acetylcholine receptors during synaptogenesis (after Letinsky and Morrison-Graham, Kullberg et al., and Schuetze)

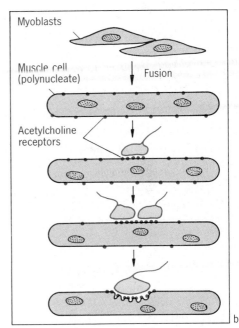

Pre- and postsynaptic membranes are restructured during synapse formation

A nerve terminal can assume two typical forms, one being a growth cone, the other a synapse. Both of these cellular specializations can release transmitter, have neurotransmitter receptors, comparable vesicular structures, and similar elements of the cytoskeleton. It is therefore not surprising that the growth cones on the tips of the outgrowing dendrites are converted into synapses during the formation of synaptic contact sites. This requires several processes at the level of the growth cones to occur. The growth cone has to recognize that it has arrived at its target. It must then stop growing and finally take on the morphological and physiological properties of a presynaptic (or postsynaptic) terminal. This requires a conversion of motile properties, cytoskeletal organization and membrane turnover in the growth cone. It has been proposed that this could all happen via a regulation of the intracellular Ca^{2+} concentration. Since the intracellular Ca^{2+} concentration can be changed by electrical activity as well as by neurotransmitters, then the formation and stability of a synapse could also be regulated by neuronal activity and transmitter release. However, the molecular details of these processes in the CNS are only just beginning to be understood.

Greater insight into the molecular mechanisms which operate in the pre- and postsynaptic membrane during synapse formation has come from experiments on the neuromuscular synapse (Fig. 7.**20**). The following facts, among others, have been established on this model system:

- Muscle cells that have not yet been innervated already have specialized membrane regions. Postsynaptic receptors for acetylcholine are present for example, and are found concentrated in certain membrane regions. These regions are distributed all over the surface of the embryonic muscle cell, but are not preferentially used by the innervating motoneurons for the formation of a synaptic terminal.
- During synapse formation the presynaptic motoneurons initiate a long-term reorganization of the postsynaptic membrane. Shortly after innervation, lateral migration leads to a concentration of the acetylcholine receptors in the subsynaptic membrane in which a density of over 10 000 receptor molecules per square micrometer can be reached. In contrast, receptor molecules disappear progressively from extrasynaptic regions. New receptor molecules with other biochemical and biophysical properties are synthesized. In the process, the embryonic form of the acetylcholine receptor is replaced by an adult form which differs in its γ-subunit. Further, there is a stabilization of acetylcholinesterase molecules in the basal lamina of the synaptic cleft. Innervation also influences the differentiation of embryonic muscle cells (the maturation of adult muscle fibers from myotubes). The type of innervating motoneuron can also determine the contractile properties of the muscle fibers.
- Several presynaptic factors cause the postsynaptic reorganization. The electrical activity of the motoneuron and presynaptic transmitter release have important roles in the regulation of postsynaptic differentiation processes. Polypeptides which are released from the presynaptic motoneuron are involved in this postsynaptic reorganization. Signals coming from the presynaptic motoneuron during innervation are assumed to act on gene expression in the muscle fiber.
- The postsynaptic cell acts reciprocally on the presynaptic terminal. The process of synapse formation is a gradual process of maturation. This is particularly true for the conversion of a growth cone into a fully functional presynaptic terminal. The biochemical, physiological, and morphological properties of the mature presynaptic terminal emerge only over the course of several days or weeks, and are significantly influenced by the properties of the postsynaptic muscle cell.

The number of synapses formed is regulated

The developmental interactions between a presynaptic and a postsynaptic cell continue well beyond the formation of a functional synapse. Both neurons use their functioning synapse to influence each other's further differentiation. At each postsynaptic cell, the correct number of synapses must be formed by the correct number of presynaptic neurons. This matching process often occurs via an overproduction of synapses followed by *elimination of supernumerary synapses* (Fig. 7.**21**).

Studies on mammalian neuromuscular synapses show that an embryonic muscle cell is generally innervated by several motoneurons. Many of the synapses initially formed are eliminated during the animal's development so that only the synaptic input from one motoneuron per muscle fiber remains. The reduction in the superfluous synapses occurs gradually during the initial phases of neonatal development. The neurons in some parasympathetic ganglia of neonatal animals are still innervated by several preganglionic axons. During the course of maturation, synapse elimination reduces the number of preganglionic axons which innervate a neuron in the ganglion. In some instances only a single presynaptic neuron remains connected with a given postsynaptic cell. The Purkinje cells of the cerebellum are innervated at first by several climbing fibers, but then a progressive reduction of these initial synapses occurs. After some time each Purkinje cell is innervated by only a single climbing fiber. Synapse elimination also occurs where presynaptic contacts are formed at electroanatomically incorrect sites on the postsynaptic cell. Thus synapses which are formed on unsuitable axonal regions of spinal motoneurons early in development are later eliminated.

What mechanisms are responsible for the developmentally-dependent transformation and degeneration of functional synaptic connections? Competition between the different innervating neurons seems to be an important factor. In many cases the process of synaptic elimination can be reduced when the corresponding number of innervating neurons is experimentally reduced. Competition between innervating neurons can occur via chemical or electrical signals. It may involve competition for a limited trophic factor, or simply for an available site on the postsynaptic cell. Examples of particularly extensive synaptic reorganization can be demonstrated in the visual and somatosensory systems of vertebrates. In many cases the synaptic reorganization seems to be largely determined by neuronal activity in the competing innervating fibers (see p. 228 ff.).

Regulation of the synaptic contact sites leads to transiently formed synapses which disappear again later. Accordingly, many axons lose synaptic contact with given postsynaptic cells. However, the number of synapses formed by the remaining presynaptic neurons can be simultaneously increased. It is almost as if the "correct" neurons were able to form more synaptic contact sites on a given postsynaptic cell following elimination of the "wrong" synapses than before. The adjustment of the correct number of synapses ensures that the remaining connections between pre- and postsynaptic neurons are not only qualitatively correct, but also quantitatively correctly weighted.

Similar processes to those involved in the elimination of transiently formed synapses lead to the elimination of dendrites, axons, or terminal arborizations. Even whole projection pathways in the embryonic CNS are transiently laid down and then removed later, for example in certain neocortical regions of mammals. However, not only synapses, dendrites, and axons are initially established in "excess" and then removed; entire neurons can also have a similar fate.

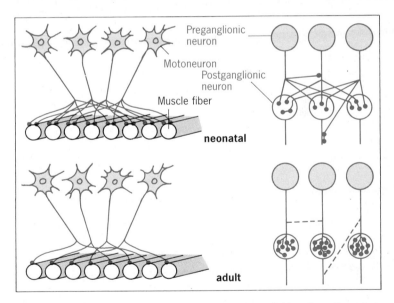

Fig. 7.21   Elimination of synapses. Diagram of the innervation process in skeletal muscle fibers (left), and ganglion cells in the parasympathetic nervous system (right), of mammals. In neonatal animals the skeletal muscle fibers as well as the postganglionic neurons are initially polyneuronally innervated. The elimination of synapses leads to the mature state in which one postsynaptic cell is only innervated by a single presynaptic neuron (after Thompson, and Purves and Lichtman)

Neurons which do not form synaptic connections can be eliminated by cell death

During the normal development of the nervous system many neurons show a remarkable behavior. They die. Developmentally determined cell death occurs in the central as well as the peripheral nervous system. In some regions of the nervous system up to 75% of all neurons die within a short period during development.

Neuronal death is *preprogrammed* in many cases, rather as if neurons in a particular developmental stage commit suicide. In the nematode *Caenorhabditis elegans,* 131 cells in the whole embryo die, most of these being neurons (Fig. 7.**22**). Cell death in this animal is

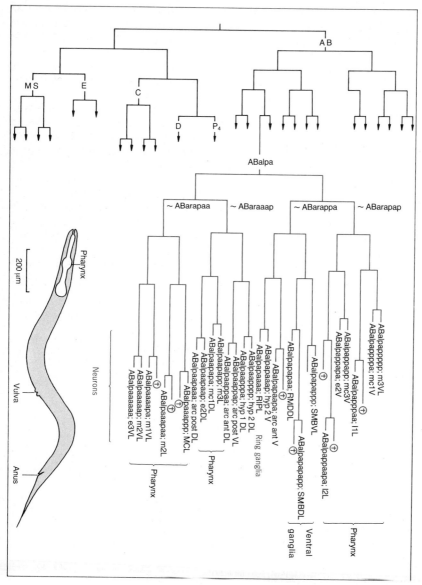

Fig. 7.**22**   Programmed cell death in a nematode. Lineage of several neurons in *Caenorhabditis*. Crosses indicate programmed neuronal cell death. Surviving neurons are identified according to the sequence of their cell divisions from progenitors, and are also given an abbreviated functional name (after Chalfie)

under the control of several identified genes. When these genes are inactivated by mutations, the neurons, which would otherwise die, remain alive and fully functional. In insects a programmed cell death occurs during neuronal adaptation to changes in peripheral organization. These changes occur in the embryo during segmental differentiation, or postembryonically during metamorphosis. In Lepidoptera for example, certain larval motoneurons die in a programmed way during the early pupal phase. Other larval motoneurons only die after the transformation to the adult butterfly. Others again survive metamorphosis but change their structure and connectivity (Fig. 7.**23**). These processes are initiated by complex interactions between hormonal signals, which in turn are regulated by the CNS.

In other cases neuronal death is associated with *competition* for the innervation of target cells. Through neuronal proliferation processes an overabundance of possible presynaptic neurons becomes available to innervate a limited number of postsynaptic target cells. During the innervation of these target cells a form of contest arises among the presynaptic cells, with the losers dying.

The extent of cell death can often be experimentally reduced either by lowering the number of competing neurons, or by making additional target cells available via transplantation. Classic experiments of this type have been carried out on the innervation of the limb buds in chick embryos and in amphibian larvae (Fig. 7.**24**). During normal development excess motoneurons are produced in the spinal cord. About half these motoneurons normally die during the establishment of neuromuscular synapses. If a limb bud is experimentally removed before the outgrowth of motoneurons, then cell death is drastically increased: almost all the ipsilateral leg motoneurons die. On the other hand, if an additional leg rudiment is transplanted onto one side of the embryo, then many more than half the ipsilateral motoneurons can be saved from death.

What is this regulation of the number of presynaptic neurons by the number of available target cells based on? It could have to do with competition for a limited number of postsynaptic binding sites. When transplantation is used to offer neurons a greater innervation area, more cells can make synaptic contacts and survive. However, there could also be competition for an important survival-promoting substance produced by the target cells. Survival of a neuron would only then be possible when there is an uptake of this substance via a

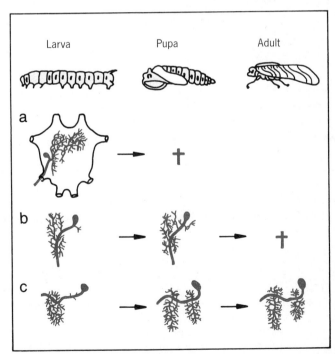

Fig. 7.**23** Cell death during metamorphosis of an insect. Larval motoneurons in the segmental ganglia of *Manduca* experience different fates during metamorphosis. **a** A motoneuron that dies in the pupa. **b** A motoneuron that dies in the adult animal. **c** A motoneuron that survives metamorphosis (after Truman)

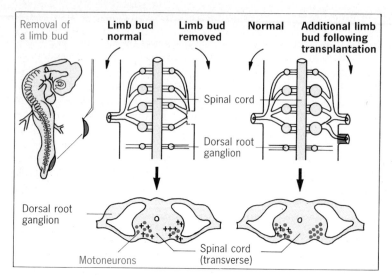

Fig. 7.**24**   Regulation of cell death in outgrowing neurons by the number of available target cells. About half of the established leg motoneurons in the spinal cord of the chick normally die. The extent of this cell death is increased when the ipsilateral limb bud is removed before innervation. The extent of cell death is reduced when an additional limb bud is transplanted to the ipsilateral side (after Hamburger)

functional synapse. Those neurons unable to establish stable synaptic contacts with post-synaptic cells would die. In this case the elimination of redundant neurons would be like death by starvation rather than murder. Activity can also contribute to cell death. The muscle cells in vertebrate embryos contract as soon as they are innervated by motoneurons, because these motoneurons propagate spontaneously generated action potentials. If neuromuscular transmission, and with it the activity of the muscle cells, is blocked in these cases, it leads to a marked reduction in the cell death that would otherwise occur among motoneurons. Finally, it is also possible that those motoneurons which die have formed the correct synapses with muscle cells, but have themselves not received the correct synapses from premotor interneurons. Whatever the mechanisms, the phenomenon of neuronal cell death is a process which is dynamic, characterized by feedback, and results in the innervating neuronal population becoming matched to the receptive capacity of the postsynaptic target cells.

The development of neuronal connectivity does not depend solely on cellular specificity

Partner finding and the formation of synapses during the development of complex neuronal projections are often not preprogrammed in a precise way. A neuronal specificity certainly is expressed which makes it easier for a neuron to form synapses with appropriate target cells. According to the chemoaffinity hypothesis, this could be based on the fact that presumptive pre- and postsynaptic neurons are labeled with corresponding chemical tags. However the process that finally leads to correct and exact synaptogenesis can be marked by provisional and even wrong growth pathways, as well as by the formation of transient synapses often far away from the final target area. Even when the correct target cells have been found there is a sorting and matching of those synapses developed in order to increase the precision of neuronal projections.

The developing nervous system is therefore a very plastic structure. The development of neuronal connectivity is characterized by an *equilibrium* between formation and elimination of synapses. The fine tuning of synaptic connections is the result of a long-term process which can extend far into the postnatal life of the animal. This process involves not only internal, neurogenic factors, but also external influences from the world of sensory experience. Studies on the ontogeny of the vertebrate visual system show this particularly clearly. It is important to understand that many developmental processes continue to be effective in postembryonic and adult life, either under normal conditions or during a regenerative response to injury.

References

General Reviews

Akam, M. 1987. The molecular basis for metameric pattern in the Drosophila embryo. Development 101: 1-22.

Anderson, H., Edwards, J. S. and Palka, J. 1980. Developmental neurobiology of invertebrates. Annu. Rev. Neurosci. 3: 97-139

Barde, Y. A. 1989. Trophic factors and neuronal survival. Neuron 2: 1525-1534.

Banerjee, U. and Zipursky, S. L. 1990. The role of cell–cell interaction in the development of the Drosophila visual system. Neuron 4: 177-187.

Bray, D. and Hollenbeck, P. J. 1988. Growth cone motility and guidance. Annu. Rev. Cell Biol. 4: 43-62.

Campos-Ortega, J. A. and Hartenstein, V. 1985. The Embryonic Development of Drosophila Melanogaster. Springer, Berlin.

Edelman, G. M. 1984. Modulation of cell adhesion during induction, histogenesis and perinatal development of the nervous system. Annu. Rev. Neurosci. 7: 339-378.

Finlay, B. L. and Sengelaub, D. R. (eds.) 1989. Development of the Vertebrate Retina. Plenum, New York.

Hall, B. K. and Hörstadius, S. 1988. The Neural Crest. Oxford, London.

Hall, Z. W. (ed.). 1992. An Introduction to Molecular Neurobiology, Sinauer, Sunderland.

Jacobson, M. 1991. Developmental Neurobiology, 3rd edition. Plenum, New York.

Keynes, R. and Lumsden, A. 1990. Segmentation and the origin of regional diversity in the vertebrate central nervous system. Neuron 2: 1-9.

Lance-Jones, C. and Landmesser, L. 1981. Pathway selection by embryonic chick motoneurones in an experimentally altered environment. Proc. R. Soc.

Landis, S. C. 1983. Neuronal growth cones. Annu. Rev. Physiol. 45: 567-580.

Landis, S. C. 1983. Neuronal Growth cones. Annu. Rev. Physiol. 45: 567-580.

Landmesser, L. 1980. The generation of neuromuscular specificity. Annu. Rev. Neurosci. 3: 279-302.

LeDouarin, N. M. 1982. The Neural Crest. Cambridge University Press, New York.

LeDouarin, N. M., Smith, J. and Le Lievre, C. S. 1982. From the neural crest to the ganglia of the peripheral nervous system. Annu. Rev. Physiol. 43: 653-671.

Marthy, H. J. (ed.) 1985. Cellular and Molecular Control of Direct Cell Interactions. Plenum, New York.

Patterson, P. H. and Purves, D. 1982. Readings in Developmental Neurobiology. Cold Spring Harbor, New York.

Pittman, R. N. 1990. Developmental roles of proteases and inhibitors. Semin. Dev. biol. 1: 65-74.

Purves, D. and Lichtman, J. W. 1985. Principles of Neural Development. Sinauer, Sunderland.

Reichardt, L. F. and Tomaselli, K. J. 1991. Extracellular matrix molecules and their receptors: Functions in neural development. Annu. Rev. Neurosci. 14: 531-570.

Rutishauser, U. and Jessell, T. M. 1988. Cell adhesion molecules in vertebrate neural development. Physiol. Rev. 68: 819-857.

Sanes, J. R. 1983. Roles of extracellular matrix in neural development. Annu. Rev. Physiol. 45: 581-600.

Sanes, J. R. 1989. Extracellular matrix molecules that influence neural development. Annu. Rev. Neurosci. 12: 491-517.

Schuetzte, S. M. and Role, L. W. 1987. Developmental regulation of nicotinic acetylcholine receptors. Annu. Rev. Neurosci. 10: 403-458.

Sharma, S. C. (ed.) 1984. Organizing Principles of Neural Development. Plenum, New York.

Stent, G. S. and Weisblat, D. A. 1985. Cell lineage in the development of invertebrate nervous systems. Annu. Rev. Neurosci. 8: 45-70.

Takeichi, M. 1990. Cadherins: A molecular family important in selective cell–cell adhesion. Annu. Rev. biochem. 59: 237-252.

Tomaselli, K. J., Neugebauer, K. M., Bixby, J. L., Lilien, J. and Reichardt, L. F. 1988. N-cadherin and integrins: Two receptor systems that mediate neuronal process outgrowth on astrocyte surfaces. Neuron 1: 33-43.

Truman, J. W. 1984. Cell death in invertebrate nervous systems. Annu. Rev. Neurosci. 7: 171-188.

Udin, S. B. and Fawcett, J. W. 1988. Formation of topographic maps. Annu. Rev. Neurosci. 11: 289-327.

Williams, R. W. and Herrup, K. 1988. The control of neuron number. Annu. Rev. Neurosci. 11: 423-454.

Yanker, B. A. and Shooter, E. M. 1982. The biology and mechanism of action of nerve growth factor. Annu. Rev. Biochem. 51: 845-868.

Original Publications

Anderson, M. J. and Cohen, M. W. 1977. Nerve-induced and spontaneous redistribution of acetylcholine receptors on cultured muscle cells. J. Physiol. 268: 757-773.

Angeletti, R. H., Hermodson, M. A. and Bradshaw, R. A. 1973. Amino acid sequences of mouse 2.5 S nerve growth factor. II. Isolation and characterization of the thermolytic and peptic peptides and the complete covalent structure. Biochemistry 12: 100-115.

Angeletti, R. H., Mercanti, D. and Bradshaw, R. A. 1973. Amino acid sequences of mouse 2.5 S nerve growth factor. I. Isolation and characterization of the soluble tryptic and chymotryptic peptides. Biochemistry 12: 90-100.

Attardi, D. G. and Sperry, R. W. 1963. Preferential selection of central pathways by regenerating optic fibers. Exp. Neurol. 7: 46-64.

Axelsson, J. and Thesleff, S. 1959. A study of supersensitivity in denervated mammalian skeletal muscle. J. Physiol. 147: 178-193.

Bandtlow, C. E., Heumann, R., Schwab, M. E. and Thoenen, H. 1987. Cellular localization of nerve growth factor synthesis by in situ hybridization. EMBO J. 6: 891-899.

Bennett, M. R., Florin, T. and Woog, R. 1974. The formation of synapses in regenerating mammalian striated muscle. J. Physiol. 238. 79-92.

Berg, D. K. and Hall, Z. W. 1975. Increased extrajunctional acetylcholine sensitivity produced by chronic postsynaptic neuromuscular blockade. J. Physiol. 244: 659-676.

Ball, E. E., Ho, R. K. and Goodman, C. S. 1985. Development of neuromuscular specificity in the grasshopper embryo: Guidance of motoneuron growth cones by muscle pioneers. J. Neurosci. 5: 1808-1819.

Bastiani, M. J., du Lac, S. and Goodman, C. S. 1986. Guidance of neuronal growth cones in the grasshopper embryo. I. Recognition of a specific axonal pathway by the pCC neuron. J. Neurosci. 6: 3518-3531.

Bastiani, M. J. and Goodman, C. S. 1986. Guidance of neuronal growth cones in the grashopper embryo. III. Recognition of specific glial pathways. J. Neurosci. 6: 3542-3551.

Bastiani, M. J., Harrelson, A. L., Snow, P. M. and Goodman, C. S. 1987. Expression of fasciclin I and II glycoproteins on subsets of axon pathways during neuronal development in the grasshopper. Cell 48: 745-755.

Bastiani, M. J., Raper, J. A. and Goodman, C. S. 1984. Pathfinding by neuronal growth cones in grasshopper embryos. III. Selective affinity of the G growth cone for the P cells within the A/P fascicle. J. Neurosci. 4: 2311-2328.

Bate, C. M. 1976. Embryogenesis of an insect nervous system. I. A map of the thoracic and abdominal neuroblasts in Locusta migratoria. J. Embryol. Exp. Morphol. 35: 107-123.

Bentley, D. and Caudy, M. 1983. Pioneer axons lose directed growth after selective killing of guidepost cells. Nature 304: 62-65.

Bentley, D. H. and Keshishian, H. 1982. Pathfinding by peripheral pioneer neurons in grasshoppers. Science 218: 1082-1088.

Betz, W. J., Caldwell, J. H. and Ribchester, R. R. 1980. The effects of partial denervation at birth on the development of muscle fibres and motor units in rat lumbrical muscle, J. Physiol. 303: 265-279.

Birks, R., Katz, B. and Miledi, R. 1960. Physiological and structural changes at the amphibian myoneural junction in the course of nerve degeneration. J. Physiol. 150: 145-168.

Bixby, J. L. and Van Essen, D. C. 1979. Competition between foreign and original nerves in adult mammalian skeletal muscle. Nature 282: 726-728.

Blochlinger, K., Bodmer, R., Jack, J., Jan, L. Y. and Jan, Y. N. 1988. Primary structure and expression of a product from cut, a locus involved in specifying sensory organ identity in Drosophila. Nature 333: 629-635.

Brenner, H. R. and Johnson, E. W. 1976. Physiological and morphological effects of post-gangli-

onic axotomy on presynaptic nerve terminals. J. Physiol. 260: 143-158.

Brenner, H. R. and Martin, A. R. 1976. Reduction in acetylcholine sensitivity of axotomized ciliary ganglion cells. J. Physiol. 260. 159-175.

Brenner, H. R. and Sakmann, B. 1983. Neurotrophic control of channel properties at neuromuscular synapses of rat muscle. J. Physiol. 337: 159-172.

Brenner. S. 1974. The genetics of Caenorhabditis elegans. Genetics 77: 71-94.

Bridgman, P. C. and Dailey, M. E. 1989. The organization of myosin and actin in rapid frozen nerve growth cones. J. Cell Biol. 108: 95-109.

Brockes, J. P. and Hall, Z. W. 1975. Acetylcholine receptors in normal and denervated rat diaphragm muscle. II. Comparison of junctional and extrajunctional receptors. Biochemistry 14: 2100-2106.

Brown, M. C., Jansen, J. K. S. and Van Essen, D. 1976. Polyneuronal innervation of skeletal muscle in new-born rats and its elimination during maturation. J. Physiol. 261: 387-422.

Burden, S. J., Sargent, P. B. and McMahan, U. J. 1979. Acetylcholine receptors in regenerating muscle accumulate at original synaptic sites in the absence of the nerve. J. Cell Biol. 82: 412-425.

Campenot, R. B. 1977. Local control of neurite development by nerve growth factor. Proc. Natl. Acad. Sci. USA 74: 4516-4519.

Caudy, M. and Bentley, D. 1986. Pioneer growth cone morphologies reveal proximal increases in substrate affinity within leg segments of grasshopper embryos. J. Neurosci. 6: 364-379.

Chang, S., Rathjen, F. G. and Raper, J. A. 1987. Extension of neurites on axons is impaired by antibodies against specific neural cell surface glycoproteins. J. Cell Biol. 104: 355-362.

Chiba, A., Shepherd, D. and Murphey, R. K. 1988. Synaptic rearrangement during postembryonic development in the cricket. Science 240: 901-905.

Cohen, M. W. 1972. The development of neuromuscular connexions in the presence of D-tubocurarine. Brain Res. 41: 457-463.

Cohen, M. W. 1980. Development of an amphibian neuromuscular junction in vivo and in culture. J. Exp. Biol. 89: 43-56.

Cohen, S. 1959. Purification and metabolic effects of a nerve-growth promotion protein from snake venom. J. Biol. Chem. 234: 1129-1137.

Cohen, S. 1960. Purification of a nerve-growth promoting protein from the mouse salivary gland and its neuro-cytotoxic antiserum. Proc. Natl. Acad. Sci. USA 46: 302-311.

Connolly, J. A., St. John, P. A. and Fischbach, G. D. 1982. Extracts of electric lobe and electric organ from Torpedo californica increase the total number as well as the number of aggregates of chick myotube acetylcholine receptors. J. Neurosci. 2: 1207-1213.

Dennis, M. J. and Miledi, R. 1974. Characteristics of transmitter release at regenerating frog neuromuscular junctions. J. Physiol. 239: 571-594.

Dennis, M. J. and Yip, J. W. 1978. Formation and elimination of foreign synapses on adult salamander muscle. J. Physiol. 274: 299-310.

Desai, C., Garriga, G. McIntire, S. L. and Horvitz, H. R. 1988. A genetic pathway for the development of the Caenorhabditis elegans HSN motor neurons. Nature 336: 638-646.

Doe, C. Q. and Goodman, C. S. 1985. Early events in insect neurogenesis. I. Development and segmental differences in the pattern of neuronal precursor cells. Devel. Biol. 111: 193-205.

Doe, C. Q. and Goodman, C. S. 1985. Early events in insect neurogenesis. II. The role of cell interactions and cell lineage in the determination of neuronal precursor cells. Devel. Biol. 111: 206-219.

Doe, C. Q., Smouse, D. and Goodman, C. S. 1988. Control of neuronal fate by the Drosophila segmentation gene even-skipped. Nature 333: 376-378.

Eide, A.-L. Jansen, J. K. D. and Ribchester, R. R. 1982. The effect of lesions in the neural crest on the formation of synaptic connexions in the embryonic chick spinal cord. J. Physiol. 324: 453-478.

Eisen, J. S., Pike, S. H. and Debu, B. 1989. The growth cones of identified motoneurons in embryonic zebrafish select appropriate pathways in the absence of specific cellular interactions. Neuron 2: 1097-1104.

Edmonson, J. C., Liem, R. K. H., Kuster, J. E. and Hatten, M. E. 1988. Astrotactin: a novel neuronal cell surface antigen that mediates neuron–astroglial interactions in cerebellar microcultures. J. Cell Biol. 106: 505-517.

Edwards, J. S. and Chen, S. 1979. Embryonic development of an insect sensory system, the abdominal cerci of Acheta domesticus. Roux's Arch. Dev. Biol. 186: 151-178.

Fischbach, G. D. and Schuetze, S. M. 1980. A postnatal decrease in acetylcholine channel open time at rat end-plates. J. Physiol. 303: 125-137.

Fontaine, B. and Changeux, J.-P. 1989. Localization of nicotinic acetylcholine receptor α-subunit transcripts during myogenesis and motor endplate development in the chick. J. Cell Biol. 108: 1025-1037.

Frank, E. and Fischbach, G. D. 1979. Early events in neuromuscular junction formation in vitro: Induction of acetylcholine receptor clusters in the postsynaptic membrane and morphology of newly formed synapses. J. Cell Biol. 83: 143-158.

Frank, E., Jansen, J. K. S., Lomo, T., and Westgaard, R. H. 1975. The interaction between foreign and original nerves innervating the soleus muscle of rats. J. Physiol. 247: 725-743.

Frank, E. and Mendelson, B. 1990. Specification of synaptic connections between sensory and motor neurons in the developing spinal cord. J. Neurobiol. 21: 33-50.

Gaze, R. M., Keating, M. J. and Chung, S. H. 1974. The evolution of the retinotectal map during development in Xenopus. Proc. R. Soc. Lond B 185: 301-330.

Ghysen, A. 1980. The projection of sensory neurons in the central nervous system of Drosophila: choice of the appropriate pathway. Devel. Biol. 78: 521-541.

Goodman, C. S., Bastiani, M. J., Doe, C. Q., du Lac, S., Helfand, S. L., Kuwada, J. Y. and Thomas, J. B. 1984. Cell recognition during neuronal development. Science 225: 1271-1279.

Goodman, C. S. and Spitzer, N. C. 1979. Embryonic development of identified neurones: Differentiation from neuroblast to neuron. Nature 280: 208-213.

Goodman, C. S., O'Shea, M., McCaman, R. E. and Spitzer, N. C. 1979. Embryonic development of identified neurons: Temporal pattern of morphological and biochemical differentiation. Science 204: 219-222.

Greene, L. A., Varon, S., Pitch, A. and Shooter, E. M. 1971. Substructure of the β subunit of mouse 7S nerve growth factor. Neurobiology 1: 37-48.

Grinvald, A. and Farber, I. C. 1981. Optical recording of calcium action potentials from growth cones of cultured neurons with a laser microbeam. Science 212: 1164-1167.

Guillery, R. W. and Kaas, J. H. 1974. The effects of monocular lid suture upon the development of the visual cortex in squirrels (Sciureus carolinensis). J. Comp. Neurol. 154: 443-452.

Guillery, R. W. and Stelzner, D. J. 1970. The differential effects of unilateral lid closure upon the monocular and binocular segments of the dorsal lateral geniculate nucleus in the cat. J. Comp. Neurol. 139: 413-422.

Gundersen, R. W. and Barrett, J. N. 1979. Neuronal chemotaxia: Chick dorsal root axons turn toward high concentrations of nerve growth factor. Science 206: 1079-1080.

Hafen, E., Basler, K., Edstroem, H. and Rubin G. M. 1987. Sevenless, a cell-specific homeotic gene of Drosophila, encodes a putative transmembrane receptor with a tyrosine kinase domain. Science 236: 55-63.

Hamburger, V. 1939. Motor and sensory hyperplasia following limb-bud transplantations in chick embryos. Physiol. Zool. 12: 268-284.

Hamburger, V. 1975. Cell death in the development of the lateral motor column of the chick embryo. J. Comp. Neurol. 160: 535-546.

Hamburger, V., Brunso-Bechtold, J. K. and Yip, J. W. 1981. Neuronal death in the spinal ganglia of the chick embryo and its reduction by nerve growth factor. J. Neurosci. 1: 60-71.

Harrelson, A. L. and Goodman, C. S. 1988. Growth cone guidance in insects: Fasciclin II is a member of the immunoglobulin superfamily. Science 242: 700-708.

Harrison, R. G. 1910. The outgrowth of the nerve fiber as a mode of protoplasmic movement. J. Exp. Zool. 9: 787-846.

Hartzell, H. C. and Fambrough, D. M. 1972. Acetylcholine receptors: Distribution and extrajunctional density in rat diaphragm after denervation correlated with acetylcholine sensitivity. J. Gen. Physiol. 60: 248-262.

Heffner, C. D., Lumsden A. G. S. and O'Leary, D. D. M. 1990. Target control of collateral extension and directional axon growth in the mammalian brain. Science 247: 217-220.

Hendry, I. A., Stöckel, K., Thoenen, H. and Iversen, L. L. 1974. The retrograde axonal transport of nerve growth factor. Brain Res. 68: 103-121.

Henrickson, C. K. and Vaughn, J. E. 1974. Fine structural relationships between neurites and radial glial processes in developing mouse spinal cord. J. Neurocytol. 3: 659-679.

Ho, R. K. and Goodman, C. S. 1982. Periperal pathways are pioneered by an array of central and peripheral neurones in grasshopper embryos. Nature 297: 404-406.

Hohn, A., Leibrock, J., Bailey, K. and Barde, Y.-A. 1990. Identification and characterization of a novel member of the nerve growth factor/brain-derived growth factor family. Nature 344: 339-341.

Hollyday, M. and Hamburger, V. 1976. Reduction of the naturally occurring motor neuron loss by enlargement of the periphery. J. Comp. Neurol. 170: 311-320.

Hollyday, M., Hamburger, V. and Farris, J. 1977. Localization of motor neuron pools supplying identified muscles in normal and supernumerary legs of chick embryo. Proc. Natl. Acad. Sci. USA 74: 3582-3586.

Hume, R. I., Role, L. W. and Fischbach, G. D. 1983. Acetylcholine release from growth cones detected with patches of acetylcholine receptor-rich membranes. Nature 305: 632-634.

Hunter, D. D., Shah, V. Merlie, J. P. and Sanes, J. R. 1989. A laminin-like adhesive protein concentrated in the synaptic cleft of the neuromuscular junction. Nature 338: 229-234.

Innocenti, G. M. 1981. Growth and reshaping of axons in the establishment of visual callosal connections. Science 212: 824-827.

Jansen, J. K. S. and Fladby, T. 1990. The perinatal reorganization of the innervation of skeletal muscle in mammals. Prog. Neurobiol. 34: 39-90.

Jessell, T. M., Siegel, R. E. and Fischbach, G. D. 1979. Induction of acetylcholine receptors on cultured skeletal muscle by a factor extracted from brain and spinal cord. Proc. Natl. Acad. Sci. USA 76: 5397-5401.

Kriegstein, A. R. 1977. Development of the nervous system of Aplysia californica. Proc. Natl. Acad. Sci. USA 74: 375-378.

Kuffler, D. P., Thompson, W. and Jansen, J. K. S. 1980. The fate of toreign endplates in cross-innervated rat soleus muscle. Proc. R. Soc. Lond. B 208: 189-222.

Kuwada, J. Y. 1986. Cell recognition by neuronal growth cones in a simple vertebrate embryo. Science 233: 740-746.

Kuwada, J. Y. and Kramer, A. P. 1983. Embryonic development of the leech nervous system. Primary axon outgrowth of identified neurons. J. Neuroscience 3: 2098-2111.

Lance-Jones, C. and Landmesser, L. 1980. Motoneurone projection patterns in the chick hind limb following early partial reversals of the spinal cord. J. Physiol. 302: 581-602.

Lond. B 214: 19-52.

Law, M. I. and Constantine-Paton, M. 1981. Anatomy and physiology of experimentally produced striped tecta. J. Neurosci. 1: 741-749.

Le Douarin, H. M. 1980. The ontogeny of the neural crest in avian embryo chimaeras. Nature 286: 663-669.

Le Douarin, N. M. 1986. Cell line segregation during peripheral nervous system ontogeny. Science 231: 1515-1522.

Leibrock, J., Lottspeich, F. Hohn, A., Hofer, M. Hengerer, B., Masiakowski, P. Thoenen, H. and Barde, Y.-A. 1989. Molecular cloning and expression of brain-derived neurotrophic factor. Nature 341: 149-152.

Letinsky, M. S., Fischbeck, K. H. and McMahan, U. J. 1976. Precision of reinnervation of original postsynaptic sites in frog muscle after a nerve crush. J. Neurocytol. 5: 691-718.

Letourneau, P. C. 1975. Cell-to-substratum adhesion and guidance of axonal elongation. Devel. Biol. 44: 92-101.

Levi-Montalcini, R. and Cohen, S. 1960. Effects of the extract of the mouse submaxillary salivary glands on the sympathetic system of mammals. Ann. N. Y. Acad. Sci. 85: 324-341.

Levine, R. B. and Truman, J. W. 1982. Metamorphosis of the insect nervous system: changes in morphology and synaptic interactions of identified neurons. Nature 299: 250-252.

Loer, C. M. and Kristan, W. B. 1989. Central synaptic inputs to identified leech neurons determined by peripheral targets. Science 244: 64-66.

Longo, A. M. and Penhoet, E. E. 1974. Nerve growth factor in rat glioma cells. Proc. Natl. Acad. Sci. USA 71: 2347-2349.

Mangold, O. 1933. Über die Induktionsfähigkeit der verschiedenen Bezirke der Neurula von Urodelen. Naturwissenschaften 21: 761-766.

McMahan, U. J., Edgington, D. R. and Kuffler, D. P. 1980. Factors that influence regeneration of the neuromuscular junction. J. Exp. Biol. 89: 31-42.

Matsumoto, S. G and Murphey, R. K. 1977. Sensory deprivation during development decreases the responsiveness of cricket giant interneurons. J. Physiol. 268: 533-548.

Meier, T., Chabaud, F. and Reichert, H. 1991. Homologous patterns in the embryonic development of the peripheral nervous system in the grasshopper Schistocerca gregaria and the fruitfly Drosophila melanogaster. Development 112: 241-251.

Meier, T. and Reichert, H. 1990. Embryonic development and evolutionary origin of the orthopteran auditory organs. J. Neurobiol. 21: 592-610.

Meier, T. and Reichert, H. 1991. Serially homologous development of the peripheral nervous system in the mouthparts of the grasshopper. J. Comp. Neurol. 305: 201-214.

Mensini-Chen, M. G., Chen, J. S. and Levi-Montalcini, R. 1978. Sympathetic nerve fibers in growth in the central nervous system of neonatal rodents upon intracerebral NGF injections. Arch. Natl. Biol. 116: 53-84.

Miledi, R. 1960. The acetycholine sensitivity of frog muscle fibres after complete or partial denervation. J. Physiol. 151: 1-23.

Miledi, R. 1960. Junctional and extra-junctional acetylcholine receptors in skeletal muscle fibres. J. Physiol. 157: 24-30.

Mills, L. R. and Kater, S. B. 1990. Neuron-specific and state-specific differences in calcium homeostasis regulate the generation and degeneration of neuronal architecture. Neuron 2: 149-163.

Murphey, R. K. 1981. The structure and development of a somatotopic map in crickets: the cercal afferent projection. Devel. Biol. 88: 236-246.

Murphey, R. K., Johnson, S. E. and Sakaguchi, D. S. 1983. Anatomy and physiology of supernumerary cercal afferents in crickets: Implication for pattern formation. J. Neurosci. 3: 312-325.

Nitkin, R. M., Smith, M. A., Magill, C., Fallon, J. R., Yao, Y.-M. M., Wallace, B. G. and McMahon, U. J. 1987. Identification of agrin, a synaptic organizing protein from Torpedo electric organ. J. Cell Biol. 105: 2471-2478.

Njå, A. and Purves, D. 1978. The effects of nerve growth factor and its antiserum on synapses in the superior cervical ganglion of the guinea-pig. J. Physiol. 277: 53-75.

Patel, N. H., Snow, P. M. and Goodman, C. S. 1987. Characterization and cloning of fasciclin III: a glycoprotein expressed on a subset of neurons and axon pathways in Drosophila. Cell 48: 975-988.

Patterson, P. H. and Chun, L. L. Y. 1977. Induction of acetylcholine synthesis in primary cultures of dissociated rat sympathetic neurons. I. Effects of conditioned medium. Devel. Biol. 56: 263-280.

Pearson, K. G., Boyan, G. S., Bastiani, M. and Goodman, C. S. 1985. Heterogeneous properties of segmentally homologous interneurones in the ventral cord of locusts. J. Comp. Neurol. 223: 133-145.

Pilar. G., Landmesser, L. and Burstein, L. 1980. Competition for survival among developing ciliary ganglion cells. J. Neurophysiol. 41: 233-254.

Purves, D. 1975. Functional and structural changes in mammalian sympathetic neurones following interruption of their axons. J. Physiol. 252: 429-463.

Purves, D. and Lichtman, J. W. 1980. Elimination of synapses in the developing nervous system. Science 210: 153-157.

Purves, D. and Sakmann, B. 1974. The effect of contractile activity on fibrillation and extrajunctional acetylcholine sensitivity in rat muscle maintained in organ culture. J. Physiol. 237: 157-182.

Purves, D. and Sakmann, B. 1974. Membrane properties underlying spontaneous activity of denervated muscle fibres. J. Physiol. 239: 125-153.

Raisman, G. and Field, P. 1973. A quantitative investigation of the development of collateral innervation after partial deafferentation of the septal nuclei. Brain Res. 50: 241-264.

Rakic, P. 1971. Neuron–glia relationship during granule cell migration in developing cerebellar cortex. A Golgi and electron-microscopic study in Macacus rhesus. J. Comp. Neurol. 141: 283-312.

Rakic, P. 1972. Mode of cell migration to the superficial layers of the fetal monkey neocortex. J. Comp. Neurol. 145: 61-83.

Rakic, P. 1977. Genesis of the dorsal lateral geniculate nucleus in the rhesus monkey: Site and time of origin, kinetics of proliferation, routes of migration and pattern of distribution of neurons. J. Comp. Neurol. 176: 23-52.

Rakic, P. 1977. Prenatal development of the visual system in rhesus monkey. Phil. Trans. R. Soc. Lond. B 278: 245-260.

Raper, J. A., Bastiani, M. and Goodman 1983. Pathfinding by neuronal growth cones in grasshopper embryos: I. Divergent choices made by the growth cones of sibling neurons. J. Neurosci. 3: 20-30.

Raper, J. A., Bastiani, M. and Goodman 1983. Pathfinding by neuronal growth cones in grasshopper embryos: II. Selective fasciculation onto specific axonal pathways. J. Neurosci. 3: 31-41.

Raper, J. A., Bastiani, M. and Goodman 1983. Pathfinding by neuronal growth cones in grasshopper embryos: IV. The effects of ablating the A and P axons upon the behavior of the G growth cone. J. Neurosci. 4: 2239-2345.

Rauschenecker, J. P. and Singer, W. 1980. Changes in the circuitry of the kitten visual cortex are gated by postsynaptic activity. Nature 280: 58-60.

Redfern, P. A. 1970. Neuromuscular transmission in newborn rats. J. Physiol. 209: 701-709.

Rotshenker, S. 1979. Synapse formation in intact innervated cutaneous-pectoris muscles of the frog following denervation of the opposite muscle. J. Physiol. 292: 535-547.

Rutishauser, U., Acheson, A., Hall, A. K., Mann, D. M. and Sunshine, J. 1988. The neural cell adhesion molecules (NCAM) as a regulator of cell–cell interactions. Science 240: 53-57.

Rutishauser, U., Grumet, M. and Edelman, G. M. 1983. Neural cell adhesion molecule mediates initial interactions between spinal cord neurons and muscle cells in culture. J. Cell Biol. 97: 145-152.

Rutishauser, U., Hoffman, S. and Edelman, G. M. 1982. Binding properties of a cell adhesion molecule from neural tissue. Proc. Natl. Acad. Sci. USA 79: 685-689.

Sanes, J. R. and Hall, Z. W. 1979. Antibodies that bind specifically to synaptic sites on muscle fiber basal lamina. J. Cell Biol. 83: 357-370.

Sanes, J. R., Marshall, L. M. and McMahan, U. J. 1978. Reinnervation of muscle fiber basal lamina removal of muscle fibers. J. Cell Biol. 78: 176-198.

Schacher, S., Kandel, E. R. and Woolley, R. 1979. Development of neurons in the abdominal ganglion of Aplysia californica. I. Axosomatic synaptic contacts. Dev. Biol. 71: 163-175.

Schmidt, J. T., Cicerone, C. M. and Easter, S. S. 1978. Expansion of the half retinal projection to the tectum in goldfish: An electrophysiological and anatomical study. J. Comp. Neurol. 177: 257-278.

Shankland, M., Bentley, D. and Goodman, C. S. 1982. Afferent innervation shapes the dendritic branching pattern of the medial giant interneuron in grasshopper embryos raised in culture. Dev. Biol. 92: 507-520.

Shatz, C. J. 1983. The prenatal development of the cat's retinogeniculate pathway. J. Neurosci. 3: 482-499.

Shatz, C. J. 1990. Impulse activity and the patterning of connections during CNS development. Neuron 5: 745-756.

Shatz, C. J. and Luskin, M. B. 1986. The relationship between the geniculocortical afferents and their cortical target cells during development of the cat's primary visual cortex. J. Neurosci. 6: 3655-3668.

Snow, P. M., Zinn, K., Harrelson, A. L., McAllister, L., Schilling, J., Bastiani, M. J., Makk, G. and Goodman, C. S. 1988. Characterization and cloning of fasciclin I and fasciclin II glycoproteins in the grasshopper. Proc. Natl. Acad. Sci. USA 85: 5291-5295.

Sperry, R. W. 1944. Optic nerve regeneration with return of vision in anurans. J. Neurophysiol. 7: 57-69.

Sperry, R. W. 1945. Restoration of vision after crossing of optic nerves and after contralateral transplantation of eye. J. Neurophysiol. 8: 15-28.

Sperry, R. W. 1963. Chemoaffinity in the orderly growth of nerve fiber patterns and connections. Proc. Natl. Acad. Sci. 50: 703-710.

Spitzer, N. C. 1982. Voltage- and stage-dependent uncoupling of Rohon-Beard neurones during embryonic development of Xenopus tadpoles. J. Physiol. 330: 145-162.

Stürmer, C. A. O. and Raymond, P. A. 1989. Developing retinotectal projection in larval goldfish. J. Comp. Neurol. 281: 630-640.

Sutter, A., Riopelle, R. J., Harris-Warrick, R. M. and Shooter, E. M. 1979. Nerve growth factor receptors characterization of two distinct classes of binding sites on chick embryo sensory ganglia cells. J. Biol. Chem. 254: 5972-5982.

Taghert, P. H. and Goodman, C. S. 1984. Cell determination and differentiation of identified serotonin-containing neurons in the grasshopper embryo. J. Neurosci. 4: 989-1000.

Taghert, P. H., Doe, C. Q. and Goodman, C. S. 1984. Cell determination and regulation during development of neuroblasts and neurons in the grasshopper embryo. Nature 307: 163-165.

Tessier-Lavigne, M., Placzek, M., Lumsden, A. G. S., Dodd, J. and Jessell, T. M. 1988. Chemotropic guidance of developing axons in the mammalian central nervous system. Nature 336: 775-778.

Thoenen, H., Bandtlow, C. and Heuman, R. 1987. The physiological function of nerve growth factor in the central nervous system: Comparison with the periphery. Rev. Physiol. Biochem. Pharmacol. 109: 146-178.

Thomas, J. B., Bastiani, M. J., Bate, M. and Goodman, C. S. 1984. From grasshopper to Drosophila: A common plan for neuronal development. Nature 310: 203-207.

Thompson, W. 1983. Synapse elimination in neonatal rat muscle is sensitive to pattern of muscle use. Nature 302: 614-616.

Trisler, D. and Collins, F. 1987. Corresponding spatial gradients of TOP molecules in the developing retina and optic tectum. Science 237: 1208-1209.

Truman J. W. 1983. Programmed cell death in the nervous system of an adult insect. J. Comp. Neurol. 216: 445-452.

Truman, J. W., Taghert, P. H., Copenhaver, P. F., Tublitz, N. J. and Schwarz, L. M. 1981. Eclosion hormonde may control all ecdyses in insects. Nature 291: 70-71.

Usdin, T. B. and Fischbach, G. D. 1986. Purification and characterization of a polypeptide from chick brain that promotes the accumulation of acetylcholine receptors in chick myotubes. J. Cell Biol. 103: 493-507.

Vassin, H., Bremer, K. A., Knust, E. and Campos-Ortega, J. A. 1987. The neurogenic gene Delta of Drosophila melanogaster is expressed in neurogenic territories and encodes a putative transmembrane protein with EGF-like repeats. EMBO J. 6: 3431-3440.

Walter, J., Henke-Fahle, S. and Bonhoeffer, F. 1987. Avoidance of posterior tectal membranes by temporal retinal axons. Development 101: 909-913.

Walter, J., Kern-Veits, B., Huf, J., Stolze, B. and Bonhoeffer, F. 1987. Recognition of position-specific properties of tectal cell membranes by retinal axons in vitro. Development 101: 685-696.

Weeks, J. C. and Truman, J. W. 1985. Independent steroid control of the fates of motoneurons and their muscles during insect metamorphosis. J. Neurosci. 5: 2290-2300.

Weeks, J. C. and Truman, J. W. 1986. Steroid control of neuron and muscle development during the metamorphosis of an insect. J. Neurobiol. 17: 249-267.

Yoon, M. 1972. Transposition of the visual projection from the nasal hemiretina onto the foreign rostral zone of the optic tectum in goldfish. Exp. Neurol. 37: 451-462.

Young, S. H. and Poo, M.-M. 1983. Spontaneous release of transmitter from growth cones of embryonic neurones. Nature 305: 634-637.

8. Maintenance and Repair

The Processes of Neuronal Homeostasis

Mechanisms for the preservation of neuronal integrity

The neuron, like no other cell, has an extensive and branched structure. Axons can be up to several meters long and yet have a diameter of only a millionth of this length. The axon terminals of neurons can branch up to 100 000 times into discrete synapses. Special mechanisms are necessary to maintain the structural and functional integrity of such cells. On the one hand, the neuron itself must ensure that there is an exchange of essential molecules between the cell body and all of its branches: the various parts of the cell must be in molecular communication. On the other hand, the morphologically ramified cell requires a certain structural stability. This stabilization is carried out by the neuron itself, as well as by specialized supporting cells.

Axonal transport is the basis for molecular communication between cell bodies and neurites

The endoplasmic reticulum and the Golgi complex are normally localized in the cell body of a neuron. Accordingly, important molecules like proteins and membrane lipids are synthesized in the cell body. These molecular building blocks are used everywhere in the cell, particularly at the synaptic terminals which can lie distant from the cell body. The biosynthesis of some transmitter substances can occur at the synapse itself, and there is also a degradation and reincorporation of membrane components at the synapse during turnover of synaptic vesicles. However, there is a constant demand for newly synthesized enzymes and membrane components. How do these synthesized cell body products reach the distant sites where they are utilized? Passive diffusion is useless here. To travel a distance of a meter in an axon by diffusion alone would take an aver-

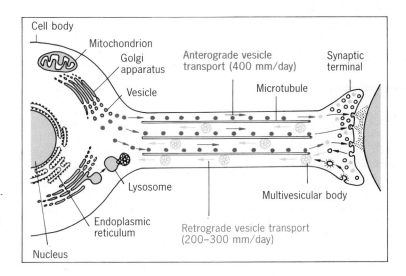

Fig. 8.1   Axonal transport. Schematic representation of anterograde and retrograde fast axonal transport. The transport process is based on the movement of vesicles along the microtubules (after Allen)

age-sized protein molecule a few decades. The neuron must therefore use active transport mechanisms that depend on metabolic processes. These are called *axonal transport processes,* but they also occur in dendrites. These axonal transport processes differ in their direction, their rate, and in the type of molecule they transport.

Axonal transport has several directional components

Microscopic examination of a living axon shows that membrane vesicles move along the axon in a relatively rapid, seemingly saltatory, fashion. Almost all the organelles in axons and dendrites are translocated by these *fast components* of axonal transport (Fig. 8.1). This transport runs in both directions: away from the cell body in the *anterograde* direction, and back from the synaptic terminals to the cell body in the *retrograde* direction. The rate of transport in the anterograde direction in mammals is about 400 mm per day. Almost all newly synthesized lipids and membrane glycoproteins, as well as some of the molecules which are secreted at the synapses, are translocated by rapid anterograde transport. In the retrograde direction the rate is about 200–300 mm per day. In this way breakdown products are returned in lysosomal organelles back to the cell body. Further, extracellular trophic substances which are taken up at the synapses, or signal molecules which signal the functional state of the synaptic terminal can also be transported back to the cell body. This process can be used to anatomically demonstrate the projection pathways of neurons. Radioactively labeled substances, or enzymes like horseradish peroxidase, can be injected near the synaptic terminal. These substances are taken up at the synapse and transported retrogradely in the axon back to the cell body. The cell body along with its axon can then be revealed anatomically using autoradiography in the case of radioactively labeled substances, or by a histological method in the case of peroxidase.

The mechanism of rapid axonal transport is based on an ATP-dependent binding and translocation of vesicles along microtubules. On an individual microtubule, vesicles of one type can move in the anterograde direction, and vesicles of another type in the retrograde direction. Two different translocation proteins are assumed to be responsible for the binding and directionally specific transport of vesicles. The microtubules therefore function to some extent as polarized guide rails. All vesicles are transported in an ongoing manner and at the same rate. However, the larger ones often seem to be impeded in their movement, giving the transport a saltatory appearance. Since the retrogradely transported vesicles are generally larger than those transported anterogradely, they are assumed to be impeded more and so are moved somewhat more slowly overall.

Apart from the fast axonal transport there is also a *slow component* with which cytoskeletal proteins and cytoplasmic enzymes are transferred anterogradely from the cell body to distant cell regions. These slow components have a rate of about 1–10 mm per day. A rate of about 1 mm per day corresponds roughly to the rate at which microtubules lengthen via polymerization of tubulin monomers. It is therefore conceivable that this slow supply of proteins from the cell body region is driven by the addition of monomers to the fibers of the cytoskeleton. However, the cytoskeletal fibers have a further important role apart from this function in transporting intracellular substances.

Neuronal structure is maintained by the cytoskeleton

The stability of the many highly branched dendrites, as well as the long and very thin axon of a neuron, could not be maintained without a supporting scaffold. Such a scaffold is found inside every neuron. It is formed by the fibrillar elements of the cytoskeleton (Fig. 8.2). The cytoskeleton consists of three types of fibrous elements: microtubules, neurofilaments and microfilaments. Together they make up about half the proteins in a neuron.

Microtubules are among the largest fibers of the neuronal cytoskeleton. They are tube-shaped polymers of tubulin units and have a diameter of about 25 nm. *Neurofilaments,* the main structural elements in the neuron, are about 10 nm in diameter. There are about ten times as many neurofilaments per cell as there are microtubules. These filaments are normally arranged parallel to the long axis of neurites. However, in degenerative diseases like senile dementia these filaments can be deposited in a spherically shaped tangle. Finally, *microfilaments* are the thinnest fiber type with a diameter of 3–5 nm. They are composed of double helices of actin monomers like the actin filaments of muscle fibers. Interestingly, microfilaments are constantly being built up and broken down. About half the actin in a neuron occurs in the nonpolymerized form. As in other cells, the microfilaments in neurons also aggregate, particularly near the cell membrane. Anchoring proteins ensure that some of these filaments are directly bound to the membrane.

Together, the fibrillar proteins in the cytoskeleton form a sort of cellular corset which supports the somewhat labile structure of the neuron from the inside. However, neurons are also "supported" from the outside, in several senses. This support comes from an important class of nonneuronal cells.

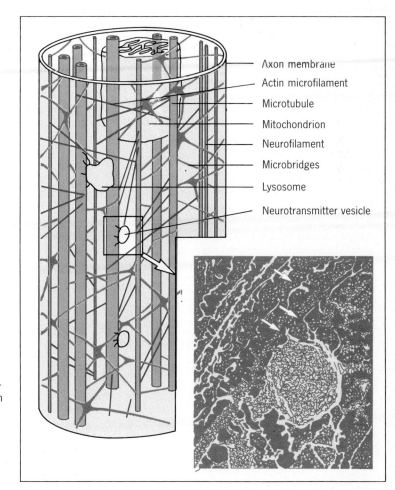

Axon membrane
Actin microfilament
Microtubule
Mitochondrion
Neurofilament
Microbridges
Lysosome
Neurotransmitter vesicle

Fig. 8.**2** Fibrillar elements of the cytoskeleton. Schematic representation of the arrangement of microtubules, neurofilaments, and microfilaments in an axon. The inset shows the ultrastructure of a vesicle which is being transported along a microtubule via coupling proteins (arrows) (after Hirokawa et al and Johnston)

Neural tissue is always composed of neurons and glia cells

Glia cells occur throughout the nervous system. They are generally small and fill almost the entire nonneuronal space. In the mammalian CNS there can be from 10 to 50 times more glia cells than neurons. Different types of glia can be distinguished in the CNS of vertebrates (Fig. 8.3). *Astrocytes* are star-shaped cells with many ramifications, and whose terminals form multiple branches between neural processes. Astrocytes are found associated with axons as well as with cell bodies. Further, they often form close connections with blood capillaries. They represent the most abundant type of glia cell. *Oligodendrocytes* are small cells whose processes wrap themselves like a lamella around several axons. In this way they myelinate the central axons and have the same function as the Schwann cells of the peripheral nervous system. *Ependymal cells* form the inner lining of cavities in the CNS. *Microglia cells* are phagocytotic cells which become active during disease or injury. A similar classification of glia cells is not unambiguously possible in invertebrates, although functional similarities in the glia cells occurring there are evident.

Glia cells play several roles in the maintenance of neurons

Glia cells probably do not generate action potentials in vivo. They have a resting potential that is almost totally determined by the potassium permeability. They can therefore respond in an electrically passive way to changes in the extracellular potassium concentration. Glia cells are often connected to one another via *gap junctions*. However, most are separated from neighboring neurons by extracellular spaces about 20 nm wide. They do not have axons, nor do they form typical synapses. Nevertheless, certain glia cells possess both receptors for neurotransmitters and transmitter-dependent ion channels. It is possible that neighboring axons influence these glia cells via nonsynaptic transmitter release. However, it is unclear if glia cells are directly involved in the rapid electrical information processing in the brain.

Despite this, glia cells carry out numerous important functions in the CNS, with the different types of glia cell often being specialized for one or the other of these functions:

- Glia cells are the mechanical support elements for the highly structured nerve cells

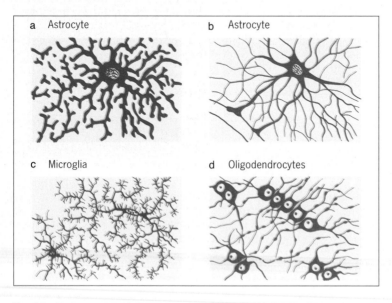

Fig. 8.**3**   Various types of glia cells in the human CNS (after Rio-Hortega)

and nerve cell tissues. In this respect they act as a type of "connective tissue" for the neuronal tissue of the brain.

- Certain glia cells establish the myelin sheath which contributes to the electrical isolation of axons. Others are involved in the spatial segregation of whole groups of neurons or axons. Even nonmyelinated single axons have a loose envelope of glia cells.
- Certain types of glia cells have a phagocytic function and so remove cell debris that arises from neuronal degeneration. In contrast to nerve cells, glia cells retain a lifelong capacity to divide and so can contribute to the formation of scar tissue in the nervous system. A perpetual capacity for division has its drawbacks: many tumors in the brain arise from glia cells.
- During development, glia cells can serve as guidance pathways or boundaries for migrating nerve cells or outgrowing axons.
- It is possible that glia cells contribute to the nutrition of nerve cells by mediating the exchange of metabolic substances between blood vessels and neurons. Strong evidence for a nutritive role for glia cells has been found in the case of retinal glia cells in the insect eye.
- It is certain that glia cells are involved in metabolic homeostasis. Glia cells can contribute to the maintenance of the K^+ concentration in the extracellular space. They act to some extent as spatial K^+ buffers by taking up excess K^+ which accumulates in the extracellular spaces following repeated neuronal discharges. Glia cells can also help to regulate the concentration of transmitter substances like glutamate and GABA in the intercellular spaces.

The composition of the extracellular medium is regulated

The biochemical composition of the extracellular medium is not only regulated by glia cells. Homeostasis is so important that an additional, overlying mechanism is also employed. This mechanism ensures that the brain has its own metabolically constant fluid environment. In vertebrates this is the *cerebrospinal fluid*. Why go to all that effort? Signal generation in neurons depends on the concentrations and movements of different ions. Changes in ionic con-

centrations in the vicinity of neurons are therefore likely to influence this signal generation. A constancy in the composition of the extracellular medium is therefore a prerequisite for a constancy in the transfer of information by nerve cells.

In contrast to the blood plasma and other body fluids, the concentrations of electrolytes, sugar, amino acids, and fatty acids in the cerebrospinal fluid are kept stable within narrow limits. Even the concentrations of hormones, antibodies, proteins, and pharmacological substances are regulated in the cerebrospinal fluid. This regulation is carried out by the endothelial cells which line the blood capillaries in the brain. On the one hand, these cells form a mechanical barrier in that they are connected to one another by *tight junctions,* and so prevent an uncontrolled leakage of molecules out of the blood circulation and into neural tissue. On the other hand, they actively transport metabolic substances. This means that endothelial cells selectively remove substances from the blood and then selectively transport them to the cerebrospinal fluid. In sum, the endothelial cells establish a *blood–brain barrier.* Once substances pass the blood–brain barrier and reach the cerebrospinal fluid they distribute themselves via diffusion throughout the intercellular spaces—the narrow gaps between glia and neurons. Since practically no part of the brain is more than 50 μm away from a blood capillary, substances can then spread passively in this way throughout the whole brain. The total diffusion time in the intercellular space is then only about 10–20 sec.

Regeneration

Degenerative processes and the extent of possible regeneration

Injuries to the nervous system can have wide-ranging consequences. In most cases parts of nerve cells which become separated from the cell body degenerate (due to a loss of essential axonal transport), and are then phagocytosed by other nonneural cells. This degeneration can activate numerous different processes in the denervated target cells and even lead to their degeneration (anterograde degeneration). The parts of the severed neuron which remain in contact with the cell body are also affected. On the one hand, the whole neuron can degenerate, in which case presynaptic cells can also be influenced (retrograde degeneration). On the other hand, regenerative changes can occur which metabolically prepare the axotomized cell for the regeneration of new neurites. This involves an increase in the size of the cell body, in the number of free polysomes, and in the synthesis of protein and RNA. Under favorable conditions regenerating neurons can form axons which can reinnervate their target cells. The capacity to regenerate, particularly in the peripheral nervous system, is amazing and can lead to the complete restoration of a missing function. However, it is important here that the cell bodies themselves are not directly damaged.

The regenerative growth of new neurons is limited

The adult nervous system is much more limited in its ability to generate new cells from existing precursor cells than other tissues and organ systems. Only very few new nerve cells are produced once the processes which occur during development have run their course. The majority of adult neurons withdraw from the mitotic cycle and are no longer capable of cell division. Exceptions are some structures where a continued replacement of neurons occurs even in the adult animal. In vertebrates the olfactory sensory cells, for example, are continually replaced by new receptor cells which then form new connections with the olfactory lobe. The limited generation of new neurons is one reason for the generally irreversible effects of injuries to the CNS.

Regenerative processes allow the formation of new neurites and synapses

Although as a rule the CNS cannot generate new neurons to replace lost ones, surviving nerve cells can form new processes. These neurites can grow out in a directed manner and form specific synaptic connections. Two cases which have been particularly well studied are the regeneration of the neuromuscular synapse, and regeneration in the visual system of lower vertebrates.

The reestablishment of a functional synaptic contact between a motoneuron and a muscle fiber is typical of the regenerative capacity of the peripheral nervous system

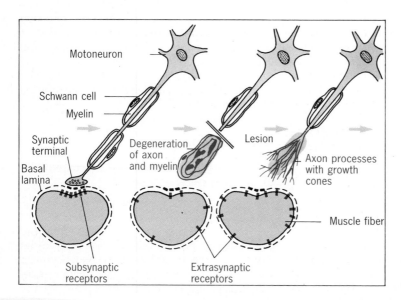

Fig. 8.4 Regeneration of a neuromuscular connection. Following axotomy the distal axon segment degenerates, while at the end of the proximal segment sprouts form, bearing growth cones which grow toward the target tissue. On contact with the target cells, synapses are mostly formed at the same sites as previous synaptic contacts. After denervation, the muscle fiber synthesizes new acetylcholine receptors which are also incorporated into extrasynaptic regions of the membrane. Following reinnervation the receptors again aggregate in the subsynaptic region (after Kelley)

(Fig. 8.4). Regeneration is made possible by specific changes in the presynaptic and postsynaptic cells. Following degeneration of the distal segment of the severed axon, new growth cones are formed on the proximal segment (the part still attached to the cell body). There is a "sprouting" of new processes. These grow at a rate of several millimeters per day toward the target tissue, and in the process often use the basal laminae of the former axonal Schwann cell sheath as guides. Having reached the denervated muscle cell, the regenerated axon generates new presynaptic terminals at the same sites as the previous synapses. Molecular labels in the extracellular matrix surrounding the muscle fibers are important here.

After denervation there are also changes on the postsynaptic (muscle fiber) side. The electrotonic properties of the membrane change. Newly synthesized acetylcholine receptors are incorporated all over the membrane, and not only at the previous subsynaptic region. The chemosensitivity of the postsynaptic membrane increases along with the increase in these extrasynaptic receptors, whose molecular properties have changed compared to the normal synaptic receptors. A state of supersensitivity arises in which the response of a muscle fiber to application of the neurotransmitter is up to 1000 times more sensitive than normal. For reasons which are not yet clear, a supersensitive muscle fiber is particularly receptive to reinnervation. This even leads to "incorrect" synapses being accepted from foreign axons, but these are then suppressed by the formation of "correct" synapses between the motoneuron and muscle. Some of this receptiveness to reinnervation could be based on the transient expression of N-CAM on the muscle surface. The supersensitivity recedes following the reestablishment of normal innervation, and the receptors of the postsynaptic membrane again aggregate in the subsynaptic region. The extracellular matrix also seems to play an important organizational role here.

A regeneration of the connections between the retina and tectum can occur in the retinotectal system of lower vertebrates following complete transection of the optic nerve (and thus of the axons of all the retinal ganglion cells). The axons of the retinal ganglion cells grow back in an orderly way to their "correct" target cells in the tectum and form new synapses there. The regenerative process leads to the reestablishment of a functionally intact visual system which indicates the formation of highly selective synaptic connections. The retinotopically correct projection is even maintained when the retina is rotated by 180° after severing the optic nerve (Fig. 8.5). Since the axons from the inverted retina project back to their original target sites, the visually guided behavior of such animals is dramatically altered—it is 180° out of alignment. A similarly dramatic regeneration of whole nerve tracts does not seem to occur in the mammalian CNS.

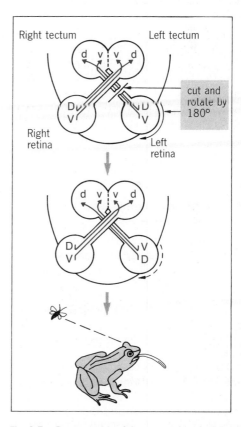

Fig. 8.5 Regeneration of the connections in the retinotectal system of the frog following transection of the optic nerve and rotation of the eye. The retinal axons of the rotated left eye regrow into the tectum and form functional connections with their original target cells. Following regeneration, the behavioral response to visual input is 180° out of alignment. d, D = dorsal, v,V = ventral (after Sperry)

Apart from the capacity to generate new synaptic connections when they are injured, intact nerve cells also have the tendency to form axon collaterals and so occupy synaptic contact sites which become free following the loss of other neurons. The freeing of synaptic contact sites on a target cell seems to stimulate neighboring axon terminals to grow out and form new presynaptic terminals. This can result in a considerable increase in the target region innervated by a neuron. A similar process occurs when a neuron's target cell is lost. In this case the affected neuron forms synapses with other, even "incorrect" and already innervated target cells, which it would normally never innervate.

These processes seem to involve the reactivation of multiple mechanisms formerly active during development. It might be possible, for example, that neurons are "programmed" to form a certain number of synapses, and that the number and location of the synapses actually formed are regulated by competition with other neurons. When neurons are lost the surviving neurons then competitively regenerate the synaptic connectivity patterns. The initiation and regulation of this process involves not only the potential presynaptic neurons, but also the active participation of the denervated target cells.

Trophic substances stimulate the outgrowth of neurites

Guiding structures seem to be important in the regenerative outgrowth of an axon toward a target tissue. But chemotactic processes are also of considerable importance. There is a range of trophic and growth promoting factors which contributes to a maintained increase in metabolic activity, to an outgrowth of neurites, and to the survival and differentiation of regenerating nerve cells.

Denervated cells release growth-promoting diffusible substances which attract the growth cones of regenerating axons. Up to now this process has been mainly studied on model systems in cell culture. In a cell culture the directed growth of some neurites can be guided by the release of small amounts of NGF from a pipette (Fig. 8.6). In other cases the behavior of growth cones can be controlled by the presence of a neurotransmitter in the cell medium.

Surface molecules on the cell membrane

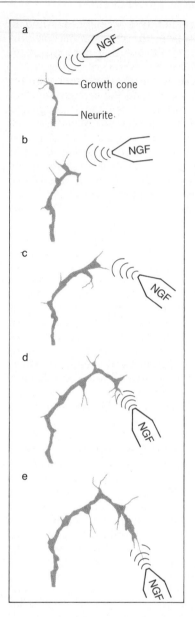

Fig. 8.**6**   Guidance of a growth cone by NGF gradients in cell culture. The growth cone of a neurite of a dorsal root ganglion cell follows the tip of a micropipette from which small amounts of NGF are released. Ninety minutes have elapsed between **a** and **e** (after Gundersen and Barret)

and on the extracellular matrix also seem to play an important role in the outgrowth of neurites. These molecules include gangliosides and glycoproteins like fibronectin and laminin. N-CAM also seems to be important for outgrowth since the addition of antibodies against N-CAM to the culture medium can prevent the bundling of axons into nerve-like aggregates. Other substances are known to be "factors" promoting regeneration but have not yet been molecularly described. It is also likely that changes in the hormonal milieu influence the regenerative outgrowth of neurons.

Transplantations allow regeneration in the central nervous system

For a long time it was believed that neurons in the mammalian CNS had lost the capacity to regenerate. No regeneration of severed nerve pathways is normally observed in the CNS of adult mammals. However, it has recently become clear that regeneration is possible under certain circumstances, even in the mammalian CNS. The role of nonneural supporting structures seems to be critical. While the Schwann cells play an important promoting function during regeneration of the peripheral nervous system, the glia cells of the CNS, by contrast, seem to hinder the regenerative outgrowth of neurites. This is firstly because after transection of a nerve pathway in the CNS, there is a

proliferation of glia cells and a migration of fibroblasts, so that a thick scar tissue forms which is then impenetrable for outgrowing axons. Secondly, growth-inhibiting myelin-associated factors are found on the astrocytes and oligodendrocytes of the adult CNS, something which does not occur among the Schwann cells. A partial regeneration of previously severed fibers can be demonstrated in the corticospinal tract of the mouse if these inhibitory factors are eliminated by *in vivo* application of blocking antibodies.

Adult nerve cells which do not normally undergo regenerative axonal growth in the CNS can sprout in some cases when a section of peripheral nerve is provided. If, for example, the medulla and spinal cord of the rat are bridged with a section of peripheral nerve, then the axons of central neurons can enter the transplanted nerve bridge from both sides and grow through to the other end (Fig. 8.7). However, they stop growing shortly after they reenter the tissue of the CNS.

Although it is difficult for adult nerve tissue in the CNS to grow regeneratively, transplanted embryonic nerve tissue can do this quite well (Fig. 8.8). Transfer of part of an embryonic nervous system, or a suspension of embryonic nerve cells, into an adult CNS can result in an outgrowth of neurites, and even the formation of synapses between transplant and host tissue.

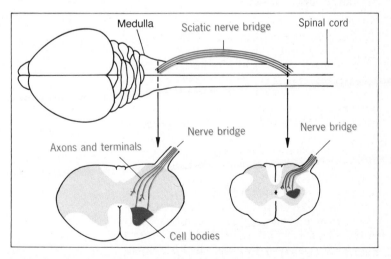

Fig. 8.**7**   Axons in the CNS can grow through a bridge made up of peripheral nerve. A bridge of peripheral nerve is implanted between the medulla and thoracic spinal cord of a rat. After some time axons from neurons of the CNS grow through the bridge from both sides (after Aguayo et al., and Fine)

In some cases the regeneration of synaptic connections can be amazingly precise. Following the transplantation of normal embryonic cerebellar tissue into the cerebellum of a mutant mouse whose Purkinje cells degenerate prematurely, the Purkinje cells of the transplanted tissue are observed to migrate into the correct layers of the host cerebellum and replace the missing Purkinje cells there. In the process they form the appropriate dendritic structures, and make correct synapses with the parallel fibers and other interneurons of the host cerebellum.

In other cases a more diffuse synapse formation results which can nevertheless have important therapeutic effects. Transplants of neurons of the substantia nigra which might lead to a reestablishment of the dopaminergic innervation of the corpus callosum are being intensively studied. Deficiencies in the substantia nigra lead to various motor disturbances in animals, and to Parkinson's disease in humans. Implanting embryonic dopaminergic nerve cells has led to an alleviation of the motor disturbances in the CNS of animals whose dopaminergic input system has been destroyed.

Adult neurons can form neurites and establish new connections even in the absence of injury

An analysis of regeneration suggests that processes like competition for synaptic contact sites might also occur in the intact adult animal. Indeed, adult neurons do actually seem to be able to continually change their structure and synaptic connections. For example, extension and retraction of dendrites are normal occurrences among neurons of the sympathetic ganglia of young adult mammals. Over a timespan of a few months, neurons in the superior cervical ganglion of the mouse show distinct changes in their dendritic geometry (Fig. 8.9). In this process, some dendritic branches are completely retracted while others are formed *de novo*. This change in dendritic morphology is probably accompanied by the formation of new sites for synaptic contact.

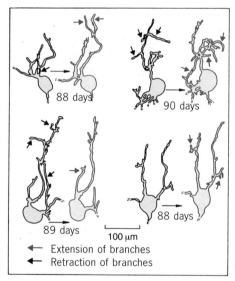

Fig. 8.**9**   Structural plasticity in adult neurons. Changes in the dendritic branching patterns of adult neurons from the superior cervical ganglion of the mouse over a time span of 3 months (after Purves et al.)

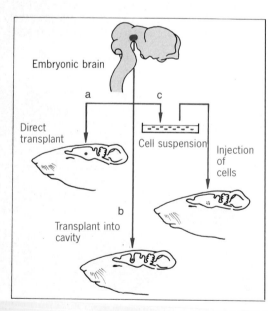

Fig. 8.**8**   Transplantation in the CNS. Tissue from the embryonic brain of a rat can be transplanted into an adult brain either as a tissue transplant or as a cell suspension (after Dunnett and Björklund)

An example of a regularly occurring reconfiguration of adult neurons occurs in the visual system of some teleosts. Both the retina and the tectum are continually growing during the lifespan of the goldfish. The retina grows in a concentric manner, while the tectum grows in a crescent shape at its caudal end. Despite these topological differences, an ordered retinotopic projection is maintained throughout life. Ganglion cells in the center of the retina for example, always project onto the current center of the tectum. In order to maintain the correct retinotectal projection during growth, and to make room for newly ingrowing axons, the terminals of the retinal ganglion cells already present on the surface of the tectum must be continually displaced. In this process old synapses are retracted and new ones formed (Fig. 8.10).

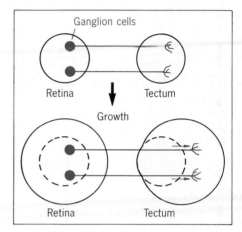

Fig. 8.**10** Displacement of the terminals of retinal ganglion cells on the growing surface of the tectum during postembryonic development in the goldfish (after Easter)

References

General Reviews

Björklund, A. and Stenvi. U. 1984. Intracerebral neural implants: Neuronal replacement and reconstruction of damaged circuits. Annu. Rev. Neurosci. 7: 279-308.

Bray, D. 1991. Cell Movements. Garland, New York.

Bray, D. and Gilbert, D. 1981. Cytoskeletal elements in neurons. Annu. Rev. Neurosci. 4: 505-523.

Bray, D., Raminsky, M. and Aguayo, A. J. 1981. Interactions between axons and their sheath cells. Annu. Rev. Neurosci. 4: 127-162.

Brown, M. C., Holland, R. L. and Hopkins, W. G. 1981. Motor nerve sprouting. Annu. Rev. Neurosci. 4: 17-42.

Bunge, R. P., Bartlett Bunge, M. and Eldrige, C. F. 1986. Linkage between axonal ensheathment and basal lamina production by schwann cells. Annu. Rev. Neurosci. 9: 305-328.

Burgoyne, R. D. (ed.) 1991. The Neuronal Cytoskeleton. Wiley-Liss, New York.

Cotman, C. E. (ed.) 1985. Synaptic Plasticity. Guilford, New York.

Gage, F. H. and Fisher, L. J. 1991. Intracerebral grafting: A tool for the neurobiologist. Neuron 6: 1-12.

Kao, C. C., Bunge, R. P. and Reier, P. J. (eds.) 1983. Spinal Cord Reconstruction. Raven, New York.

Matus, A. 1988. Microtubule-associated proteins: Their potential role in determining neuronal morphology. Annu. Rev. Neurosci. 11: 29-44.

Mjorell, P. (ed.) 1984. Myelin. 2nd edition, Plenum, New York.

Nicholls, J. G. (ed.) 1982. Repair and Regeneration of the Nervous System. Springer, Berlin.

Vallee, R. B. and Bloom, G. S. 1991. Mechanisms of fast and slow axonal transport. Annu. Rev. Neurosci. 14: 59-92.

Yurek, D. M. and Sladek, J. R. 1990. Dopamine cell replacement: Parkinson's disease. Annu. Rev. Neurosci. 13: 415-440.

Zafar, I. (ed.) 1986. Axoplasmic Transport. CRC Press, Boca Raton.

Original Publications

Aguayo, A. J., Bray, G. M. and Perkins, S. C. 1979. Axon–Schwann cell relationships in neuropathies of mutant mice. Ann. N. Y. Acad, Sci. 317: 512-531.

Aguayo, A. J., Charron, L. and Bray, G. M. 1976. Potential of Schwann cells from unmyelinated nerves to produce myelin: A quantitative ultrastructural and radiographic study. J. Neurocytol. 5: 565-573.

Aguayo, A. J., Dickson, R., Trecarten, J., Attiwell, M., Bray, G. M. and Richardson, P. 1978. Ensheathment and myelination of regenerating PNS fibres by transplanted optic nerve glia. Neurosci. Let. 9: 97-104.

Aguayo, A. J., Kasarjian, J., Skamene, E., Kongshavn, P. and Bray, G. M. 1977. Myelination of mouse axons by Schwann cells transplanted from normal and abnormal human nerves. Nature 268: 753-755.

Benfey, M. and Aguayo, A. J. 1982. Extensive elongation of axons from rat brain into peripheral nerve grafts. Nature 296: 150-152.

Bignami, A. and Dahl, D. 1974. Astrocyte-specific protein and neuroglial differentiation: An immunoflourescence study with antibodies to the glial fibrillary acidic protein. J. Comp. Neurol. 153: 27-38.

Bittner, G. D. 1981. Trophic interactions of CNS giant axons in crayfish. Comp. Biochem. Physiol. 68A: 299-306.

Björklund, A., Dunnett, S. B., Stenevi, U., Lewis, N. E. and Iversen, S. D. 1980. Reinnervation of the denervated striatum by substantia nigra transplants: Functional consequences as revealed by pharmacological and sensorimotor testing. Brain. Res. 199: 307-333.

Bowery, N. G., Brown, D. A., White, R. D. and Yamini, G. 1979. (^{3}H)-γ-Aminobutyric acid uptake into neuroglial cells of rat superior cervical sympathetic ganglia. J. Physiol. 293: 51-74.

Bray, B. M., Villegas-Pérez, M. P., Vidal-Sanz, M. and Aguayo, A. J. 1987. The use of peripheral nerve grafts to enhance neuronal survival, promote growth and permit terminal reconnections in the central nervous system of adult rats. J. Exp. Biol. 132: 5-19.

Brightman, M. W., Klatzo, I., Olsson, Y. and Reese, T. S. 1970. The blood–brain barrier to proteins under normal and pathological conditions. J. Neurol. Sci. 10: 215-239.

Brockes, J. P., Fryxell, K. J. and Lemke, G. E. 1981. Studies on cultured Schwann cells: The induction of myelin synthesis, and the control of their proliferation by a new growth factor. J. Exp. Biol. 95: 215-230.

Bundgaard, M. and Cserr, H. F. 1981. A glial blood–brain barrier in elasmobranches. Brain Res. 226: 61-73.

Caroni, P., and Schwab, M. E. 1988. Two membrane protein fractions from rat central myelin with inhibitory properties for neurite growth and fibroblast spreading. J. Cell Biol. 106: 1281-1288.

Caroni, P., and Schwab, M. E. 1988. Antibody against myelin-associated inhibitor of neurite growth neutralizes nonpermissive substrate properties of CNS white matter. Neuron 1: 85-96.

Cohen, M. W. 1970. The contribution by glial cells to surface recordings from the optic nerve of an amphibian. J. Physiol. 210: 565-580.

Cohen, M. W., Gerschenfeld, H. M. and Kuffler, S. W. 1968. Ionic environment of neurones and glial cells in the brain of an amphibian. J. Physiol. 197: 363-380.

Coles, J. A. and Tsacopoulos, M. 1981. Ionic and possible metabolic interactions between sensory neurones and glial cells in the retina of the honeybee drone. J. Exp. Biol. 95: 75-92.

Cserr, H. and Rall, D. P. 1967. Regulation of cerebro-spinal fluid (K⁺) in the spiny dogfish, Squalus acanthias. Comp. Biochem. Physiol. 21: 431-434.

Currie, D. N. and Kelly, J. S. 1981. Glial versus neuronal uptake of glutamate. J. Exp. Biol. 95: 181-193.

David, S. and Aguayo, A. J. 1981. Axonal elongation into peripheral nervous system "Bridges" after central nervous system injury in adult rats. Science 214: 931-933.

Dennis, M. J. and Miledi, R. 1974. Electrically induced release of acetylcholine from denervated Schwann cells. J. Physiol. 237: 431-452.

Droz, B., Di Giamberardino, L., Koenig, N. J., Boyenval, J. and Hassig, R. 1978. Axon–myelin transfer of phospholipid components in the course of their axonal transport as visualized by radio-autography. Brain Res. 155: 347-353.

Dunnett, S. B. and Björklund, A. 1987. Mechanisms of function of neural grafts in the adult mammalian brain. J. Exp. Biol. 132: 265-289.

Easter, S. S. Jr., Rusoff, A. C. and Kish, P. E. 1981. The growth and organization of the optic nerve and tract in juvenile and adult goldfish. J. Neurosci. 1: 793-811.

Elliott, E. J. and Muller, K. J. 1983. Sprouting and regeneration of sensory axons after destruction of ensheathing glial cells in the leech central nervous system. J. Neurosci. 3: 1994-2006.

Gainer, H., Tasaki, I. and Lasek, R. J. 1977. Evidence for the glia–neuron protein transfer hypothesis from intracellular perfusion studies of squid giant axons. J. Cell Biol. 74: 524-530.

Grafstein, B. and Forman, D. S. 1980. Intracellular transport in neurons. Physiol. Rev. 60: 1167-1283.

Gundersen, R. W. and Barrett, J. N. 1980. Characterization of the turning response of dorsal root neurites toward nerve growth factor. J. Cell Biol. 87: 546-554.

Gutnick, M. J., Connors, B. W. and Ransom, B. R. 1981. Dye-coupling between glial cells in the guinea pig neocortical slice. Brain Res. 213: 486-492.

Hoy, R., Bittner, G. D. and Kennedy, D. 1967. Regeneration in crustacean motoneurons: Evidence for axonal fusion. Science 156: 251-252.

Kuffler, S. W. 1967. Neuroglial cells: Physiological properties and a potassium mediated effect of neuronal activity on the glial membrane potential. Proc. R. Soc. Lond. B 168: 1-21.

Kuffler, S. W., Nicholls, J. G. and Orkand, R. K. 1966. Physiological properties of glial cells in the central nervous system of amphibia. J. Neurophysiol. 29: 768-787.

Kuffler, S. W. and Potter, D. D. 1964. Glia in the leech central nervous system: Physiological properties and neuron–glia relationship. J. Neurophysiol. 27: 290-320.

Landis, D. M. and Reese, T. S. 1981. Membrane structure in mammalian astrocytes: A review of freeze-structure studies on adult, developing, reactive and cultured astrocytes. J. Exp. Biol. 95: 35-48.

Lane, N. J. 1981. Invertebrate neuroglia-junctional structure and development. J. Exp. Biol. 95: 7-33.

Lasek, R. J., Gainer, H. and Barker, J. L. 1977. Cell-to-cell transfer of glial proteins to the sqid giant axon. J. Cell Biol. 74: 501-523.

Lasek, R. J. and Tytell, M. A. 1981. Macromolecular transfer from glia to the axon. J. Exp. Biol. 95: 153-165.

Levitt, P. and Rakic, P. 1980. Immunoperoxidase localization of glial fibrillary acidic protein in radial glial cells and astrocytes of the developing rhesus monkey brain. J. Comp. Neurol. 193: 815-840.

Livingston, R. B., Pfenninger, K., Moor, H. and Akert, K. 1973. Specialized paranodal and inter-paranodal glial–axonal junctions in the peripheral and central nervous system: A freeze-etching study. Brain Res. 58: 1-24.

Lund, R. D. and Lund, J. S. 1973. Reorganization of the retinotectal pathway in rats after neonatal retinal lesions. Exp. Neurol. 40: 377-390.

McIntosh, J. R. and Porter, M. E. 1989. Enzymes for microtubule-dependent motility. J. Biol. Chem. Sci. 264: 6001-6004.

Newman, E. A. 1986. High potassium conductance in astrocyte endfeet. Science 233: 453-454.

Nicholls, J. G. and Kuffler, S. W. 1964. Extracellular space as a pathway for exchange between blood and neurons in the central nervous system of the leech: Ionic composition of glial cells and neurons. J. Neurophysiol. 27: 645-671.

Nicholls, J. G. and Kuffler, S. W. 1965. Na and K content of glial cells and neurons determined by flame photometry in the central nervous system of the leech. J. Neurophysiol. 28: 519-525.

Orkand, P. M., Bracho, H. and Orkand, R. K. 1973. Glial metabolism: Alteration by potassium levels comparable to those during neural activity. Brain Res. 55: 467-471.

Orkand, R. K., Nicholls, J. G. and Kuffler, S. W. 1966. Effect of nerve impulses on the membrane potential of glial cells in the central nervous system of amphibia. J. Neurophysiol. 29: 788-806.

Orkand, R. K., Orkand, P. M. and Tang, C.-M. 1881. Membrane properties of neuroglia in the optic nerve of Necturus. J. Exp. Biol. 95: 49-59.

Palka, J. and Edwards, J. S. 1974. The cerci and abdominal giant fibers of the house cricket Acheta domesticus. II. Regeneration and effects of chronic deprivation. Proc. R. Soc. Lond. B 185: 105-121.

Paton, J. A. and Nottebohm, R. N. 1984. Neurons generated in the adult brain are recruited into functional circuits. Science 225: 1046-1048.

Pentreath, V. M. and Kai-Kai, M. A. 1982. Significance of the potassium signal from neurones to glial cells. Nature 295: 59-61.

Peracchia, C. 1981. Direct communication between axons and glia cells in crayfish. Nature 290: 597-598.

Purves, D., Thompson, W. and Yip, J. W. 1981. Reinnervation of ganglia transplanted to the neck from different levels of the guinea-pig sympathetic chain. J. Physiol. 313: 49-63.

Raff, M. C. 1989. Glial cell diversification in the rat optic nerve. Science 243: 1450-1455.

Ransom, B. R. and Goldring, S. 1973. Slow depolarization in cells presumed to be glia in cerebral cortex of cat. J. Neurophysiol. 36: 869-878.

Rawlins, F. 1973. A time-sequence autoradiographic study of the in vivo incorporation of [1,2-^{3}H] cholesterol into peripheral nerve myelin. J. Cell Biol. 58: 42-53.

Reese, T. S. and Karnovsky, M. J. 1967. Fine structural localization of a blood–brain barrier to exogenous peroxidase. J. Cell Biol. 34: 207-217.

Richardson, P. M., McGuiness, U. M. and Aguayo, A. J. 1980. Axons from CNS neurones regenerate into PNS grafts. Nature 284: 264-265.

Salem, R. D., Hammerschlag, R., Bracho, H. and Orkand, R. K. 1975. Influence of potassium ions on accumulation and metabolism of [^{14}C]-glucose by glial cells. Brain Res. 86: 499-503.

Schmidt, R. H., Björklund, A. and Stenevi, U. 1981. Intracerebral grafting of dissociated CNS tissue suspensions: A new approach for neuronal transplantation to deep brain sites. Brain Res. 218: 347-356.

Schnell, L. and Schwab, M. E. 1990. Axonal regeneration in the rat spinal cord produced by an antibody against myelin-associated neurite growth inhibitors. Nature 343: 269-272.

Schon, F. and Kelly, J. S. 1974. Autoradiographic localization of [^{3}H]GABA and [^{3}H] glutamate over satellite glial cells. Brain Res. 66: 275-288.

Schwab, M. E. 1990. Myelin-associated inhibitors of neurite growth. Exp. Neurol. 109: 2-5.

Scott, S. A. 1975. Persistence of foreign innervation on reinnervated goldfish extraocular muscles. Science 189: 644-646.

Scott, S. A. and Muller, K. J. 1980. Synapse regeneration and signals for directed growth in the central nervous system of the leech. Dev. Biol. 80: 345-363.

Skene, J. H. P. and Shooter, E. M. 1983. Denervated sheath cells secrete a new protein after nerve injury. Proc. Natl. Acad. Sci. USA 80: 4169-4173.

Skene, J. H. P. and Willard, M. 1981. Characteristics of growth-associated polypeptides in regenerating toad retinal ganglion cell axons. J. Neurosci. 1: 419-426.

Steward, O., Cotman, C. W. and Lynch, G. S. 1973. Reestablishment of electrophysiologically functional entorhinal cortical input to the dentate gyrus deafferented by ipsilateral entorhinal lesions: Innervation by the contralateral entorhinal cortex. Exp. Brain Res. 18: 396-414.

Stone, L. S. and Zaur, I. S. 1940. Reimplantation and transplantation of adult eyes in the salamander (Triturus viridescens) with return of vision. J. Exp. Zool. 85: 243-269.

Syková, E. 1981. K$^+$ changes in the extracellular space of the spinal cord and their physiological role. J. Exp. Biol. 95: 93-109.

Syková, E., Shirayev, B., Kriz, N. and Vycklický L. 1976. Accumulation of extracellular potassium in the spinal cord of frog. Brain Res. 106: 413-417.

Takato, M. and Goldring, S. 1979. Intracellular marking with Lucifer Yellow CH and horseradish peroxidase of cells electrophysiologically characterized as glia in the cerebral cortex of the cat. J. Comp. Neurol. 186: 173-188.

Tang, C. M., Cohen, M. W. and Orkand, R. K. 1980. Electrogenic pumps in axons and neuroglia and extracellular potassium homeostasis. Brain Res. 194: 283-286.

Tang, C.-M., Strichartz, G. R. and Orkand, R. K. 1979. Sodium channels in axons and glial cells of the optic nerve of Necturus maculosa. J. Gen. Physiol. 74: 629-642.

Van Essen, D. and Jansen, J. K. 1974. Reinnervation of rat diaphragm during perfusion with α-bungarotoxin. Acta Physiol. Scand. 91: 571-573.

Villegas, J. 1981. Schwann-cell relationships in the giant nerve fibre of the squid. J. Exp. Biol. 95: 135-151.

Wallace, B. G., Adal, M. and Nicholls, J. G. 1977. Regeneration of synaptic connexions of sensory neurones in leech ganglia in culture. Proc. R. Soc. Lond. B 199: 567-585.

Zeuthen, T. and Wright, E. M. 1981. Epithelial potassium transport: Tracer and electrophysiological studies in choroid plexus. J. Membr. Biol. 60: 105-128.

9. Processes Dependent on Experience

Plasticity

The extent to which sensory experience influences the brain

The notion that the nervous system is a rigid, hard-wired functional unit, and is therefore more like a collection of integrated circuits than living tissue, does not correspond to reality. Many regions of the brain can change structurally and functionally, depending on sensory experience. Certain neuronal systems are even critically dependent on sensory information from the environment to become correctly configured during postnatal development. The mechanisms mediating this *developmentally based plasticity* can remain active long after the early postnatal phase. The stability of fully developed synapses is constantly affected by experience, as are some of the neuronal connectivity patterns, even in the mature brain. Since every animal experiences different environmental influences, experience-dependent neuronal plasticity also contributes to individuality.

Many processes in neuronal development depend on experience

Genetic and epigenetic information guides the development of the nervous system during embryogenesis. In many cases this information is sufficient to construct a system with the necessary precision. In other situations this is not the case, and additional information must be available for further development of a fully functional brain. Where could this information originate? Beyond a certain developmental stage environmental information provided by sensory organs is available to the nervous system. Could sensory signals be incorporated as organizing elements in the developmental process? The answer is yes, provided that

- the surroundings in which the animal develops are sufficiently differentiated,
- interactions with the surroundings are possible at the appropriate developmental

stages, and
- the sensory signals perceived match the intrinsic response properties of the nerve cells concerned.

When sensory signals fit into the neurogenetic framework, they can in fact influence the functional and structural development of certain parts of the nervous system. Developmental processes which are guided by sensory experience can select and consolidate appropriate connections from the repertoire of neuronal connectivity provided by embryonic development, while disconnecting other inappropriate connections. These changes can be very important for the *self-organization* of sensory systems.

The fact that sensory experience can regulate and modify neuronal connections can be demonstrated in different systems, and in a range of animals including invertebrates and vertebrates. In insects plasticity marks the development of certain neurons in the CNS. Neurons in the corpora pedunculata of *Drosophila* are restructured postembryonically, and sensory experience can intervene in the restructuring process. Anatomical, physiological, and biochemical effects of sensory experience can all be demonstrated at the neuronal level. In vertebrates, auditory experience can be important for the development and maintenance of acoustic recognition. In the early postnatal development of owls, humans, and guinea pigs, there is a limited period during which sensory experience has long-lasting effects on neuronal mechanisms for sound localization. In this phase, the neuronal computational system is plastically matched to the individual acoustic properties of the head and ears of each animal. An experience-dependent fine tuning may be continually active in the adult animal and so contribute to maintaining the precision of the system.

Developmental processes dependent on experience also mark many aspects of social behavior. In humans, as in other primates, severe disturbances in normal social experience can lead to long-term defects in behavior. The mechanisms responsible for these processes are still largely unknown.

Visual experience leads to plastic changes in the central visual system

One of the best examples of development-dependent plasticity is the formation of neuronal binocularity in the mammalian visual cortex (Fig. 9.1). Most neurons in the primary visual cortex of a monkey that has grown up under normal conditions respond to appropriate stimulation of each of the two eyes. This binocularity of the cortical neurons is important for three-dimensional vision. A synchronous and balanced activation of the visual pathways arising from both eyes is necessary during a certain *critical phase* in postnatal development for neuronal binocularity to occur. This happens more or less automatically when the animal can see normally.

If, however, the synchrony of the normal visual input is disturbed during the critical developmental phase, for example by an induced strabismus (squint), then the binocularity of the neurons in the visual cortex cannot be established. This is surprising because in strabismus both eyes are stimulated equally and the animal can see normally with each eye. Nevertheless, the fact that the corresponding regions of both retinas did not simultaneously perceive exactly the same image during a critical developmental phase is already enough to cause serious, and in many cases irreversible, visual defects. This is evidence for the fact that balanced

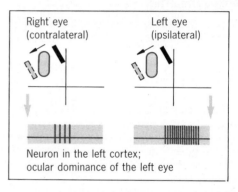

Fig. 9.**1a**   Neuronal binocularity and ocular dominance in the primate visual cortex. Response of a typical neuron in the left half of the visual cortex to a moving bar of light. The neuron responds better when the stimulus is perceived by the ipsilateral eye. In this schema the visual fields (oval) for the right and left eyes are represented separately

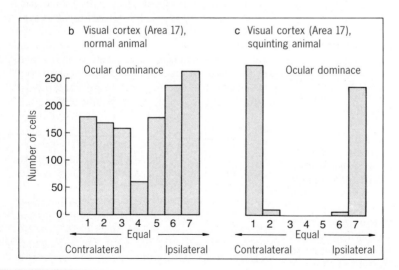

Fig. 9.**1b**   Distribution of ocular dominance in the visual cortex. Cells in groups 1 and 7 receive information from only one eye. All other cells receive input from both eyes. In groups 2,3 and 5,6 the input from one eye dominates. In group 4 both eyes have about the same influence. **c** Effect on ocular dominance in the visual cortex of an induced strabismus during the critical phase in development. The majority of cells are supplied with information from one eye or the other, but not from both eyes (after Hubel and Wiesel)

activation of the visual pathways from both eyes during a certain postnatal developmental stage is critical for the formation of binocularity.

Direct experimental evidence for this comes from studies on cats. In these experiments all the action potentials evoked by the retina were first blocked by the application of tetrodotoxin (TTX). Both the optic nerves were then selectively stimulated with implanted electrodes during the critical phase. When the electrical stimulation of the two nerves was performed synchronously, then binocularity formed in the neurons of the visual cortex and was also maintained later. However, when the electrical stimulation of the two nerves was carried out asynchronously, then most of the cortical neurons could only be activated later by one of the two eyes. Studies at the level of individual neurons have shown that only about 200–400 milliseconds at most are allowed to elapse between the two stimuli if neuronal binocularity is to occur.

Sensory deprivation can lead to severe disturbances of the nervous system

When we consider the disturbances which are caused in the visual system as a result of relatively small imbalances in stimulation, then it is not surprising that visual deprivation during postnatal development can have serious consequences. For example, if an eye in a monkey remains closed for the time between birth and 6 months of age, then the animal will be permanently functionally blind in this eye. And this despite the fact that the neurons of the retina and lateral geniculate function normally for the most part. The cause of this serious visual disturbance is to be found in the visual cortex. Hardly any neurons there respond to stimulation of the affected eye following deprivation. By contrast, almost all the neurons of the visual cortex can be activated by stimulation of the eye which remained open. This can be confirmed by functional neuroanatomical studies which reveal the ocular dominance bands in

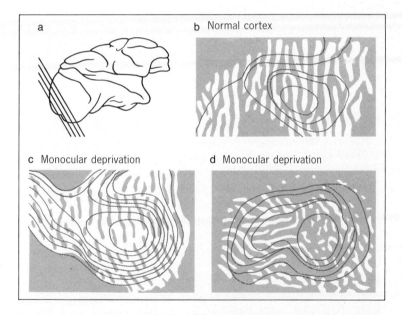

Fig. 9.**2**   Changes in the ocular dominance bands during visual deprivation. **a** Sections through the visual cortex of a monkey in which the visual pathway from the right eye was radioactively labeled 10 days earlier. The sections are processed for autoradiography and the labeled tissue regions displayed as light areas using dark-field microscopy. **b** The ocular dominance bands of a normal animal are equally large. The light bands represent the terminals of geniculocortical afferents which transmit input from the labeled right eye. The dark bands represent the afferents which transmit input from the other eye. **c** Ocular dominance bands in an 8-month-old animal whose left (unlabeled) eye was closed at 2 weeks of age. The light bands have expanded considerably since almost all the input to the visual cortex now comes from the right eye. **d** Ocular dominance bands in an 18-month-old animal whose right (labeled) eye was closed at 2 weeks of age. The dark bands have expanded considerably, since almost all the input to the visual cortex now originates from the left eye (after Hubel et al.)

the animal deprived of input to one eye (Fig. 9.2). Whereas in a normal animal the alternating ocular dominance bands of both eyes are about equally large, in a visually deprived animal the ocular dominance bands of the open eye have expanded considerably, at the cost of those of the closed eye, which have almost disappeared. Some change in ocular dominance can be seen at the level of individual neurons within hours of monocular deprivation. The beginnings of a complete loss of input from the deprived eye can already be detected after 12 hours.

The effects which result from closure of an eye during a certain developmental phase are not related, in the first instance, to the lack of stimulation of this eye. It is much more likely that the closed eye is at a disadvantage compared with the open one in terms of stimulation, and that this leads to the loss of cortical function. Thus, one is dealing here with *competitive processes*. This is consistent with the observation that the consequences of closing both eyes are much less severe than the closing of just one. In fact the ocular dominance bands remain anatomically correctly segregated in animals deprived of the use of both eyes, provided the deprivation does not last for months.

This is also consistent with the fact that the effects of a monocular deprivation during the critical period can be reversed: provided that the deprivation has not lasted too long, and that once the closed eye is opened, the eye that was formerly open is closed for the appropriate duration.

The critical phase for the experience-dependent formation of cortical bands does not proceed homogeneously. During the most intensive period, one week of visual deprivation in one eye is already sufficient to cause a complete loss of vision in this eye. The critical phase also seems to occur at several stages in the different parts of the visual system. However, monocular or binocular deprivation has hardly any effect on the visual system if it occurs after the critical developmental phase.

The self-organization of the visual cortex is activity-dependent

How does the altered neuronal competition resulting from monocular deprivation during the critical phase lead to the dramatic decrease in the number of neurons driven by the deprived eye, and so to the striking changes in ocular dominance bands? In a monkey, ocular-dominance bands are already present in rudi-

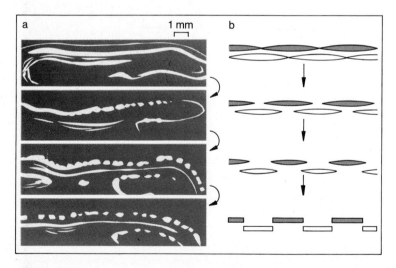

Fig. 9.**3**   Postnatal development of the ocular dominance bands in the cat. **a** Autoradiographic representation of the distribution of geniculocortical afferents which transmit the input from one eye. Different developmental stages (2, 3, 5, 13 weeks) are shown. If the animal can see normally, the ocular dominance bands develop progressively during the period under study. **b** Model to explain the postnatal formation of ocular dominance bands under normal developmental conditions. The temporal sequence for the segregation of geniculocortical afferents which transmit input from the right eye (shaded structures), and those which transmit input from the left eye (light structures), is shown. The extensive overlapping which is still present shortly after birth declines with increasing age (after LeVay et al., and Hubel et al.)

mentary form at birth. The axon terminals of the (monocularly driven) afferent neurons from the lateral geniculate are already present in cortical layer IVc. However, they have not yet segregated according to their current monocular input. The branches coming from an axon still cover a region corresponding to several mature ocular dominance bands. Appropriately, these "perinatal" ocular dominance bands still overlap to a considerable extent.

After birth, competitive interactions lead to a gradual formation of the segregated ocular dominance bands (Fig. 9.3). This involves the laterally extended branches of the afferent neurons retracting to the area of a single cortical band. This process of competition-induced retraction depends on the proper activation of the visual system. Thus, when the visual input from one eye is disrupted because of monocular deprivation, the afferent terminals of those neurons driven by the deprived eye retract abnormally far, and then supply only a small area of the ocular dominance bands that normally develop. By contrast, those neurons driven by the open eye retain all of their extended terminal field. These terminal branches not only do not retract, but somewhat later

they even spread further, sending axon terminals into those neighboring cortical regions no longer occupied by the afferent fibers of the other visual channel. These processes do not occur if all the neuronal activity in both visual pathways is blocked by injection of TTX. Then the terminal regions of the different monocularly supplied afferents in layer IVc retain their extensive overlap, and ocular dominance bands cannot develop further.

Apart from these changes in the extent of the cortical bands, microanatomical processes also occur during the self-organization of the visual cortex. The extension and retraction of afferent terminals are partly related to the formation and breakdown of sites of synaptic contact. Furthermore, there is also good evidence that the synaptic efficacy of intracortical neurons can change in an experience-dependent way even when no change in the anatomical distribution of axon terminals is apparent.

The assumption that properly formed ocular dominance bands develop as a result of competition between two groups of afferent fibers for the same terminal region is supported by experimental manipulations on animals which do not normally form ocular dom-

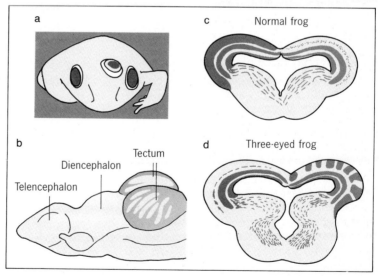

Fig. 9.**4**   Ocular dominance bands in a frog are induced by transplantation of a third eye. **a** A frog in which a third eye rudiment has been embryonically transplanted onto the side of the head. **b** The brain of such a three-eyed frog. Dark bands on the left half of the tectum are the stained afferents from the transplanted third eye. **c** Normal frog. Autoradiographic representation of the retinotectal afferents from the contralateral eye in the right tectal half (left side of figure). No bands have formed. **d** Three-eyed frog. The left tectal half is innervated by the contralateral eye and the third eye. Autoradiographic representation of the retinotectal afferents from the contralateral eye in the left tectal half (right side of figure). Tectal bands have formed (after Constantine-Paton)

inance bands. In the frog, each half of the tectum is innervated exclusively by retinal ganglion cells from the contralateral eye. Accordingly, binocularly driven neurons are rarely found in the tectum. If a third eye rudiment is implanted into a frog embryo, then the retinal ganglion cells of this eye project into the same contralateral half of the tectum as those of the normally situated eye. Interactions between the retinal ganglion cells of the two ipsilateral eyes then occur, and ocular dominance bands form during development (Fig. 9.4). The neurons in these alternating tectal bands are then preferentially driven by either the normal or the supernumerary eye. Even here the formation of cortical bands is activity-dependent; the formation of bands is suppressed when neuronal activity is blocked by the application of TTX.

The principle of associative synaptogenesis

The binocular neurons of the mature visual cortex have identical receptive fields in both retinas, and receive information in the same way from the same region of the visual field. Therefore during neurogenesis, millions of afferent neurons have to be organized so that only those afferent fibers driven by precisely corresponding retinal regions project onto common target cells. The problem that arises, however, is that during embryonic development it is impossible to predict which retinal regions of both eyes will precisely correspond to one another in the mature visual system. This depends on the different head and eye dimensions of different individuals. How can this problem be solved? One elegant solution would be to compare the electrical activity in the afferent nerve fibers from the two eyes during normal vision. Neurons driven by corresponding retinal loci would then fire in a highly correlated way, since by definition they would be excited by the same optical stimulus. A developmental mechanism would therefore be required to selectively consolidate those retinal afferent inputs which transmit highly correlated activity patterns.

Many experiments on the visual system have led to theories on consolidating mechanisms. Some of these ideas are formulated in the concept of *associative synaptogenesis*. This assumes that an increase or decrease in synaptic stability (or synaptic efficacy) depends on the temporal correlation of activity in presynaptic and postsynaptic cells. Thus the following rule for synaptic modification might apply: the efficacy of a given synapse is increased if the activity in the presynaptic and postsynaptic cells is highly temporally correlated, and it is decreased if the postsynaptic cell is active and the presynaptic cell is inactive (Fig. 9.5a). This modification rule leads directly to the result that two or more converging nerve fibers must be active synchronously for them to remain connected to the same postsynaptic target cell. As soon as the presynaptic cells are active at different times, they will begin to compete with one another. The synapse of the presynaptic cell which activates the postsynaptic cell more, will then be stabilized at the expense of the other, inactive, presynaptic cells (Fig. 9.5b).

The concept of associative synaptogenesis is particularly attractive because it would lead to the experience-dependent formation of neuronal connections which respond to commonly occurring coupled stimulus patterns. The causal relationship between highly associated external sensory impressions could, by associative synaptogenesis, be reflected in the neuronal connectivity of the resulting nervous system. During the course of its development, the brain could in this self-organizatory way become capable of perceiving the specific properties of the outside world.

The question of *which* neuronal mechanisms might be responsible for an associative synaptogenesis cannot be answered with certainty at the moment. Several lines of evidence point to *NMDA receptor channels* in postsynaptic cells as being important for neuronal plasticity, at least in the visual cortex. There are several reasons for this.

— NMDA receptor channels are especially common in the neonatal visual cortex. Their frequency decreases later.
— Perfusion with selective antagonists of the NMDA receptor channel prevents activity-dependent remodeling from occurring in the primary visual cortex, without affecting the responses of cortical neurons to light.
— Long-term changes in the response properties of cortical neurons can be achieved by pairing visual stimuli and localized perfusion with NMDA receptor agonists and other neuromodulators.

— The properties of the NMDA receptor channel are especially well suited for assessing the temporal association between pre- and postsynaptic activity. These include the fact that an increased Ca^{2+} permeability of the postsynaptic membrane can only be achieved when the presynaptically released neurotransmitter *and* a postsynaptic depolarization occur simultaneously (see Fig. 3.**18**).

What is certain is that the process of associative synaptogenesis in the visual system cannot depend solely on the temporal pattern of incoming afferent signals. Further neuronal constraints must be satisfied. In the formation of ocular dominance bands, for example, the associative mechanism should only be active when both eyes fixate a specific target, and not just when they are moved in an uncoordinated way. Additional, largely unknown, neuronal control mechanisms therefore also must be involved in these plastic events.

Plasticity is also present in the adult nervous system

In the visual system, plasticity seems to be restricted to a relatively short postnatal period. In other systems, new sensory experiences can influence nervous system architecture in the adult animal as well. This is seen most clearly in the somatosensory system of primates. In this system the topographically organized cortical representations of specific peripheral body parts can be changed by sensory input, throughout the life of the animal.

This plasticity is most obvious when some of the mechanosensory input is completely blocked (Fig. 9.**6**). If, for example, one of the nerves supplying the hand of a monkey is severed, systematic changes occur in that particular cortical field in which the now denervated hand region was represented. Shortly after denervation a rudimentary representation of the hand regions bordering the denervated region appears in one part of this cortical region. This cortical representation, which is not apparent under normal conditions, is assumed to be "unmasked" by denervation.

If no regeneration of the severed nerve occurs, then in the following weeks the sensory projections of the neighboring hand regions gradually take over the denervated cortical region. In this way a partially ordered somato-

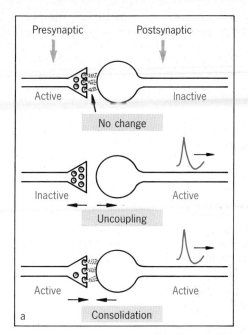

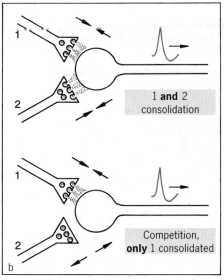

Fig. 9.**5a,b** Model for the activity-dependent modification of synaptic connections in the visual system. **a** Rules for synaptic modification. No change when the presynaptic cell is active and the postsynaptic cell is inactive. Synaptic destabilization when the postsynaptic cell is active and the presynaptic cell is inactive. Synaptic consolidation when the presynaptic and the postsynaptic cells are active simultaneously. **b** Selective stabilization of convergent input synapses occurs when their activity is temporally correlated. Competition between the converging input synapses occurs when their activity is not temporally correlated (after Singer)

topic representation with structured receptive fields is established for these hand regions. With time, further topographic reorganization follows. Projection areas which previously lay completely outside the denervated region, shift into it. Similar processes occur after amputation of a finger. The representational area in the somatosensory cortex that has become vacant is taken over by neighboring finger and hand regions.

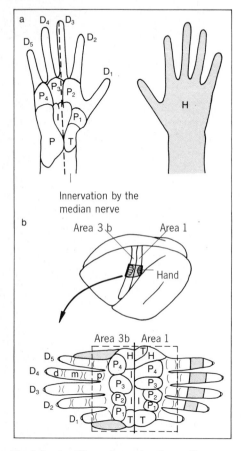

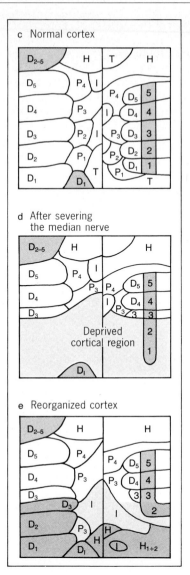

Fig. 9.**6b-e**   Normal cortex, schematic inset from **b. d** Sensory deprivation after severing the median nerve. The same illustration as in **c**, but shortly after sectioning the median nerve. There is no mechanosensory input to that part of the cortex representing the hand region innervated by the median nerve. **e** Reorganization of the cortex after two months. A large part of the deprived cortical region is activated by stimulation of the dorsal side of the hand (dark regions). The representation of the P_3, P_4 and I regions of the ventral side of the hand innervated by the ulnar nerve have expanded. All the reorganized regions are topographically structured (after Merzenich and Kaas)

Fig. 9.**6a, b**   Effect of severing the median nerve on the representation of the hand in the somatosensory cortex of the adult monkey. **a** The ventral side (light) and the dorsal side (dark) of the monkey's hand. D_1, D_2, D_3, D_4, D_5, P_1, P_2, P_3, P_4, P, I, and T refer to different regions of the ventral side. H refers to the whole dorsal side. The radial half of the ventral side of the hand is innervated by the median nerve. The ulnar half of the ventral side is innervated by the ulnar nerve. The dorsal side is innervated by the ulnar and the radial nerves. **b** Schematic illustrating the topographic representation of the hand in areas 3b and 1 of the somatosensory cortex. Cortical regions which represent the dorsal side of the hand are shown dark

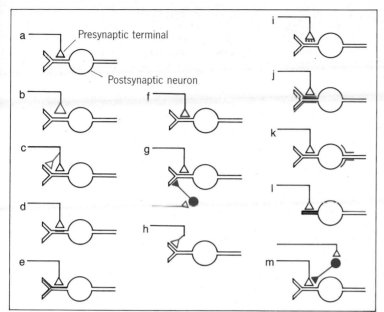

Fig. 9.**7** Hypothetical model for plasticity in the somatosensory cortex. **a** Synaptic connection between a presynaptic and a postsynaptic cell before the plastic change. Possible plasticity mechanisms are. **b** Enlargement of the terminal. **c** Sprouting of the terminal. **d** Changes in the postsynaptic receptors. **e** Changes in dendritic conductances. **f** Contraction of the synaptic cleft. **g** Postsynaptic disinhibition. **h** Displacement of the terminal along the dendrite. **i** Increased transmitter release. **j** Changes in dendritic fine structure. **k** Changes in the impulse initiating zone. **l** Dendritic retraction. **m** Disinhibition of an excitatory terminal (after Devor)

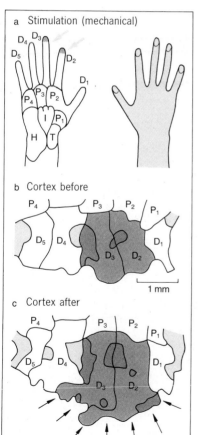

Fig. 9.**8** Changes in the cortical representation of the hand after maintained selective finger stimulation in an adult monkey. **a** Mechanical stimulation of fingers D_2 and D_3 for several months (1–2 hours daily). Representation of the ventral and dorsal sides of the hand as in Figure 9.**6**. **b** Cortical representation of the hand in area 3b of a normal monkey before the selective stimulation. **c** Cortical representation of the hand in area 3b of the same animal several months after the selective stimulation. The representations of fingers D_2 and D_3 at the sites corresponding to the stimulated fingers have enlarged (arrows) (after Jenkins and Merzenich)

The somatosensory projections in the brain of the adult monkey are therefore *dynamic;* projections can expand into functionally deprived regions. This indicates that in the adult animal there is an ongoing competition for certain cortical regions, and that this competition is dependent on sensory inputs. These processes are assumed to occur not only in the cortex, but also in the subcortical centers of the somatosensory system. The cellular mechanisms responsible for these plastic processes are not yet clearly understood. Several possible mechanisms are shown schematically in Figure 9.7.

Experiments in which animals with completely intact innervation are induced to preferentially stimulate a particular hand region show that the topographic organization of the cortical system can be changed with use. If a monkey is trained to employ only its middle finger in a repetitive exercise, there is an expansion in the representation of this finger in the somatosensory cortex (Fig. 9.**8**). It is still not clear if this experience-dependent modification of topographically organized representations is caused by a change in the effectiveness of latent, already established connections, or by the formation of new synaptic connections.

These results indicate that experience is continually restructuring the response-specificity of certain regions in the somatosensory cortex, and that dynamic processes modify the topography of cortical maps throughout life. This sort of plasticity could be a general property of the cortex and play an important role in the acquisition of certain sensorimotor skills. What is interesting is that these activity-dependent, reorganizational, processes are in principle similar to learning processes. It is an attractive hypothesis to assume that there is a continuum between the plastic self-organization which matches the elements of the nervous system to one another and to environmental influences, and the learning processes, which also occur in the mature individual.

Learning Processes

Learning as an ongoing form of neuronal differentiation

We are what we are mainly because of what we have learned. From learning processes, we obtain information about ourselves and about causality in the surrounding world. Via learning, the brain can acquire new capabilities and information during a lifetime, quite apart from those capabilities it has gained in the course of the millions of years of its evolutionary history. In many respects learning can be seen as a late form of neuronal differentiation which continues over the entire lifetime. Even today, Cajal's suggestion that developmental and learning processes are to some extent based on the same mechanisms–namely on changes in the effectiveness of synaptic connections–is true, though in a somewhat modified form. Plastic changes at certain synapses are important events in learning and memory. Fortuitously, precisely these sorts of events can be studied at the cellular and molecular level.

Learning is an adaptive behavioral change based on experience

Everyone knows that learning does not necessarily show up as a change in behavior. However, an accurate documentation and study of learning processes is generally only possible from behavioral observation. In this sense the diversity of different behaviors is reflected in a diversity of different learning modes. Nevertheless, two main types of learning processes can be distinguished. *Nonassociative learning* results in behavioral changes in response to the presentation of a single type of stimulus. The temporal pairing of different stimuli is unimportant here. By contrast, in *associative learning* an animal makes a connection between different stimuli or behavioral states. Both forms of learning occur in invertebrates and vertebrates.

Habituation and *sensitization* are widespread forms of nonassociative learning. Both can last for minutes, hours, or days, depending on the stimulus configuration used. In habituation, a behavioral response to a stimulus that initially has a certain novelty value diminishes on repeated presentation of that stimulus, i.e. stimulus repetition leads to a reduction in a stimulus-dependent behavioral response. In most instances the strength of the response decreases without there being a qualitative change. Habituation is probably the simplest form of learning. In this way an animal learns to "ignore" stimuli which have lost their urgency or novelty. Sensitization is a somewhat more complex learning process during which many behavioral responses can be strengthened in a long-lasting way by a very intense or painful stimulus. Sensitization leads to animals becoming "aware" of stimuli which would otherwise be classed as unimportant. Although even a previously habituated behavioral response can be rapidly restored by sensitization (dishabituation), sensitization is not simply the inverse of habituation. In contrast to habituation, sensitization influences not only isolated and relatively specific neuronal pathways, but a variety of neuronal circuits.

Associative learning serves to establish a causal relationship between different stimuli or events. In the *classical conditioning* described by Pavlov, a relationship is established between a "conditioned" stimulus, which produces little or no response, and an "unconditioned" stimulus which always results in a clear response (Fig. 9.9). In classical conditioning, the repeated and temporally precise coupling of the conditioned stimulus to the unconditioned stimulus which immediately follows

produces a long-term association between the two stimuli. Afterward, the presentation of the conditioned stimulus alone can lead to the release of the behavioral response. As a result of associative learning the nervous system is in a position to link causes and effects to one another. It has achieved the capacity to detect elementary causal relationships.

Classical conditioning is not the only form of associative learning. In *operant conditioning* an animal learns how to solve a particular problem following the principle of trial and error. This type of associative learning generally depends on an adequate reward or punishment. Another form of associative learning can occur when an animal becomes ill from eating poisoned food. In this *food aversion learning* the animal can establish an association, often after only a single trial, between food consumed and a sickness which might occur hours later, and so learn to avoid this particular food in the future. The particular efficiency of food aversion learning indicates that most nervous systems have an inherent capacity to establish certain associations more easily than others. Even a simple garden snail can learn and maintain food aversion after a single trial.

A range of further more *"complex" learning processes* are also known, and these include

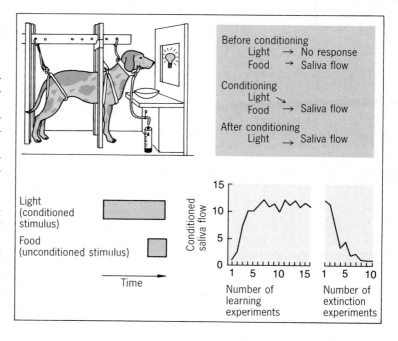

Fig. 9.**9** Classical conditioning according to Pavlov. A light or sound stimulus as a conditioned stimulus is presented temporally correlated with food as an unconditioned stimulus. The presentation of light alone, which before conditioning produced no response, produces the same response as food after conditioning (top). The conditioning is most effective when the conditioned stimulus is presented shortly before the unconditioned stimulus (lower left). The conditioned response (saliva flow) is learned rapidly. If, after conditioning, the light stimulus is repeatedly presented without simultaneous presentation of food, there is a decline (extinction) in the conditioned response (lower right)(after Hilgard et al.)

Before conditioning
Light → No response
Food → Saliva flow

Conditioning
Light ↘
Food → Saliva flow

After conditioning
Light → Saliva flow

Light (conditioned stimulus)

Food (unconditioned stimulus)

Time

Conditioned saliva flow

Number of learning experiments

Number of extinction experiments

imprinting, latent learning, and learning by observation. In *imprinting,* which generally occurs only during a critical developmental phase, particular social forms of behavior important for species preservation are learned (recognition of one's parents, learning of a species-specific communication form etc.). *Latent learning* can lead to the acquisition of certain abilities like running error-free through a maze without any obvious reward or punishment. *Learning by observation* enables an animal to learn a particular action more quickly by observing the act being performed by another, experienced, animal.

Memory is the storage and recall of experiences

Memory, the ability to store and recall information about previous experiences, is essential for learning. Memory is widespread in the animal kingdom; relatively simple animals like platyhelminths can learn and store what they have learned in a memory. In higher animals like molluscs, arthropods and vertebrates, the formation of memory seems to proceed in several stages (Fig. 9.**10**). The first stage involves the representation of the information to be learned in the neuronal circuitry of the nervous system. In the second stage this information is registered and stored in the brain. One assumes that the contents are first stored in a labile *short-term memory.* A range of dynamic, neuronal plasticity mechanisms are probably involved in this short-term storage. The stored information is then transferred to a *long-term memory.* This long-term storage is probably based on lasting functional or structural changes in the nervous system. As long as the information is in the short-term memory it can be easily forgotten, and is also more susceptible to neuronal disturbances. Information storage is more permanent and robust following transfer to the long-term memory. The third stage of memory can be considered to be the recall of stored information. As we know only too well, neuronal memory is not 100% permanent. In general there is a gradual loss either of the stored information itself, or of the capacity to recall this information.

Synaptic plasticity can be the basis of simple learning and memory processes

Several elementary learning processes, especially habituation and sensitization, have been successfully studied at the cellular level, and most comprehensively in the marine mollusc *Aplysia* (Fig. 9.**11a**). This animal possesses a gill as a respiratory organ, which apart from respiratory pumping movements, can also carry out a defensive withdrawal reflex. Lightly touching the siphon associated with the gill leads to the gill as well as the siphon being withdrawn into the mantle cavity. The neuronal network which mediates this reflex consists on the one hand of monosynaptic excitatory connections between mechanosensory receptor cells and the motoneurons of the gill and siphon, and on the other hand of polysynaptic connections from the mechanosensory receptor cells which converge on the motoneurons via excitatory and inhibitory interneurons.

The gill withdrawal reflex habituates on repeated stimulation, and this habituation can last for a short (hours) or long (weeks) time depending on the stimulus configuration. A systematic study of the neurons in the circuit for the gill withdrawal reflex has shown that the habituation is at least partly based on homosynaptic depression both at the synapses between sensory neurons and motoneurons, and at those between sensory neurons and interneurons (Fig. 9.**11b**). The EPSPs which the sensory neurons evoke in the motoneurons and interneurons decrease on repeated activation of the

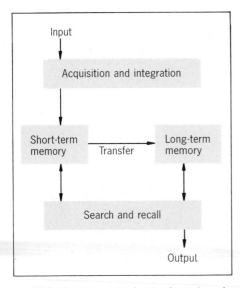

Fig. 9.**10**　General model for the formation of memory, considerably simplified (after Menzel)

sensory cells, that is, on repeated stimulation. As a consequence, the number of action potentials generated per stimulus in the motoneurons also decreases on repeated stimulation, which results in an habituation of the behavioral response. Similar synaptic processes have been observed during habituation in the mechanosensory systems of the crayfish and cockroach.

The gill withdrawal reflex of *Aplysia* also displays sensitization. The gill withdrawal reflex initiated by weak tactile stimulation is persistently greater in amplitude and time course when it follows a strong mechanical or electrical stimulation of the head or tail. A mechanism for this sensitization has been described at the neuronal level (Fig. 9.**11c**). It again has to do with a changed signal transfer at the synapses between the sensory neurons and the postsynaptic motoneurons and interneurons of the gill and siphon. The sensitizing stimuli excite certain facilitating interneurons, which in turn form synapses with the presynaptic terminals of the sensory neurons. The activation of the facilitating interneurons initiates molecular reaction cascades in the presynaptic sensory terminals, which then result in a lasting increase in the amount of transmitter that can be released from the sensory neurons. Thus, the sensitization of the gill withdrawal reflex is based at least partly on a heterosynaptic facilitation. Further important functional mechanisms in sensitization include changes in the excitability of the postsynaptic motoneurons, as well as the coordinated recruitment of certain interneurons into a reflex circuit. These changes probably contribute most to sensitization, but it is not yet clear how they arise.

Particularly long-lasting forms of habituation and sensitization can be generated in *Aplysia* if appropriate stimulus parameters are used. Some of these behavioral modifications can last up to weeks, and structural as well as functional changes are observed in the sensory synapses concerned. An analysis of the active zones in the presynaptic terminals of the sensory neurons shows that both the overall number of active zones and their spatial distribu-

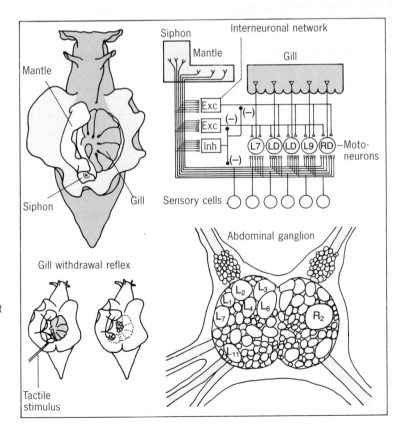

Fig. 9.**11a** Habituation and sensitization of the gill withdrawal reflex in *Aplysia*. Contact causes the gill to be withdrawn into the mantle cavity (left). Simplified circuit diagram for the withdrawal reflex as well as the position in the abdominal ganglion of some of the neurons involved in the reflex (right)

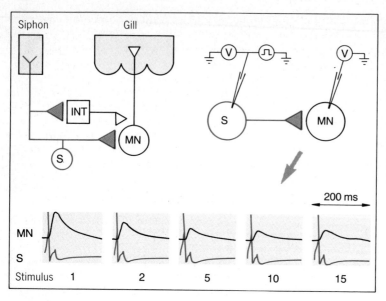

Fig. 9.**11b** Mechanisms for habituation. The site of habituation at the synapses between sensory cells and postsynaptic motoneurons and interneurons (top left). Intracellular stimulation and recording allow the study of synaptic transmission between a sensory cell and a motoneuron (top right). Selective repetitive stimulation of the sensory cell leads to a decline in the EPSP in the postsynaptic motoneuron (bottom)

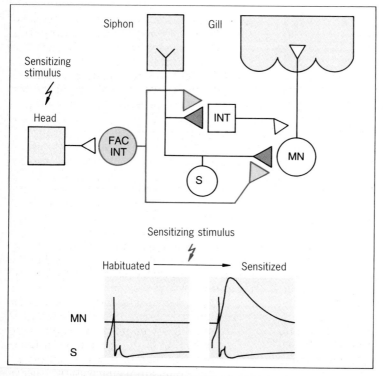

Fig. 9.**11c** Mechanisms for sensitization. The sensitizing stimulus activates interneurons which facilitate the synaptic transmission between sensory cells and postsynaptic motoneurons and interneurons (top). A habituated response can be restored by sensitization (bottom). The synaptic transmission between sensory cell and motoneuron, which is strongly attenuated in a habituated animal, can be restored by sensitization. S = sensory cell, MN = motoneuron, FAC INT = facilitating interneuron, INT = interneuronal network (after Kandel)

tion are greatly reduced in long term habituation, but greatly increased in long term sensitization. These long term behavioral changes seem to involve not only changes in signal transmission at the active synapses, but also effect the number of active synapses. Thus, functional synaptic plasticity is accompanied by structural synaptic plasticity.

A particularly interesting form of synaptic plasticity occurs in the hippocampus of the vertebrate brain. The hippocampus plays an important role in the development of certain learning and memory capabilities, and is phylogenetically a very old part of the cerebral cortex. Like other cortical structures it possesses a relatively stereotyped, repetitive, microarchitecture. It receives its inputs from the entorhinal cortex, from the septum, and from the contralateral hippocampus. The two most important pathways for internal information transfer within the hippocampus are the mossy fibers which project from the granule cells, and the Schaffer collaterals of the pyramidal cells in the CA3 region (Fig. 9.12a).

Experiments have shown that many synapses in the hippocampus have a special form of plasticity termed *long-term potentiation* or LTP. LTP can be produced, for example, by high-frequency stimulation for a few seconds of the fibers coming from the entorhinal cortex. If these input fibers are subsequently activated by single test stimuli, then postsynaptic potentials, which are now much larger than before the high-frequency stimulation, are observed in many neurons of the hippocampus. What is special about this postsynaptic potentiation is that it can last for an amazingly long time. Depending on the stimulus conditions, LTP which lasts for hours, days or weeks can be evoked in the pyramidal and granule cells of the hippocampus (Fig. 9.12b).

In order to evoke LTP the inducing stimulus strength must exceed a critical threshold level. This can occur either by the activation of a sufficiently large number of presynaptic fibers from the same input pathway, or by the simultaneous activation of presynaptic fibers of different input pathways. An interesting phenomenon is observed when when a group of weakly excitatory fibers which are not in a position to evoke LTP alone, is activated together with a group of strongly excitatory fibers. If both groups of fibers project onto the same postsynaptic cell, then associative excit-

atory interactions can occur (Fig. 9.12c). LTP is evoked by the simultaneous activation of the weak *and* the strongly excitatory fibers, and this amplifies the synaptic transmission of both fiber types in a long-lasting manner. In this way a synaptic facilitation of the weakly excitatory fibers results. Since this facilitating property is observed only during temporally synchronous activation of the two input channels, LTP is considered an interesting model mechanism for associative learning.

Associative learning has a cellular basis

What do we know about the neuronal basis of associative learning? Studies on several systems show that simple forms of associative learning can be based on changes in existing neuronal connections. Consider for example the gill withdrawal reflex of *Aplysia* when it undergoes classical conditioning (Fig. 9.13a). In the course of conditioning one can take advantage of the fact that the withdrawal reflex can be initiated by stimulation of the siphon as well as the mantle. During the training phase, a tactile stimulation of one of these sensory structures is temporally paired with an intense electrical shock to the tail, while tactile stimulation of the other sensory structure occurs without a temporally paired electrical shock. In the test phase following successful conditioning, a stronger withdrawal reflex is elicited by mechanical stimulation of the structure whose stimulation was paired with an electric shock, than is elicited by stimulation of the structure which was not.

For associative learning to occur, there must be a convergence at the neuronal level between the pathways which mediate the conditioned stimulus (tactile contact) and the unconditioned stimulus (electroshock). An analysis of the neuronal elements involved in the response shows that such a convergence occurs at the level of the mechanosensory neurons (Fig. 9.13b). As a result of the electric shocks there is a heterosynaptic facilitation of all mechanosensory neurons. However, there is a strengthening of the facilitation in those mechanosensory neurons in which sensory excitation was temporally paired with the electroshock, and which were, thus, active immediately before firing of the facilitatory interneurons. In other words: the extent of heterosynaptic facilitation in the sensory neurons is ac-

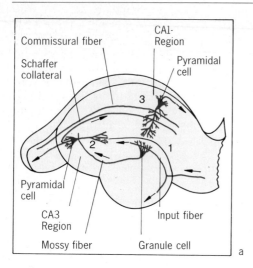

Commissural fiber

Schaffer collateral

CA1-Region

Pyramidal cell

3

Pyramidal cell

CA3 Region

Mossy fiber

2

1

Input fiber

Granule cell

a

Fig. 9.**12**   LTP in the hippocampus. **a** Simplified diagram of the most important excitatory pathways which display LTP. The connections between input fibers and granule cells (1), mossy fibers and pyramidal cells (2), and Schaffer collaterals and pyramidal cells (3), are shown for individual neurons. **b** LTP in the CA1 region. A measure of the EPSP amplitude in the dendrites of the pyramidal cells is plotted against time. The time of tetanic stimulation is given by the arrow. Insets show the EPSPs before, and 90 minutes after, the initiation of LTP. **c** Associative properties of LTP. Schematic representation of the convergence of weakly and strongly excitatory fibers onto the same target cell. Following prior tetanic stimulation, the weakly excitatory fibers evoke an EPSP which is not larger than before tetanus, while the strongly excitatory fibers evoke an EPSP which is much larger than before tetanus. Following prior simultaneous tetanic stimulation of the weakly *and* strongly excitatory fibers, a test stimulation of *either* evokes an EPSP which is much larger than before tetanus (after Nicoll et al.)

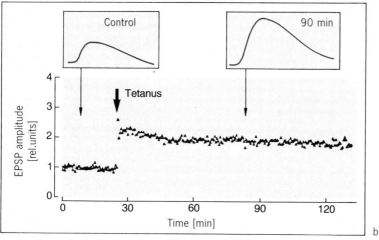

Control

90 min

Tetanus

EPSP amplitude [rel.units]

4

3

2

1

0

0   30   60   90   120

Time [min]

b

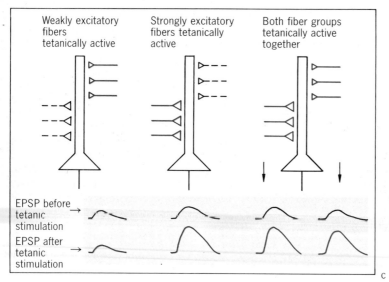

Weakly excitatory fibers tetanically active

Strongly excitatory fibers tetanically active

Both fiber groups tetanically active together

EPSP before tetanic stimulation →

EPSP after tetanic stimulation →

c

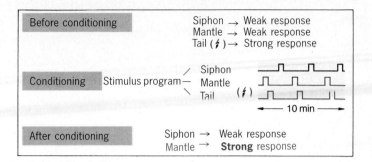

Fig. 9.**13a**   Classical conditioning of the gill withdrawal reflex in *Aplysia*. **a** Arrangement of the training and test phases. In the training phase mechanical stimulation of the mantle (conditioned stimulus) is temporally coupled to electrical stimulation of the tail (unconditioned stimulus); mechanical stimulation of the siphon (control stimulus) on the other hand, is not temporally coupled to electrical stimulation of the tail

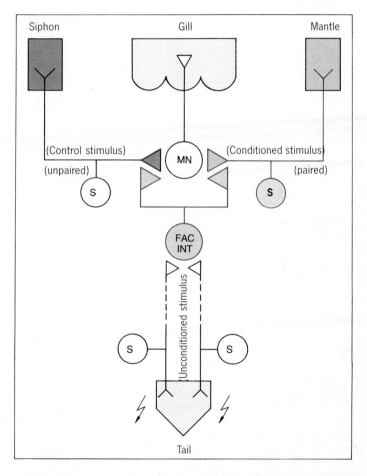

Fig. 9.**13**   Simplified circuit diagram for conditioning. A convergence of the pathways which transmit the unconditioned stimulus and those which transmit the conditioned stimulus occurs at the level of the mechanosensory cells. During conditioning a long-term amplification of synaptic transmission is elicited in those mechanosensory neurons which were active immediately before the facilitatory interneurons. S = sensory cell, MN = motoneuron, FAC INT = facilitating interneuron (after Kandel)

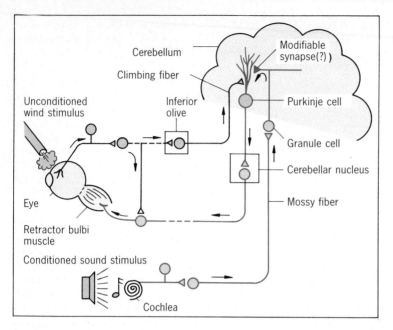

Fig. 9.**14**   Classical conditioning of the eyeblink reflex in the rabbit. Simplified representation of the neuronal circuits involved. A wind stimulus leads to the activation of motoneurons which mediate the blink response. Following repeated temporal pairing of the wind stimulus (unconditioned stimulus) and a sound stimulus (conditioned stimulus), the motoneurons can be activated by the sound stimulus alone. The cerebellum and cerebellar nuclei are involved in the conditioning. A convergence of information from the unconditioned and conditioned stimuli could occur at the level of the Purkinje cells (after Gellman and Miles)

tivity dependent. The extent to which other cellular mechanisms, for instance at the level of interneurons and motoneurons, contribute to conditioning of the gill withdrawal reflex, is still open.

Cellular studies on associative learning in vertebrates are presently focused mainly on the cerebellum, hippocampus, and cortex. The role of the cerebellum in classical conditioning, for example, is being investigated in studies on the eyeblink reflex of the rabbit (Fig. 9.**14**). In these learning experiments the eyeblink reflex, which is initially elicited in the naive animal by wind stimulation of the cornea, can be elicited by an auditory stimulus following successful conditioning. It appears that the cerebellum, and several cerebellar nuclei in particular, are important for the acquisition of this conditioned behavioral response. Some researchers even suggest that, within the cerebellum, the unconditioned stimulus might be reflected in the activity of the climbing fibers, and the conditioned stimulus in the activity of

the mossy fibers. The cerebellum is assumed to be similarly important for the learning of many other motor responses.

Model systems provide details about the molecular basis of learning

To date, there is no complete molecular analysis of a learning process. However, remarkable advances in the cellular and molecular analyses of simple learning processes have been achieved in a range of model systems. Several of the mechanisms for habituation, sensitization, and classical conditioning have been studied in the gill withdrawal reflex of *Aplysia*. This was possible because one and the same synaptic effector site is involved in all three processes.

A molecular analysis of habituation in *Aplysia* has revealed mechanisms which are responsible for the decrease in presynaptic transmitter release during homosynaptic depression (Fig. 9.**15a,b**). One of these mechanisms is the maintained inactivation of certain Ca^{2+} channels in the presynaptic sensory terminal. This inactivation of Ca^{2+} channels during habituation results in fewer and fewer Ca^{2+} ions flowing into the presynaptic terminal on repetitive initiation of action potentials. This causes a decrease in the number of transmitter quanta which are released per presynaptic action potential. As a result of the decreasing transmitter release the amplitude of the EPSPs evoked in the postsynaptic neurons is reduced, so that the excitation in these motoneurons and interneurons decreases.

A reaction cascade has been discovered to be part of the molecular basis for the presynaptic facilitation which occurs during the sensitization of the gill withdrawal reflex (Fig. 9.15c). The binding of the facilitating transmitter to receptors in the presynaptic sensory terminal activates, via a G protein an adenylate cyclase, which then causes an increase in the intracellular cAMP concentration. The increase in cAMP activates at least two further processes. First, there is an increased mobilization of transmitter vesicles via several biochemical intermediate steps. Second, a cAMP-dependent activation of protein kinases results

in a phosphorylation, and thereby inactivation, of a certain class of K^+ channel in the presynaptic membrane. As a result, action potentials in the presynaptic terminal are lengthened in duration (slowed repolarization because of a reduced K^+ permeability). This produces an increased Ca^{2+} influx with every action potential in the presynaptic terminal, and this in turn causes an increase in the number of transmitter quanta which are released per action potential.

The mechanisms of activity-dependent facilitation which are important in the conditioning of the gill reflex, are probably linked to those which occur during sensitization. There is evidence that the initiation of a heterosynaptic facilitation in the presynaptic terminal can lead to an *additional* increase in the synthesis of cAMP, if the facilitation occurs immediately after an action potential has invaded the presynaptic terminal. This increased cAMP synthesis probably occurs because the Ca^{2+} influx into the presynaptic terminal associated with the action potential stimulates adenylate cyclase via Ca^{2+}-calmodulin binding. A facilitation occurring immediately after this stimulation process would further stimulate the al-

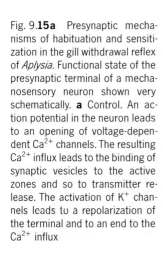

Fig. 9.**15a** Presynaptic mechanisms of habituation and sensitization in the gill withdrawal reflex of *Aplysia*. Functional state of the presynaptic terminal of a mechanosensory neuron shown very schematically. **a** Control. An action potential in the neuron leads to an opening of voltage-dependent Ca^{2+} channels. The resulting Ca^{2+} influx leads to the binding of synaptic vesicles to the active zones and so to transmitter release. The activation of K^+ channels leads to a repolarization of the terminal and to an end to the Ca^{2+} influx

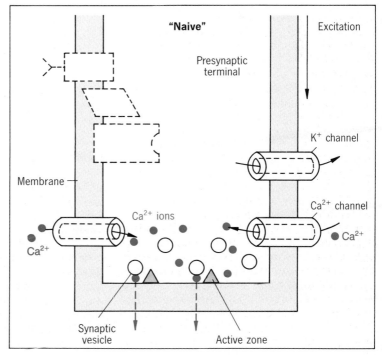

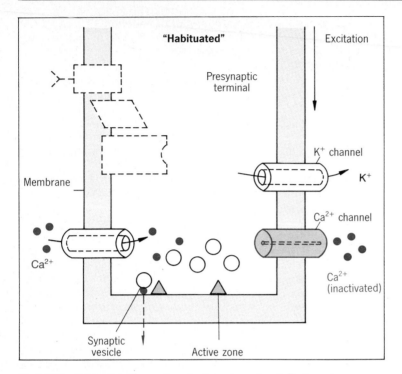

Fig. 9.**15b**   Habituation. The number of voltage-dependent Ca^{2+} channels that can be activated is reduced. The Ca^{2+} influx evoked by an action potential is correspondingly smaller. Only a few synaptic vesicles bind to the active zones and contribute to transmitter release

ready induced adenylate cyclase. As a result of a molecular convergence of (conditioned) sensory and (unconditioned) facilitatory stimulation at the level of adenylate cyclase, this would produce a greatly increased cAMP concentration, which could in turn cause increased activity-dependent facilitation.

Although it is still not clear if LTP really is involved in associative learning, the molecular basis of this phenomenon is being intensively studied. At present both presynaptic and postsynaptic mechanisms for the generation of LTP are being discussed. On the presynaptic side, a long term increase in the release of the transmitter glutamate may occur. This increase in transmitter release might be based on a phosphorylation of certain presynaptic proteins, similar to the situation in the sensory neurons of *Aplysia*. On the postsynaptic side, activation of proteases could occur during LTP, and these might then uncover more glutamate receptors in the postsynaptic membrane. However, a further postsynaptic mechanism might also be important.

A range of studies indicate, namely, that the membrane potential of the postsynaptic cell must reach a certain level of depolarization for associative LTP to occur. The reason for this seems to lie in the properties of the voltage-dependent NMDA receptor channels in the postsynaptic membrane. According to this idea, the strength of the depolarization in the postsynaptic cell evoked by the tetanic stimulation of the strongly exciting input fibers, would lead to removal of the Mg^{2+} block of the NMDA receptor channels. An increased Ca^{2+} influx into the cell could then occur via the transmitter-activated receptor channel. Ca^{2+} would act as a second messenger in the postsynaptic cell, and initiate a range of other molecular chains which, in turn, could lead to a long lasting heightened postsynaptic sensitivity. The temporal coincidence of presynaptic transmitter release and postsynaptic depolarization would be critical in this process. Both presynaptic and postsynaptic mechanisms are probably involved in the generation of LTP in the hippocampus. Postsynaptic changes could

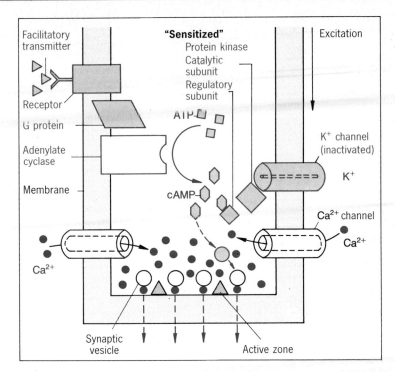

Fig. 9.**15c**   Sensitization. Facilitatory transmitter binds to the receptors which, via intermediate molecular reaction cascades, increase the mobilization of synaptic vesicles and also activate protein kinases, which in turn inactivate certain voltage-dependent K⁺ channels. The inactivation of the K^+ channels leads to a temporal lengthening of the action potential in the synaptic terminal, thereby increasing the Ca^{2+} influx, and so effecting an increase in the amount of transmitter released per action potential (after Kandel)

even feedback onto the presynaptic terminals. Finally, there is evidence that changes in the morphology of synaptic connections are important for long-term changes in synaptic transmission in the hippocampus.

The controversy over whether learning mechanisms must involve a coincidence of pre- and postsynaptic signals as postulated by Hebb, or whether an activity-dependent presynaptic facilitation is more important, currently seems to be resolving itself. It must be recognized that the neuronal plasticity which is important for learning is not based exclusively on a single molecular mechanism. The cell biology of neurons offers numerous synergistically acting mechanisms which could be involved in altering and consolidating signal transfer processes. It would be surprising if this diversity of cellular mechanisms were not utilized for the generation of the various learning processes occurring in the nervous system.

Memory: how is information stored?

Memory is still a mysterious phenomenon. Nevertheless the analysis of simple learning allows some conclusions to be drawn, at least about short-term memory.

— Memory functions can occur at identified synaptic sites; they are not inherently dependent on learning circuits distributed over a large expanse of the nervous system.
— Information storage does not require any dramatic restructuring in the nervous system. Changes in the transmission properties of already existing synaptic connections are sufficient for certain memory functions; neurons and neuronal synapses do not necessarily have to be newly formed or eliminated.
— The existence of new types of biophysical mechanisms do not have to be postulated specifically for memory processes. For example, the modulation of K⁺ channels which is

widespread in the nervous system can be utilized for the storage of certain informational components.

We still know very little about the mechanisms for long-term memory. There is evidence that changes in the structure of synapses and in the pattern of fine dendritic arborizations are important for the establishment of long-term memory. This interpretation is supported by the finding that inhibitors of protein synthesis disturb the storage of information in long-term memory, without influencing short-term memory. Maybe second messengers like Ca^{2+} or cAMP will supply the long sought-after link between short-term and long-term memory.

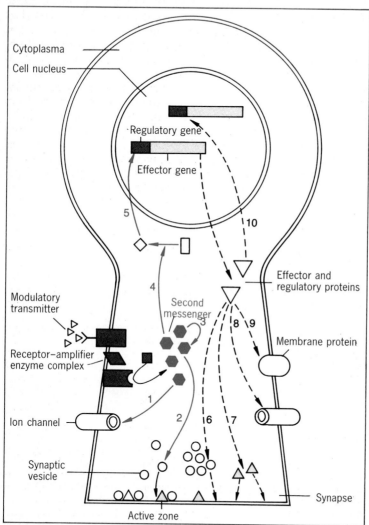

Fig. 9.**16**   Model of the possible molecular mechanisms for the formation of memory. A modulatory transmitter initiates memory-forming processes by activating a receptor–amplifier complex which produces intracellular second messenger molecules. The second messenger molecules can then initiate the following, rather short-term, processes: changes in the permeability of ion channels (1), modification of the vesicular transmitter release (2), autocatalytic formation of further second messenger molecules (3), activation of regulatory factors (4) which intervene in gene regulation (5). The resulting newly synthesized effector and regulator proteins can then initiate the following, more long-term, processes: mobilization of synaptic vesicles (6), formation of further, new active zones (7), synthesis and incorporation of new ion channels into the membrane (8), morphological expansion of the synaptic terminal (9), long-term regulation of differentiation genes (10) (after Kandel)

On the one hand such second messengers could contribute to the initiation of the local cellular changes which are apparently important for short-term memory. On the other hand, they could also be involved as a sort of molecular connection to the gene and protein regulation postulated for long-term memory (Fig. 9.16).

Memory: where is information stored?

Clearly, plasticity is not limited to a particular class of neuron. As we have seen, the critical experience-dependent changes can take place at the level of sensory neurons, interneurons and motoneurons. It is also significant that memorized information is not stored exclusively in a restricted neuronal structure. Even simple learning generally involves several parallel information channels. This would allow the storage of learned information to occur at various sites in the brain.

Although there does not seem to be a generally applicable site for the storage of learned information, there are several learning abilities which can be dramatically disturbed by specific lesions in the brain. Lesion experiments in cephalopods indicate that a visual memory is established in the optic lobes, while the memory for tactile learning is largely stored in the frontal and subfrontal brain lobes. In vertebrates, the cerebellum plays important roles in the learning of coordinated motor performance. In humans, the hippocampus and associated structures in the temporal brain lobes are critical for transferring information from short-term into long-term memory. Patients in whom these brain regions are destroyed still have a functional short-term memory, but are no longer able to transfer learned information into their long-term memory. However, information already present in long-term memory can still be recalled by these patients. This shows that the hippocampus is involved in the uptake and consolidation of learned information, but that a long-term memory is formed in other, still uninvestigated, structures.

References

General Reviews

Boothe, R. G., Dobson, V. and Teller, D. Y. 1985. Postnatal development of vision in human and nonhuman primates. Annu. Rev. Neurosci. 8: 495-546.

Brazier, M. A. B. (ed.) 1979. Brain Mechanisms in Memory and Learning. Raven, New York.

Carew, T. J. and Sahley, C. L. 1986. Invertebrate learning and memory; from behavior to molecules. Annu. Rev. Neurosci. 9: 435-487.

Changeux, J. P. and Konishi, M. (eds.) 1987. The Neural and Molecular Bases of Learning. Wiley, New York.

Cohen, M. J. and Spitzer, N. C. 1985. Comparative Neurobiology: Modes of Communication in the Nervous System. Wiley, New York.

Cotman, C. W. 1988. Excitatory amino acid neurotransmission: NMDA receptors and Hebb-type synaptic plasticity. Annu. Rev. Neurosci. 11: 61-80.

Dudai, Y. 1988. Neurogenetic dissection of learning and short-term memory in Drosophila. Annu. Rev. Neurosci. 11: 537-564.

Dudai, Y. 1989. The Neurobiology of Memory: Concepts, Findings, Trends. Oxford University Press, Oxford.

Hebb, D. O. 1949. The Organization of Behavior: A Neurophysiological Theory. Wiley, New York.

Ito, M. 1989. Long-term depression. Annu. Rev. Neurosci. 12: 85-102.

Kandel, E. R. 1976. Cellular Basis of Behavior. Freeman, San Francisco.

Kandel, E. R., Schwartz, J. H. and Jessel, T. M. (eds.) 1991. Principles of Neural Science, 3rd edition. Elsevier, New York.

Lynch, G. 1986. Synapses, Circuits, and the Beginnings of Memory. MIT Press, Cambridge.

Lynch, G., McGaugh, J. L. and Weinberger, N. M. (eds.) 1984. Neurobiology of Learning and Memory. Guilford, New York.

Marler, P. and Terrace, H. (eds.) 1984. Biology of Learning. Springer, Berlin.

McGaugh, J. L. 1989. Involvement of hormonal and neuromodulatory systems in the regulation of memory storage. Annu. Rev. Neurosci. 12: 255-288.

Rakic, P. and Singer, W. (eds.) 1988. Neurobiology of Neocortex. Wiley, New York.

Rauschenecker, J. P. and Marler, P. (eds.) 1987. Imprinting and Cortical Plasticity. Wiley, New York.

Rescorla, R. A. 1988. Behavior studies of pavlovian conditioning. Annu. Rev. Neurosci. 11: 329-352.

Schwartz, J. H. and Greenberg, S. M. 1987. Molecular mechanisms for memory: second-messenger induced modifications of protein kinases in nerve cells. Annu. Rev. Neurosci. 10: 459-476.

Teyler, T. J. and DiScenna, P. 1987. Long-term potentiation. Annu. Rev. Neurosci. 10: 131-162.

Thompson, R. F., Berger, T. W. and Madden, J. 1983. Cellular processes of learning and memory. Annu. Rev. Neurosci. 6: 447-491.

Thorpe, W. H. 1963. Learning and Instinct in Animals. Harvard University Press, Cambridge.

Woody, C. D. 1982. Memory, Learning, and Higher Function. Springer, Berlin.

Woody, C. D., Alkon, D. L. and McGaugh, J. L. (eds.) 1988. Cellular Mechanisms of Conditioning and Behavioral Plasticity. Plenum, New York.

Zucker, R. S. 1989. Short-term synaptic plasticity. Annu. Rev. Neurosci. 12: 13-32.

Original Publications

Abraham, W. C., Bliss, T. V. P. and Goddard, G. V. 1985. Heterosynaptic changes accompany longterm but not short-term potentiation of the perforant path in the anaesthetized rat. J. Physiol. 363: 335-349.

Alkon, D. L. 1979. Voltage-dependent calcium and potassium ion conductances: a contingency mechanism for an associative learning model. Science 205: 810-816.

Andersen, P., Silfrenius, H., Sundong, S. H. and Sveen, O. 1980. A comparison of distal and proximal dendrite synapses on CA1 pyramids in guinea pig hippocampal slices in vitro. J. Physiol. 307: 273-299.

Andersen, P. Sundberg, S. H., Sveen O. and Wigström, H 1977. Specific longlasting potentiation of synaptic transmission in hippocampal slices. Nature 266: 736-737.

Alvarey-Buylla, A. and Nottebohm, F. 1988. Migration of young neurons in adult avian brain. Nature 335: 353-354.

Artola, A. and Singer, W. 1987. Long-term potentiation and NMDA receptors in rat visual cortex. Nature, 330: 649-652.

Baer, M. F., Kleinschmidt, A., Gu, Q. and Singer, W. 1990. Disruption of experience-dependent synaptic modifications in striate cortex by infusion of an NMDA receptor antagonist. J. Neurosci. 10: 909-925.

Bailey, C. H. and Chen, M. 1983. Morphological basis of long-term habituation and sensitization in Aplysia. Science 220: 91-93.

Bailey, C. H. and Chen, M. 1988. Long-term memory in Aplysia modulates the total number of varicosities of single identified sensory neurons. Proc. Natl. Acad. Sci. USA 85: 2373-2377.

Blakemore, C. and Van Sluyters, R. C. 1974. Reversal of the physiological effects of monocular deprivation in kittens: Further evidence for a sensitive period. J. Physiol. 237: 195-216.

Bliss, T. V. P. and Lømo, T. 1973. Long-lasting potentiation of synaptic transmission in the dentate area of the anaesthetized rabbit following stimulation of the perforant path. J. Physiol. 232: 331-356.

Byrne, J., Castellucci, V. F. and Kandel, E. R. 1974. Receptive fields and response properties of mechano receptor neurons innervating siphon skin and mantle shelf in Aplysia. J. Neurophysiol. 37: 1041-1064.

Byrne, J., Castellucci, V. F. and Kandel, E. R. 1978. Contribution of individual mechanoreceptor sensory neurons to defensive gill withdrawal reflex in Aplysia. J. Neurophysiol. 37: 1041-1064.

Carew, T. J. and Kandel, E. R. 1973. Acquisition and retention of long-term habituation in Aplysia: correlation of behavioural and cellular processes. Science 182: 1158-1160.

Carew, T. J., Castellucci, V. F. and Kandel, E. R. 1979. Sensitization in Aplysia: Rapid restoration of transmission in synapses inactivated by long-term habituation. Science 205: 417-419.

Carew, T. J., Hawkins, R. D. and Kandel, E. R. 1983. Differential classical conditioning of a defensive withdrawal reflex in Aplysia. Science 219: 397-400.

Carew, T. J., Hawkins, R. D., Abrams, T. W. and Kandel, E. R. 1984. A test of Hebb's postulate at identified synapses which mediate classical conditioning in Aplysia. J. Neurosci. 4: 1217-1224.

Carew, T. J., Pinsker, H. M. and Kandel, E. R. 1972. Long-term habituation of a defensive withdrawal reflex in Aplysia. Science 175: 451-454.

Castellucci, V. F., Carew, T. J. and Kandel, E. R. 1978. Cellular analysis of long-term habituation of the gill-withdrawal reflex of Aplysia californica. Science 202: 1306-1308.

Castellucci, V. F., Kandel, E. R., Schwartz, J. H., Wilson, F. D., Nairn, A. C. and Greengard, P. 1980. Intracellular injection of the catalytic subunit of cyclic AMP-dependent protein kinase simulates facilitation of transmitter release underlying behavioral sensitization in Aplysia. Proc. Natl. Acad. Sci. USA 77: 7492-7496.

Chen, C. N., Denome, S. and Davis, R. L. 1986. Molecular analysis of cDNA clones and the corresponding genomic coding sequences of the Drosophila dunce$^+$ gene, the structural gene for cAMP phosphodiesterase. Proc. Natl. Acad. Sci. USA 83: 9313-9317.

Chow, K. L., Mathers, L. H. and Spear, P. D. 1973. Spreading of uncrossed retinal projection in superior colliculus of neonatally enucleated rabbits. J. Comp. Neurol. 151: 307-322.

Clark, S. A., Allard, T., Jenkins, W. M. and Merzenich, M. M. 1988. Receptive fields in the body-surface map in adult cortex defined by temporally correlated inputs. Nature 332: 444-445.

Cleland, B. G., Dubin, M. W. and Levick, W. R. 1971. Sustained and transient projection in superior colliculus of neonatally enucleated rabbits. J. Physiol. 217: 473-496.

Clinde, H. T. and Constantine-Paton, M. 1990. NMDA receptor agonist and antagonists alter retinal ganglion cell arbor structure in the developing frog retinotectal projection. J. Neurosci. 10: 1197-1216.

Cynader, M. and Mitchell, D. E. 1977. Monocular astigmatism effects on kitten visual cortex development. Nature 270: 177-178

Cynader, M. and Mitchell, D. E. 1980. Prolonged sensitivity to monocular deprivation in dark-reared cats. J. Neurophysiol. 43: 1026-1040.

Delaney, K. and Gelperin, A. 1986. Postingestive food-aversion learning to amino acid deficient diets by the terrestrial slug Limax maximus. J. Comp. Physiol. 159: 281-295.

Dudai, Y., Jan, Y.-M., Byers, D. Quinn, W. G. and Benzer, S. 1976. Dunce, a mutant of Drosophila deficient in learning. Proc. Natl. Acad. Sci. USA 73: 1684-1688.

Frost, W. N., Castellucci, V. F., Hawkins, R. D. and Kandel, E. R. 1985. Monosynaptic connections from the sensory neurons participate in the storage of long-term memory for sensitization of the gill- and siphon-withdrawal reflex in Aplysia. Proc. Natl. Acad. Sci. USA 82: 8266-8269.

Galli, L. and Maffei, L. 1988. Spontaneous impulse activity of rat retinal ganglion cells in prenatal life. Science 242: 90-91.

Gilbert, C. D. and Wiesel, T. N. 1983. Clustered intrinsic connections in cat visual cortex. J. Neurosci. 3: 1116-1133.

Greenberg, S. M., Castellucci, V. F., Bayley, H. and Schwarz, J. H. 1987. A molecular mechanism for long-term sensitization in Aplysia. Nature 329: 62-65.

Hawkins, R. D., Abrams, T. W., Carew, T. J. and Kandel, E. R. 1983. A cellular mechanism of classical conditioning in Aplysia. Activity-dependent amplification of presynaptic facilitation. Science 219: 400-405.

Held, R. and Bauer, J. A. 1974. Development of sensorially guided reaching in infant monkeys. Brain Res. 71: 265-271.

Hubel, D. H. and Wiesel, T. N. 1963. Receptive fields of cells in striate cortex of very young, visually inexperienced kittens. J. Neurophysiol. 26: 994-1002.

Hubel, D. H. and Wiesel, T. N. 1965. Binocular interaction in striate cortex of kittens reared with artificial squint. J. Neurophysiol. 28: 1041-1059.

Hubel, D. H. and Wiesel, T. N. 1970. The period of susceptibility to the physiological effects of unilateral eye closure in kittens. J. Physiol. 206: 419-436.

Hubel, D. H., Wiesel, T. N. and LeVay, S. 1977. Plasticity of ocular dominance columns in monkey striate cortex. Phil. Trans. R. Soc. Lond. B 278: 377-409.

Jacobson, S. G., Mohindra, J. and Held, R. 1981. Development of visual acuity in infants with congenital cataracts. Br. J. Opthalmol. 65: 727-735.

Kasamatsu, T., Pettigrew, J. D. and Ary, M. 1981. Cortical recovery from effects of monocular deprivation: Acceleration with norepinephrine and suppression with 6-hydroxydopamine. J. Neurophysiol. 45: 254-266.

Knudsen, E. I., Knudsen, P. F. and Esterly, S. D. 1982. Early auditory experience modifies sound localization in barn owls. Nature 295: 238-240.

Lashley, K. S. 1950. In search of the engram. Symp. Soc. Exp. Biol. 4: 454-482.

LeVay, S. and Ferster, D. 1977. Relay cell classes in the lateral geniculate nucleus of the cat and the effects of visual deprivation. J. Comp. Neurol. 172: 563-584.

LeVay, S., Stryker, M. P. and Shatz, C. J. 1978. Ocular dominance columns and their development in layer IV of the cat's visual cortex: A quantitative study. J. Comp. Neurol. 179: 223-244.

LeVay, S., Wiesel, T. N. and Hubel, D. H. 1980. The development of ocular dominance columns in normal and visually deprived monkeys. J. Comp. Neurol. 191: 1-51.

Malinow, R., Madison, D. V. and Tsien, R. W. 1988. Persistent protein kinase activity underlying long-term potentiation. Nature 335: 820-824.

Merzenich, M. M., Kaas, J. H., Wall, J., Nelson, R. J., Sur, M. and Felleman, D. 1983. Topographic reorganization of somatosensory cortical areas 3B and 1 in adult monkeys following restricted deafferentation. Neuroscience 8: 33-55.

Merzenich, M. M., Kaas, J. H., Wall, J., Sur, M., Nelson, R. J. and Felleman, D. 1983. Progression of change following median nerve section in the cortical representation of the hand in areas 3b and 1 in adult owl and squirrel monkeys. Neuroscience 10: 639-665.

Merzenich, M. M., Nelson, R. J., Stryker, M. P., Cynander, M. S., Schoppmann, A. and Zook, J. M. 1984. Somatosensory cortical map changes following digit amputation in adult monkeys. J. Comp. Neurol. 224: 591-605.

Montarolo, P. G., Goelet, P., Castellucci, V. F., Morgan, J., Kandel, E. R. and Schacher, S. 1986. A critical period for macromolecular synthesis in long-term heterosynaptic facilitation in Aplysia. Science 234: 1249-1254.

Morris, R. G. M., Anderson, E., Lynch, G. S. and Baudry, M. 1986. Selective impairment of learning and blockade of long-term potentiation by an N-methy-D-aspartate receptor antagonist, AP5. Nature 319: 774-776.

Mower, G. D., Christen, W. G. and Caplan, C. J. 1983. Very brief visual experience eliminates plasticity in the cat visual cortex. Science 221: 178-180.

Pons, T. P., Garraghty, P. E. and Mishkin, M. 1988. Lesion-induced plasticity in the second somatosensory cortex of adult macaques. Proc. Natl. Acad. Sci. USA 85: 5279-5281.

Rakic, P. 1976. Prenatal genesis of connections subserving ocular dominance in the rhesus monkey. Nature 261: 467-471.

Riesen, A. H. and Aarons, L. 1959. Visual movement and intensity discrimination in cats after early deprivation of pattern vision. J. Comp. Physiol. Psychol. 52: 142-149.

Schacher, S., Castellucci, V. F. and Kandel, E. R. 1988. cAMP evokes long-term facilitation in Aplysia sensory neurons that requires new protein synthesis. Science 240: 1667-1669.

Siegelbaum, S, A., Camardo, J. S. and Kandel, E. R. 1982. Serotonin and cyclic AMP close single K^+ channels in Aplysia sensory neurones. Nature 299: 413-417.

Shatz, C. J. and Kliot, M. J. 1982. Prenatal misrouting of the retinogeniculate pathway in Siamese cats. Nature 300: 525-529.

Shatz, C. J. and Stryker, M. P. 1978. Ocular dominance in layer IV of the cat's visual cortex and the effects of monocular deprivation. J. Physiol. 281: 267-283.

Sherk, H. and Stryker, M. P. 1976. Quantitative study of cortical orientation selectivity in visually inexperienced kitten. J. Neurophysiol. 39: 63-70.

Sheman, S. M. and Stone, J. 1973. Physiological normality of the retina in visually deprived cats. Brain Res. 60: 224-230.

Squire, L. R. and Butters, N. (eds.) 1984. Neuropsychology of Memory. Guilford, New York.

Sweatt, J. D. and Kandel, E. R. 1989. Persistent and transcriptionally-dependent increase in protein phosphorylation in long-term facilitation of Aplysia sensory neurons. Nature 339: 51-54.

Stent, G. S. 1973. A physiological mechanism for Hebb's postulate of learning. Proc. Natl. Acad. Sci. USA 70: 997-1001.

Stryker, M. P. and Harris, W. A. 1986. Binocular impulse blockade prevents the formation of ocular dominance columns in cat visual cortex. J. Neurosci. 6: 2117-2133.

Technau, G. 1984. Fiber number in the mushroom bodies of adult Drosophila melanogaster depends on age, sex and experience. J. Neurogenet. 1: 113-126.

Thompson, R. F. 1986. The neurobiology of learning and memory. Science 233: 941-947.

Van Sluyters, R. C and Levitt, F. B. 1980. Experimental strabismus in the kitten. J. Neurophysiol. 43: 686-699.

Walters, E. T. and Byrne, J. H. 1983. Associative conditioning of single sensory neurons suggests a celular mechanism for learning. Science 219: 405-408.

Wiesel, T. N. 1982. The postnatal development of the visual cortex and the influence of environment. Nature 299: 583-591.

Wiesel, T. N. and Hubel, D. H. 1963. Effects of visual deprivation on morphology and physiology of cells in the cat's lateral geniculate body. J. Neurophysiol. 26: 978-993.

Wiesel, T. H. and Hubel, D. H. 1963. Single-cell responses in striate cortex of kittens deprived of vision in one eye. J. Neurophysiol. 26: 1003-1017.

Wiesel, T. N. and Hubel, D. H. 1965. Comparison of the effects of unilateral and bilateral eye closure on cortical unit responses in kittens. J. Neurophysiol. 28: 1029-1040.

Wiesel, T. H. and Hubel, D. H. 1965. Extent of recovery from the effects of visual deprivation in kittens. J. Neurophysiol. 28: 1060-1072.

Wiesel, T. N. and Hubel, D. H. 1974. Ordered arrangement of orientation columns in monkeys lacking visual experience. J. Comp. Neurol. 158: 307-318.

Wong-Riley, M. 1979. Changes in the visual system of monocularly sutured or enucleated cats demonstrable with cytochrome oxidase histochemistry. Brain Res. 177: 11-28.

Zola-Morgan, S., Squire, L. R. and Amaral, D. G. 1986. Human amnesia and the medial temporal region: Enduring memory impairment following a bilateral lesion limited to field CA1 of the hippocampus. J. Neusosci. 6: 2950-2967.

Index